Research on Virology and Cytopathology

Research on Virology and Cytopathology

Published by iConcept Press

Research on Virology and Cytopathology

Publisher: iConcept Press Ltd.

ISBN: 978-1-922227-70-6

Printed in the United States of America

𝓲Concept
Press Ltd.

www.iconceptpress.com

Contents

Preface

Research on Cytopathology is a book presenting the information and practical applications of clinical cytology in determining the etiology, diagnosis, prognosis and therapeutic options of benign and malignant disease. Committed to bridging the gap between cytopathology and surgical pathology, this book stresses the value of clinical-pathological correlations, as well as the correlation between cytological and histological findings.

There are totally 10 chapters in this book. Chapter 1 discusses the emergence of a highly divergent Encephalomyocarditis Virus (EMCV) in Singapore where encephalomyocarditis viral infections are a concern for industries that keep animals such as zoos and farms. Chapter 2 examines the roles of known cell adhesion molecules (CAMs) in synapse formation, and reviews the participation of these CAMs in brain disorders. Chapter 3 reviews different types of tumor vessels in gastric cancer, their morphology and clinical importance. It also considers a new hypothesis of cavitary type of angiogenesis that possibly plays a key role in the tumor progression. Chapter 4 shows the impact of tumor regression in rectal cancer therapy decision tree. It is worth to note that survival in patients with locally advanced rectal cancer treated with chemoradiation followed by surgery depends of tumor response to neoadjuvant therapeutic .

Chapter 5 proposes the use of MR imaging and new catheters/devices in cardiovascular interventions. It discusses the new MR sequences, local therapeutic delivery or treating methods and tissue ablation of cardiovascular diseases. Chapter 6 brings the results of a five-year investigation about the influence of phytotherapy on the size and secretion activity of macroprolactinomas. It also demonstrates the efficiency of phytotherapy in macroprolactinoma tumour mass downsizing. It shows the implementation of phytotherapy as a novel treatment modality of this tumour cluster. Chapter 7 discusses the differential diagnosis of brain calcifications in relation to the possible psychiatric presentations reported in the recent literature. In addition, it also discusses clinical features diagnosis and possible pattern of presentation to psychiatry. Chapter 8 aims to clarify the main positioning errors during a radiograph's performance to increase the knowledge of professionals who work with this technique in order to avoid mistakes in diagnosis of oral pathologies through this complementary exam.

Chapter 9 presents the past and current situation regarding the HIV epidemic in

Pakistan. It examines the phylogenetic evidence indicating the routes of HIV transmission, and the bridging of infection across various high risk groups. Chapter 10 shows how the changing population immune-genetic pressures might affect HIV subtype A epidemic dynamics, genomic variability and epitope diversity, and steer immuno-evolution of this subtype in new directions.

Editing and publishing a book is never an easy task. Each chapter in this book has gone through a peer review, a selection and an editing process so as to guarantee its quality. Without the supports and contributions of the authors and reviewers, this book can never be able to complete. We would like to thank all of the authors in this book and all of the reviewers who participated in the reviewing process: Hassan Alizadeh, Neilane Bertoni, Arturo Carta, Raphael Richard Ciuman, S. R. Clegg, Laura Fanea, M. Fukumoto, Craig J. Goergen, Hiroshi Harada, M.J. Hosie, Nam Kyu Kim, Nam Kyu Kim, Joji Kitayama, SeungWon Kwon, Xiaoming Li, Adhemar Longatto-Filho, Xin-Ming Ma, Sobia Manzoor, Linda J. Metheny-Barlow, Asieh Zamani Naser, Shanmuga Vadivoo Natarajan, Wensheng Pan, AS Panchbhai, Duk-Woo Park, Sabri Saeed Sanabani, Joachim Scholz-Starke, P P Sedghizadeh, Masoud Shabani, Woo Keun Song, Christian Stockmann, Ramesh Teegala, Jose V. Torres, Chris Verhofstede, Yanning Yang, Ali Yilmaz, S-J Yoon, Bo Yu, Cheng-Chia Yu, Yinhua Yu and Kwok-Yung Yuen. We hope that you, the reader, will find this book interesting and useful. Any advices please feel free and are always welcome to tell us.

iConcept Press Editorial Office
June 2017

Chapter 1

Emergence of a Highly Divergent Encephalomyocarditis Virus from Nonhu-man Primates in Singapore

Koon-Wui Guy Lee[1], Dawn Su-Yin Yeo[1], Pui-San Wong[1],
Myint Zu Myaing[2], Eliza Chua[2], Serena Oh[3], Richard Sugrue[2],
Boon-Huan Tan[1]

1 Introduction and Global Distribution

The encephalomyocarditis virus (EMCV) belongs to the Cardiovirus genus within the *Picornaviridae* family, and has infected a wide range of animals worldwide (see Figure 1). First isolated in 1945 from a male gibbon in Miami, Florida, the virus has since then been reported to cause deaths in an increasingly wide range of mammals, such as several other non-human primates, rodents, pigs, elephants, and tigers (reviewed by Carocci & Bakkali-Kassimi, 2012; Liu et al., 2013; Masek-Hammerman et al., 2012; Knowles et al., 1998; Grobler et al., 1995; Kin et al., 1989; Citino et al., 1988). There have been several reports describing EMCV as the etiological agent of viral myocarditis in captive primates. These primates included semi-wild bonobos, baboons, chimpanzees, lemurs, rhesus macques, and orang utans (Masek-Hammerman et al., 2012; Jones et al., 2011; Canelli et al., 2010; Citino et al., 1998; Reddacliff et al., 1997; Hubbard et al., 1992). EMCV infection was also implicated in the deaths of various animals in Audubon Park Zoo, New Orleans, in 1985 (Wells et al., 1989); and in elephants in a Florida zoo in 1997 (Simpson et al., 1977). Outside the United States, sporadic outbreaks of EMCV involving

[1] Detection and Diagnostics Laboratory, DMERI, DSO National Laboratories, Singapore.
[2] School of Biological Sciences, National Technological University, Singapore.
[3] Wildlife Reserves Singapore, Singapore.

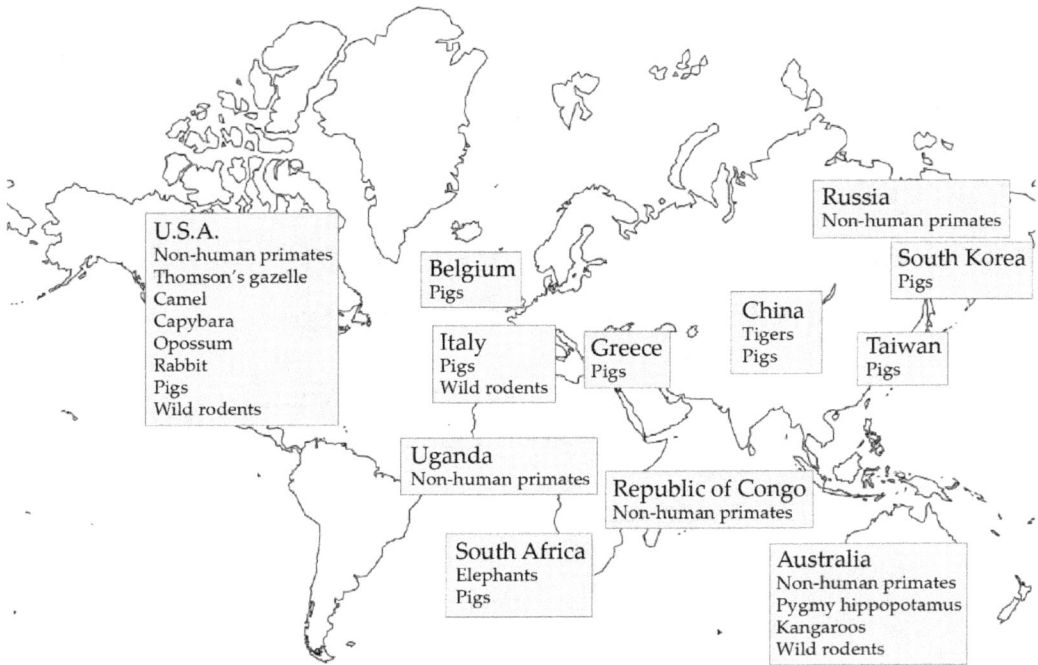

Figure 1: Encephalomyocarditis virus infections in animals around the world. This figure highlights EMCV infection as a worldwide problem for a large range of mammals. World outline adapted from www.outline-world-map.com.

a variety of zoo animals had occurred in Taronga Zoo in Australia from 1987 to 1995 (Reddacliff et al., 1997); in free-living elephants in Kruger National Park, South Africa between 1993 and 1994 (van Sandwyk et al., 2013; Grobler et al., 1995); and in an Italian zoo affecting 15 different primates between 2006 and 2008 (Canelli et al., 2010). EMCV infections were reported in Russia from monkeys bred from the Sukhumi Breeding Center in 1974 as well as in the Adler Breeding Center since 2001 (Krylova & Dzhikidze, 2005). The virus has also been recognized as a porcine pathogen, with infections in European pigs associated with sudden deaths and reproductive failure (Maurice et al., 2005; Koenen et al., 1997; Joo, 1992; Paschaleri-Papadopoulou et al., 1990; Sidoli et al., 1989). In Asia, EMCV was isolated from pigs in South Korea and implicated as the cause of reproductive failure in pigs in Taiwan (Hu et al., 1993; Park et al., 1992).

2   Genetic and Biophysical Properties

The EMCV virions are small, non-enveloped and spherical, with a diameter of approximately 28 to 30 nm (Carocci & Bakkali- Kassimi, 2012; Lipton et al., 2006). They have a single-stranded, positive-sense RNA genome that is approximately 7.6 kb in length and contain a large opening reading frame (ORF) (see Figure 2). The ORF encodes for a polyprotein that comprises both non-structural and structural elements divided into three primary precursor molecules, namely P1, P2 and P3, encoding for 11 distinct proteins. The structural proteins VP4, VP2, VP3 and VP1 make up the viral capsid and are encoded in the P1 region towards the 5'-end of the genome. Non-structural proteins are derived from the P2 and P3 regions and are encoded towards the 3'-end of the genome, the largest of which is the RNA-dependent RNA polymerase (3Dpol). In addition, EMCV genome codes for an L (Leader) protein at the N-terminus of their polyproteins. The genomic RNA also contains a highly structured 5'-UTR (untranslated region) that includes an internal ribosome entry site (IRES) from which viral protein translation is initiated in a cap-independent manner. The shorter 3'-UTR terminates with a heterogeneous poly(A) tail that is known to be involved in the binding process of the viral replicase complex (Carocci & Bakkali-Kassimi, 2012).

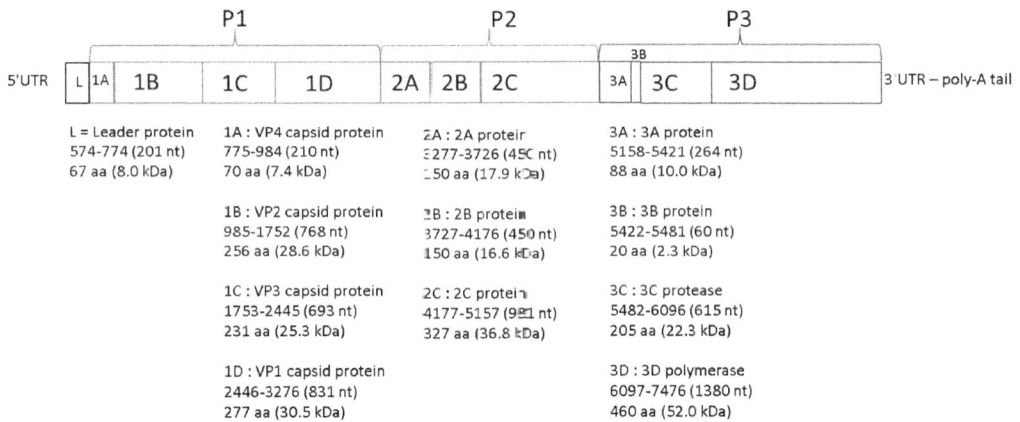

| 5'UTR | L | 1A | 1B | 1C | 1D | 2A | 2B | 2C | 3A | 3B | 3C | 3D | 3'UTR – poly-A tail |

L = Leader protein
574-774 (201 nt)
67 aa (8.0 kDa)

1A : VP4 capsid protein
775-984 (210 nt)
70 aa (7.4 kDa)

2A : 2A protein
2277-3726 (450 nt)
150 aa (17.9 kDa)

3A : 3A protein
5158-5421 (264 nt)
88 aa (10.0 kDa)

1B : VP2 capsid protein
985-1752 (768 nt)
256 aa (28.6 kDa)

2B : 2B protein
3727-4176 (450 nt)
150 aa (16.6 kDa)

3B : 3B protein
5422-5481 (60 nt)
20 aa (2.3 kDa)

1C : VP3 capsid protein
1753-2445 (693 nt)
231 aa (25.3 kDa)

2C : 2C protein
4177-5157 (981 nt)
327 aa (36.8 kDa)

3C : 3C protease
5482-6096 (615 nt)
205 aa (22.3 kDa)

1D : VP1 capsid protein
2446-3276 (831 nt)
277 aa (30.5 kDa)

3D : 3D polymerase
6097-7476 (1380 nt)
460 aa (52.0 kDa)

Figure 2: Schematic diagram depicting the genomic organization of the Encephalomyocarditis virus (EMCV) strain SingM100-02 (NCBI GenBank accession number: KC310737) (Yeo et al., 2013). Positions of the various genes on the genome are listed here, followed by size of the gene in nucleotides (nt) and the gene product size in amino acids (aa) and mass in kilo daltons (kDa). The total genomic length for this strain is 7630 nt. UTR refers to untranslated region. L codes for the leader protein. P1, P2 and P3 code for primary percursor proteins before cleavage into their various protein components as described in this figure. P1 comprises 1A, 1B, 1C and 1D, which code for the capsid proteins VP4, VP2, VP3 and VP1 respectively. P2 and P3 proteins comprise non-structural proteins associated with replication: 2A, 2B and 2C for P2, and 3A, 3B, 3C protease and 3D RNA-dependent RNA polymerase (3D pol) for P3. The EMCV genome has a poly-A tail at its 3' end.

The basic building block for the EMCV capsid is a protomer which consists of one copy of VP1, VP2, VP3 and VP4 subunits each (Carocci & Bakkali- Kassimi, 2012; Lipton et al., 2006). VP1, VP2 and VP3 are capsid subunits on the virion surface whereas VP4 is an internal capsid subunit. The five protomers assemble into a pentamer and the icosa-hedral capsid is formed by 12 pentamers, and virion particles are approximately 30 nm in diameter. Figure 3 depicts the schematic diagram of the virus particle as well as elec tron micrographs of actual viruses (Yeo at al., 2013). Of these four capsid proteins, the VP1 is the major antigenic subunit and would be a good potential target molecule for vaccine development (Suh et al., 2001; Sin et al., 1997). The structure of the EMCV cap-sid is compact and impermeable to certain high electron density molecules, conferring the virions a measure of resistance to certain harsh chemical and physical conditions (Lipton et al., 2006). EMCV has been described to be insensitive to chloroform, ether, and deoxycholate (Lipton et al., 2006). They remain infective at 4°C for weeks and are stable at freezing temperatures for years. They are not affected by a wide pH range of pH 3–10, as well as being more resistant to detergents than lipid-containing viruses (Speir, 1962; Lipton et al., 2006). They are, however, susceptible to 70% ethanol, UV ra-diation and temperatures above 50°C (Lipton et al., 2006).

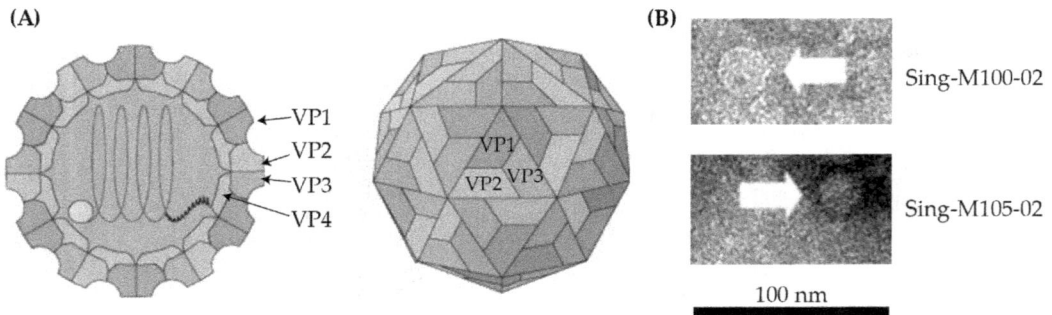

Figure 3: (A) Capsid structure of a Picornavirus (Swiss Institute of Bioinformatics, 2008), and (B) electron micrographs of Encephalomyocarditis virus (EMCV) par-ticles of Sing-M100-02 and Sing-M105-02 strains identified by white arrows. The Picornavirus capsid, as depicted on (A), is an icosahedron made up of 60 identical protomers. Each protomer consists of a single copy of VP1, VP2, VP3 & VP4 sub-units. VP1 is the most antigenic subunit; VP4 is internal. Arrows on (B) show EMCV particles as seen through electron microscopy.

3   Pathogenesis and Virulence

Laboratory study on piglets suggests that the tonsils of infected animals are likely the portal of entry, as well as the organ for viral persistence, during natural infection (Gelmetti et al., 2006). In the process of pathogenesis, EMCV can be isolated from many organs, such as palatine glands, pancreas, liver, kidney, spleen, and mesenteric lymph nodes (Papaioannou et al., 2003; LaRue et al., 2003). The initial phase of myocarditis oc-curs when EMCV infection progresses to the heart tissue. The virus then replicates ag-gressively in the cytoplasm of myocardiocytes, leading to a secondary viraemia, where the myocarditis condition becomes multifocal, with abundant inflammation of the infected tissue. Oro-nasal inoculation with 4ml of 10^3 TCID$_{50}$/ml in experimental pigs results in sudden deaths between 24 to 78 hour post-infection (Gelmetti et al., 2006). Necrosis of tissue and inflammation can be observed for cardiac and brain tissues, ultimately leading to fatality due to congestive cardiac failure. No inflammatory or degenerative conditions have been observed for other tissues during the disease progression, thus demonstrating that infection of the heart represents the late stage of pathogenesis for EMCV infection (Gelmetti et al., 2006; LaRue et al., 2003).

3.1   EMCV and Animal Infections

EMCV infections are a concern for industries that keep animals, such as zoos and farms, because they cause outbreaks of fatal cases either without predictive antecedent symptoms, or presenting with mild and non-specific clinical symptoms. Limited serological studies suggest that EMCV virulence is strain-to-host specific, and our study on susceptible orang utans in Singapore suggest fatality of approximately one third of naturally infected animals in captivity (Yeo et al., 2013; Canelli et al., 2010; Krylova & Dzhikidze, 2005). Clinical symptoms presented in naturally infected primates in captivity may present as dyspnea, lack of physical coordination, lethargy, weakness and malaise, eventually death in 12 to 24 hours (Masek-Hammerman et al., 2012; Canelli et al., 2010). Fetal losses due to EMCV infections have been documented in pregnant sows (Maurice et al., 2007; Kassimi et al., 2002). In laboratory conditions, experimental EMCV infection can be used to induce diabetes in hamsters, mice and gerbils, viral orchitis in hamsters and mice, limb paralysis, myocarditis, encephalitis and sialodacryoadenitis in mice (Carocci & Bakkali- Kassimi, 2012; Doi, 2011).

3.2   EMCV and Human Infections

Although the potential for EMCV to cross the species barrier has been demonstrated as seen from the various zoo outbreaks described above, human cases have been rare. Sporadic human EMCV infections and disease have been documented by virus isolation from different specimen types such as serum, stool samples, cerebrospinal fluid and throat washings (Gajdusek, 1955; Dick et al., 1948). A more recent study describing the etiology of acute febrile disease in locations across South America concluded that there is evidence supporting a role for EMCV in human infection and febrile illness (Oberste et al., 2009). However, the extent of the effect of EMCV on human health is still largely unknown because the disease is so infrequent in humans.

4   Epizootiology at the Singapore Zoological Gardens

Unique strains of EMCV have been identified in primates that died abruptly due to myocarditis at the Singapore Zoological Gardens. The disease was characterized by sudden deaths with cardiac congestion or lesions of the cardiac tissue identified at post-mortem.

Investigation of these deaths took place during two periods, that of 2001–2002 and 2013. Prior to the cases of viral myocarditis during 2001–2002, there had been no reported cases for this disease, and the investigation was the first in Singapore (Yeo et al., 2013). Apart from EMCV, there has been some evidence of the Coxsackie B viruses as a possible cause for animal viral myocarditis elsewhere in the world. One report described Coxsackie B4 virus as the etiological agent of fatal myocarditis in a female orang utan at the Okinawan Zoo in 1999 (Miyagi et al., 1999), whereas another reported a fatal myocarditis case in a chimpanzee at Copenhagen Zoo, Denmark, in 2010 due to Coxsackie B3 virus (Nielsen et al., 2012). However these reports are uncommon and EMCV remained the major cause of viral myocarditis in animals worldwide. This prompted our investigation to focus on EMCV diagnosis. Our investigations identified a novel lineage of EMCV strains to be the etiological agents.

4.1   The 2001–2002 Investigative Study

The 2001–2002 cases of viral myocarditis in the Singapore Zoological Gardens took place over an estimated period of 8 months, and occurred in orang utans of various ages, as well as sporadically among other zoo animals. There were altogether four deaths in the orang utan cohort, two adults and two juveniles, caused by acute myocarditis characterized by abnormalities of cardiac tissue observed at necropsy. Other animals, two zebras, one spider monkey, one guanaco, and two capybaras also died of similar clinical signs. One other adult orang utan displayed respiratory problems but recovered with intensive supportive therapy. Reverse-transcription polymerase chain reaction (RT-PCR) with EMCV specific primers against the VP3/VP1 capsid region and 3Dpol region on samples from the heart and lung necropsy tissues collected from the two juvenile orang utans that died were positive (Yeo et al., 2013). The electron micrographs on isolates revealed numerous small round virus particles with smooth appearances in the range of 20 to 30 nm (see Figure 3B). The morphology and size observed are consistent with virus members belonging to the family of *Picornaviridae* (Knowles et al., 2012). In addition, virus-infected Vero cells showed positive immunofluorescence to polyclonal antiserum raised to EMCV (Yeo et al., 2013). Put together, the data indicated that the etiological agent of the myocarditis cases in the Singapore zoo was an EMCV.

4.1.1   Investigating the Prevalence of Exposure and Potential Reservoir for EMCV Transmission

In order to investigate whether other zoo animals had been exposed to the Singapore EMCV strain, a serological survey was conducted. Sera were collected from a variety of zoo animals, in particular animals residing near the orang utans, and titrated for EMCV-neutralizing antibodies (see Table 1). A selection of capybaras (80%), chimpanzees (31%) and orang utans (50%) exhibited neutralizing antibody titers to the local strain, strongly indicating that they had been exposed to the virus. In total, 22 of 122 zoological animals (18%) exhibited neutralizing antibody titers to isolate of a local strain Sing-M105-02 (Yeo et al., 2013).

Primates	Summarized results of serological tests for EMCV
Agile gibbons	0 of 6 agile gibbons tested were positive
Capucin Jito	0 of 1 capucin jito tested were positive
Chimpanzees	4 of 13 chimpanzees tested were positive (31%)
Colobus monkeys	0 of 3 colobuses tested were positive
Gibbons	1 of 21 gibbons tested was positive (5%)
Howler monkeys	0 of 2 howler monkeys tested were positive
Japanese monkeys	0 of 2 Japanese monkeys tested were positive
Lemur	0 of 2 lemurs tested were positive
Mandrill	0 of 2 mandrills tested were positive
Orang utans	7 of 14 orag utans tested were positive (50%)
Patas monkey	0 of 1 patas tested were positive
Pig tail macaques	0 of 2 pig tail macaques tested were positive
Siamang	0 of 3 siamangs tested were positive
Slow loris	0 of 1 slow loris tested were positive
Spider monkeys	0 of 5 spider monkeys tested were positive
White nose gueron	0 of 4 white nosed guerons tested were positive
Capybaras	8 of 10 capybaras tested were positive (80%)
Wild rats	2 of 2 wild rats tested were positive (100%)
Cape hunting dog	0 of 1 cape hunting dog tested were positive
Racoon	0 of 1 raccoon tested were positive
Komodo dragons	0 of 2 komodo dragons tested were positive

Table 1: Summarized results for serological study performed on different animals from the Singapore Zoological Gardens during the 2001–2002 investigative study (Yeo et al., 2013). Percentages are given only to those yielding some positive serological results. Neutralizing antibodies from blood samples were detected using the Sing-M105-02 isolate.

Wild rodents have been considered to be the primary host reservoir and disseminators of EMCV, and they have been implicated in other zoological outbreaks of EMCV (Canelli et al., 2010; Reddacliff et al., 1997; Grobler et al., 1995; Zimmerman, 1994, Hubbard et al., 1992; Wells et al., 1989). These reports prompted the initiation of a rodent control program as a control measure for the management of the myocarditis cases at the Singapore Zoological Gardens. Captured wild rodents in this program would then be investigated for evidence that these were part of the epizootiology for the EMCV disease. Only two wild rats were caught, and both of these demonstrated high titres of neutralizing antibodies to a Singapore strain. High percentage positive serology result was also obtained from the other rodent population that was sampled: the capybara, of which 8 out of 10 were positive (see Table 2). Put together these results suggest that the virus is sustained by circulation among the rodents of this locality.

Gene	Primer name	Sequence (5' to 3')	Nucleotide Position[a]	PCR Product Size[b]	Reference
3Dpol	EMCV-RP1	CCC TAC CTC ACG GAA TGG GGC AAA G	7422–7398	286	Koenen et al., 1997
	EMCV-RP2	GGT GAG AGC AAG CCT CGC AAA GAC AG	7137–7162		
VP1	GUYVP1-F	CGT ACC CAC CTG GCT GTC CG	2339–2358	977	This study
	GUYVP1-R	GTC AAG TGG GTT TGC AGC TC	3315–3296		
VP3	GUYVP3-F	GGT TAT CGC TGT GGT GGC TC	1626–1645	1052	This study
	GUYVP3-R1	CAT ACT GTG GTC CTG GTG TC	2677–2658		

[a]Nucleotide Position based on Sing- M100-02 (NCBI GenBank accession number: KC310737).
[b]PCR product size in nucleotides (nt).

Table 2: Details of primers used or designed in this study to investigate the 2013 cases of myocarditis among primates at the Singapore Zoological Gardens. The three target genes on this table refer to those of the Encephalomyocarditis virus: 3Dpol refers to the 3D polymerase gene, VP1 refers to the VP1 capsid protein gene and VP3 refers to the VP3 capsid protein genes respectively. EMCV-RP1 and EMCV-RP2 primers were also used in our 2001–2002 investigative study (Yeo et al., 2013).

4.2   The 2013 Investigative Study

In 2013, we investigated the deaths of four non-human primates that occurred again in the Singapore Zoological Gardens, this time 11 years after the first series of cases. This 2013 investigative study has not been reported elsewhere. The first case occurred in September 2013, when a cotton-top tamarin (*Saguinus oedipus*) suffered a sudden fatality. The primate was previously healthy. Abnormalities of the cardiac tissue observed at post-mortem indicated congestion of the heart, but no other indicative abonormalities in its physical condition were observed. Within a fortnight, a hamadryas baboon (*Papio hamadryas*), one squirrel monkey (*Saimiri sciureus*) and one pygmy marmoset (*Cebuella pygmaea*) were found dead, similarly with congestive heart, and no prior clinical signs of ill health. Heart and brain necropsy samples were collected from the hamadryas baboon, squirrel monkey and pygmy marmoset, whereas only heart tissue was collected from the cotton-top tamarin. EMCV was detected via RT-PCR for the heart tissues of the cotton-top tamarin and the hamadryas baboon. EMCV was not detected in the brain tissue of the same hamadryas baboon, or in all tissue samples collected from the squirrel monkey and pygmy marmoset. This is the first report to describe infection of EMCV in a cotton-top tamarin.

5 Evolutionary Diversity

Structural proteins have been shown to be suitable for phylogenetic analyses within different genera and species of picornaviruses (Norder et al., 2001; McMinn et al., 2001; Haydon et al., 2001; Oberste et al., 2001; Santti et al., 2000; Mulders et al., 2000; Oberste et al., 2000; Brown et al., 1999; Oberste et al., 1999; Zimmerman, 1994). Furthermore, analysis using the VP1 capsid could lead to the discovery of a novel variant such as the discovery reported for Hepatitis A (Costa-Mattioli et al., 2002). The picornaviral polymerases or 3Dpol genes, on the other hand, are well conserved during evolution, and have been used as a common marker for comparisons between genera in phylogenetic studies (Koonin, 1991; Rodrigo & Dopazo, 1995; Palmberg et al., 1984). They can also be used to determine the degree of variation between the newly isolated viruses with existing EMCV strains. For example in Foot-and-Mouth-Disease viruses, high sequence divergence found in the 3Dpol regions is an indication of the virus strains diverging from the same isolate (Villaverde et al., 1988). Therefore, the 3Dpol region, being relatively conserved, is the preferred region for initial diagnostic testing due to its conserved nature, whereas the VP1 and VP3 capsid genes are variable regions of the virus, and are therefore more favourable for strain-typing (Lin et al., 2012; Zhang et al., 2007; Denis et al., 2006; Koenen et al., 1997; Krishnaswamy & Rossman, 1990).

In our 2001–2002 investigation, we used two published EMCV primer sets, P1/P2 (targeting the 3Dpol gene) for the initial detection of virus, and P9/P10 (targeting the capsid VP3/VP1 gene) for the determination of the virus genus and species (Koenen et al., 1997). These primer sets had been tested on a wide variety of EMCV isolates from different geographic locations, different host species, and at different times (Koenen et al., 1999; Vanderhallen & Koenen, 1998; Vanderhallen & Koenen, 1997). EMCV was detected in samples from the heart necropsy tissue of the first juvenile orang utan, and lung necropsy tissues of the second juvenile orang utan (Yeo et al., 2013). Other primers were used for subsequent full genome assembly and sequencing by primer walking (Yeo et al., 2013). Our straintyping RT-PCR in our 2001–2002 investigation at the Singapore Zoological Gardens revealed the emergence of a novel lineage of EMCV strains that are highly divergent from other reported strains.

Having demonstrated that the Singapore EMCV strains, Sing-M100-02 (NCBI GenBank accession number: KC310737) and Sing-M105-02 (NCBI GenBank accession number: KC310738), belonged to a unique phylogenetic lineage, we directed investigative efforts for the 2013 outbreak by diagnosing for EMCV, then performed straintyping via the VP1 and VP3 genes. In the investigation for the recent 2013 outbreak, extracted tissue samples were tested first with PCR detecting for the EMCV 3Dpol region. In sequencing the VP1 and VP3 genes and performing a phylogenetic comparison, we identified two new strains, designated Sing M106-13 and Sing M107-13. These strains were closely related to Sing-M100-02 and Sing-M105-02, adding to the number of members to lineage D of the EMCV phylogeny (van Sandwyk et al., 2013; Yeo et al., 2013). Sing M106-13 (this study) was identified from heart tissue of the deceased cotton-top tamarin, while the Sing M107-13 (this study) was identified from the heart tissue of the deceased hamadryas baboon. EMCV was not detected in tissue samples collected from the other animals.

Methodology for the 2013 investigative study is as follows. 10mg of tissue of each sample was homogenized in 3ml PBS by handheld mechanical tissue grinder while kept on ice to minimize generation of heat. The homogenate was centrifuged at 1000rpm to remove debris. 80µl of the resultant supernatant was used for genetic material extraction. Extraction procedure is as described in the QIAamp® DNA Kit (Qiagen, Germany). Briefly, samples were treated with proteinase K for 1 hour before application to the extraction column, and finally eluted in 100µl elution buffer. RT-PCR for the EMCV 3D poymerase gene was used as the initial screening method because this gene is known to be the most conserved region of the virus. Primers are described on Table 1 while cycling conditions have been described by Koenen et al (Koenen et al., 1997). To straintype the positive specimens, primers have been designed in this study to amplify the entire length of the VP1 and VP3 genes (see Table 2 for primer details). Thermal cycling conditions of the PCR for the VP1 gene are as follows: cDNA synthesis at 50°C for 30 min, initial denaturation step at 94°C for 5 min, 35 cycles of 94°C for 30 s, 55°C for 30 s and 72°C for 2 min, and a final extension step of 72°C for 10 min. Thermal cycling conditions of the PCR for the VP3 gene are as follows: cDNA synthesis at 50°C for 30 min, initial denaturation step at 95°C for 5 min, 35 cycles of 95°C for 30 s, 50°C for 30 s and 72°C for 2 min, and a final extension step of 72°C for 10 min. Expected PCR product sizes are detailed on Table 2. PCR fragments were visualized on 2% agarose gel. Primers for PCR were also used for sequencing of the products by Sanger's sequencing. Forward and reverse sequences were used as confirmation of the correct sequencing result. The VP1 and VP3 gene sequences from EMCV strains identified in this study were aligned against the VP1 and VP3 of other strains using the MegAlign program (DNASTAR, USA) with the Clustal W method.

5.1   Analysis of L, P1, P2 and P3 ORF

For the 2002 investigative study, we analysed fully sequenced EMCV and Theilovirus strains in our phylogenetic trees to demonstrate the divergence of the Singapore species in the genus Cardiovirus, as well as to emphasize the diversity and clustering of various EMCV strains (Yeo et al., 2013). Our phylogenetic analyses showed branching of the EMCV strains into four main lineages, A, B, C and D, at the nucleotide level in the VP1 and 3Dpol regions, as well as for the entire ORF. Lineages A, B and C concurred with similar clusterings of EMCV strains as described previously (van Sandwyk et al., 2013; Koenen et al., 1999; Denis et al., 2006). The Singapore strains detected in our study clustered separately as a distinct group by themselves in a novel lineage D (Yeo et al., 2013). The EMCV isolate RD1338 also clustered by itself in lineage E, highly distinct from the lineage D and other EMCV in lineages A, B and C (Philipps et al., 2012). By this method, we determined a novel lineage of EMCV, and designated the virus identified from the heart tissue of first juvenile orang utan deceased in 2002 to be Sing-M105-02 and that from the lung tissues of the second deceased juvenile orang utan was designated Sing-M100-02 (Yeo et al., 2013). In comparing the different coding regions across the entire ORF (namely L, P1, P2 and P3), and also the 3'-UTR region, we note that nucleotide sequence identities were all below 80% for the P1, P2 and P3 regions between our isolates and existing EMCV strains, demonstrating the high divergence of the Sing-M105-02 and Sing-M100-02 isolates. The phylogenetic analyses based on complete virus gene sequences (as compared to partial gene sequences) afforded us increased confidence that the Sing-M105-02 and Sing-M100-02 isolates constituted a divergent group of EMCV variants, as they clustered distinctly away from the other lineages of EMCV strains (see Figure 4). This high degree of divergence within the EMCV species is perhaps not surprising, since viruses with RNA genomes are generally reported to have a high rate of mutation (Domingo & Holland, 1997; Domingo, 2000; Lauring & Andino, 2010).

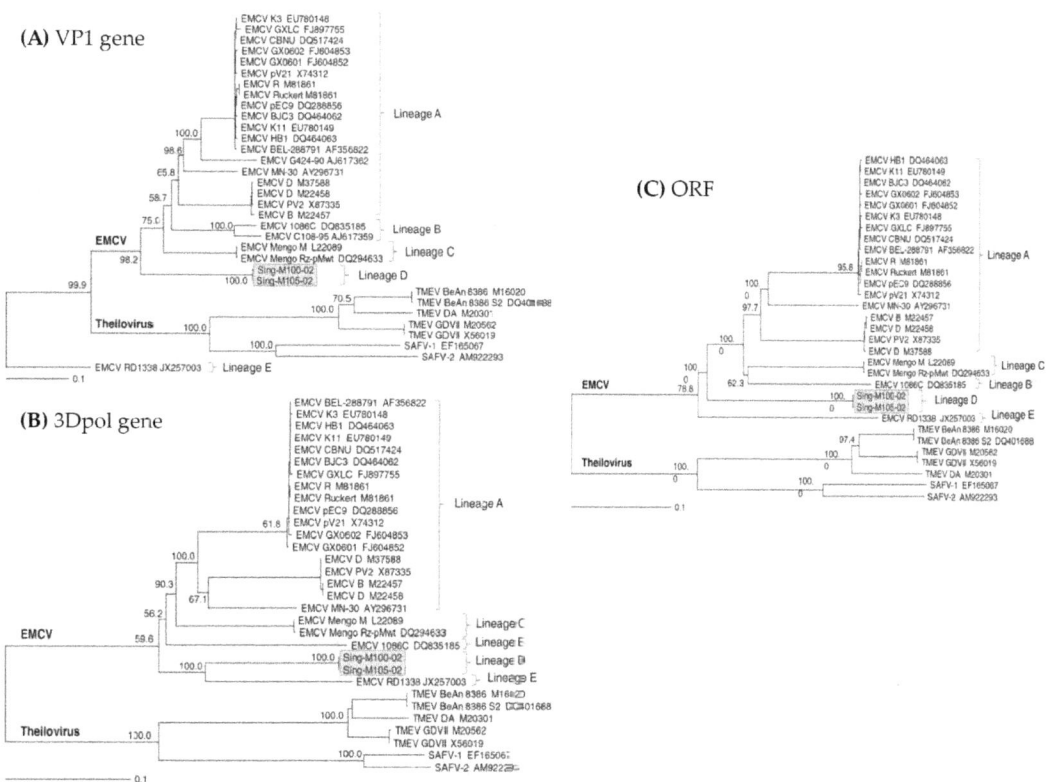

Figure 4: Phylogenetic trees constructed in the 2001–2002 investigation for the full genes encoding (A) VP1 capsid protein, (B) 3D polymerase (3Dpol), and (C) open reading frame (ORF) of Encephalomyocarditis viruses (EMCV) and Theiloviruses based on their nucleotide sequences (adapted from Yeo et al., 2013). TMEV refers to Theiler's murine encephalomyelitis virus. SAFV refers to Saffold virus. Isolate names are followed by their NCBI GenBank accession number. Blue colour highlights the EMCV strains identified during our 2001–2002 investigation. Trees are constructed with the DNASTAR (U.S.A.) program, with bootstrap analyses set at 1000 trials.

5.2   Analysis of the 3Dpol Sequence

In the conserved 3Dpol region, the extent of sequence identities between the Sing-M100-02 and Sing-M105-02 isolates and other EMCV strains ranged from 76.4% to 80.9% at nucleotide level and 79.4% to 90.5% at amino acid level. 3Dpol sequence comparison for Sing-M105-02 and Sing-M100-02 isolates with existing EMCV strains showed a maximum divergence of 24.6% and 11.3% at the nucleotide and amino acid levels respectively (Yeo et al., 2013). These results provide evidence that these strains are indeed highly divergent variants of EMCV, consistent with the other genetic and amino acid analyses performed for these strains (Yeo et al., 2013).

5.3   Analyses of Capsid Proteins VP1 and VP3

5.3.1   VP 1 Anaysis

The VP1 gene is 831 nucleotides in length, and translates to a product of 277 amino acids. Sing-M105-02 and Sing-M100-02 strains identified in our 2001–2002 investigative study share 99.9% identity in their VP1 genes (see Figure 5). When the genomes of these two strains were compared with the existing cardioviruses, the lowest sequence relationships were observed in the VP1 capsid region (as opposed to other genes). Percentage identities ranged from 61.2% to 73.6% at nucleotide level and 66.1% to 87.0% at amino acid level (Yeo et al., 2013). In addition, amino acid alignment for VP1 gene of Sing-M105-02 and Sing-M100-02 against other EMCV strains showed considerable variation in two putative neutralization antigenic sites in the gene, providing further evidence that these viral isolates represent a divergent group of EMCV, now designated as lineage D (Yeo et al., 2013). In examining the amino acid sequence alignment, we observed significant differences in the BC-loop and loop I regions in the VP1 capsid of the Sing-M105-02 and Sing-M100-02 isolates with other EMCV (see Figure 6). The BC-loop and loop I regions of the VP1 capsid protein are two putative neutralizing antigenic sites proposed in the EMCV Mengo virus strain (Luo et al., 1987; Boege et al., 1991).

In our 2013 investigative study, genetic comparative analysis of the VP1 gene between Sing M106-13 and Sing M107-13 shows that they share 99.8% homology to each other. Phylogenetic analysis of the VP1 gene of these strains against other EMCV and Theiloviruses shows Sing M106-13 and Sing M107-13 to be under Lineage D (see Figure 7). These two strains have high percentage homology to the other members of lineage D with a range of 94.8% to 94.9% identity (see Figure 5). Next closest in identity are EMCV strains from lineages A and B, with ranges of 72.6% to 74%, and 72.9% to 73.2% respectively. Slightly further in genetic identity are EMCV strains from lineage C, with a range of 70.6% to 71.6% homology. The two strains identified in this study are furthest from the lineage E and the theilovirus strains, at 62.2% to 62.3% and 51.9% to 53.8% homology respectively. Mutations on the VP1 gene can be significant, since the mouse model of EMCV has shown that the difference between diabetogenic and non-diabetogenic EMCV variants can differ by only a single amino acid mutation on VP1 (Nelsen-Salz et al., 1996). The VP1 capsid protein has two putative neutralizing antigenic sites known as the BC-loop and loop I reported in studies on mengovirus (Scraba, 1990). Amino acid

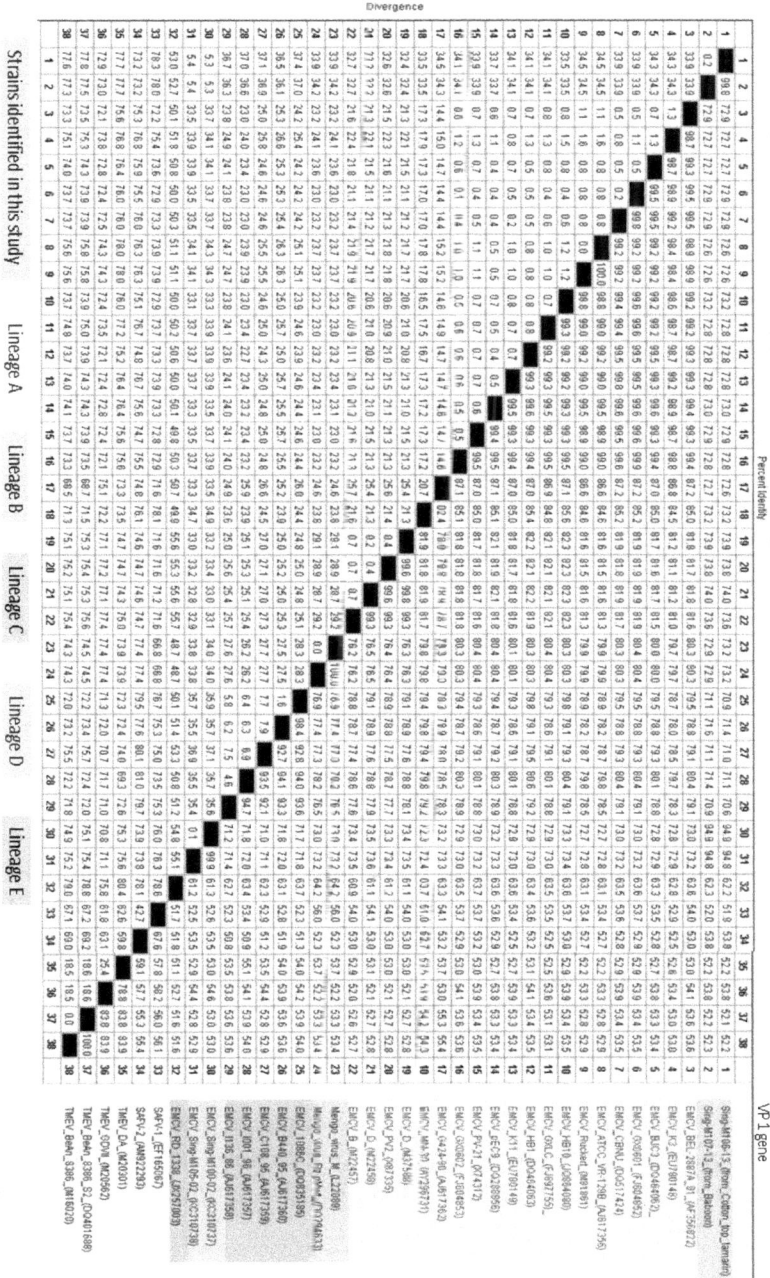

Figure 5: Chart for percentage divergence and identity of the VP1 gene for Encephalomyocarditis viruses (EMCV) and Theiloviruses based on nucleotide sequences. TMEV refers to Theiler's murine encephalomyelitis virus. SAFV refers to Saffold virus. Isolate names are followed by their NCBI GenBank accession number. EMCV strains are colour coded to highlight their lineages, except for the strains identified in this study, highlighted blue. Data was analysed by the DNASTAR program (U.S.A.)

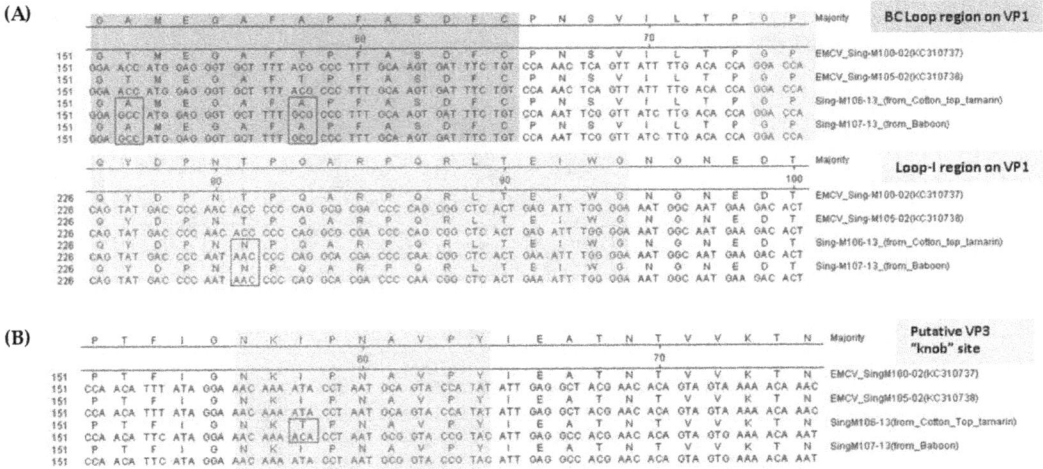

Figure 6: Amino acid mutations of Encephalomyocarditis virus lineage D strains identified in this study occurring on antigenic sites. (A) refers to a portion of the VP1 gene while (B) refers to a portion of the VP3 gene. Blue colour highlights the BC Loop region, green colour highlights the Loop-I region, and pink colour highlights the VP3 "knob" site. The boxed regions highlight positions of antigenic shift in comparison of the novel strains against the Sing-M100-02 (NCBI GenBank accession number KC310737) and SingM-105-02 (NCBI GenBank accession number KC310738) strains. Sing-M106-13 was detected from the deceased cotton-top tamarin and Sing-M107-13 was detected from the deceased hamadryas baboon. Numbers on the left margin refer to the positions of nucleotides on the respective gene, whereas numbers on the top refer to the amino acid positions of the respective gene. Data was analysed by the MegAlign program (DNASTAR, U.S.A.).

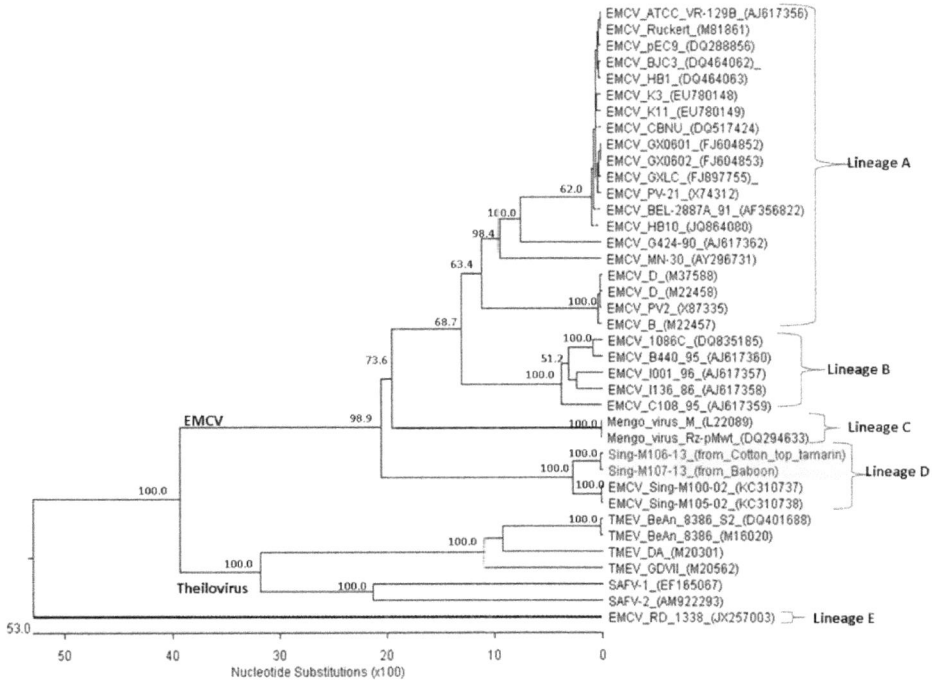

Figure 7A: Phylogenetic trees constructed in the 2013 outbreak investigation for the full genes encoding VP1 and (B) VP3 capsid proteins of Encephalomyocarditis viruses (EMCV) and Theiloviruses based on their nucleotide sequences. TMEV refers to Theiler's murine encephalomyelitis virus. SAFV refers to Saffold virus. Isolate names are followed by their NCBI GenBank accession number. Purple colour highlights the EMCV strains identified in this study. Sing-M106-13 was detected from the deceased cotton-top tamarin and Sing-M107-13 was detected from the deceased hamadryas baboon. Trees are constructed with the DNASTAR (U.S.A.) program, with bootstrap analyses set at 1000 trials.

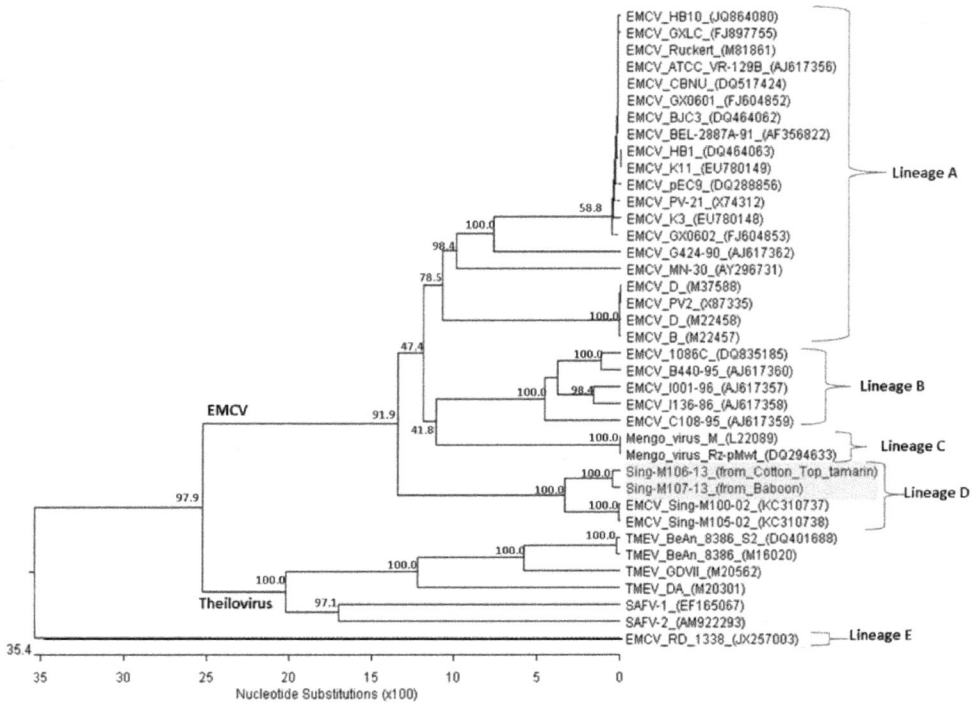

Figure 7B: Phylogenetic trees constructed in the 2013 outbreak investigation for the full genes encoding VP3 capsid proteins of Encephalomyocarditis viruses (EMCV) and Theiloviruses based on their nucleotide sequences. TMEV refers to Theiler's murine encephalomyelitis virus. SAFV refers to Saffold virus. Isolate names are followed by their NCBI GenBank accession number. Purple colour highlights the EMCV strains identified in this study. Sing-M106-13 was detected from the deceased cotton-top tamarin and Sing-M107-13 was detected from the deceased hamadryas baboon. Trees are constructed with the DNASTAR (U.S.A.) program, with bootstrap analyses set at 1000 trials.

sequence analysis among the strains of EMCV in lineage D shows that there are four amino acid changes in the two strains identified in this study when compared to Sing M100-02 and Sing M105-02 (analysis data not shown). Of these four amino acid mutations, two occurred within the BC-loop and one in the loop I (see Figure 6). Interestingly, this amounts to 75% (3 of 4) mutations at the amino acid level in VP1 occurring on antigenic regions over a period of 11 years. Since these are antigenic region of the virus, mutations of these amino acids on these regions could likely have an effect on the virulence of these strains in their infected hosts (Phillips et al., 2012).

5.3.2   VP 3 Analysis

The VP3 gene is 693 nucleotides in length and translates to a product of 231 amino acids. A genetic comparative analysis of the VP3 gene shows that Sing-M105-02 and Sing-M100-02 share 99.9% identity to each other, while Sing M106-13 and Sing M107-13 share 99.1% homology to each other (see Figure 8). Phylogenetic analysis of the VP3 gene of these strains against other EMCV and Theiloviruses shows Sing M106-13 and Sing M107-13 to be under Lineage D (see Figure 5). These two strains have high percentage homology to the other members of lineage D with a range of 93.5% to 94.0% identity (see Figure 8). Next closest in identity are EMCV strains from lineage B, with a range of 79.0% to 79.2%. Slightly further in genetic identity are EMCV strains from lineages A and C, with ranges of 76.2% to 78.0% and 76.3% to 76.9% homology. The two strains identified in this study are furthest from the lineage E and the theilovirus strains, at 71.3% to 71.4% and 61.0% to 62.5% homology respectively. Amino acid sequence analysis among the four strains of EMCV in lineage D shows that there are three amino acid changes in the two strains identified in this study when compared to Sing M100-02 and Sing M105-02 (analysis data not shown). While none of these mutations fall into the putative receptor attachment site, an amino acid mutation on residue 58 of the VP3 gene of SingM106-13 falls on an immunogenic site, a protrusive structure on the capsid known as the VP3 "knob" (see Figure 6; Phillips et al., 2012; Kobasa et al., 1995; Boege et al., 1991; Krishnaswamy and Rossman, 1990) Mutation on this site is known to affect the degree of neuro-virulence of Theiler's murine encephalomyelitis virus (TMEV) infections in rodents (Lipton et al., 2007). Collectively, the mutations identified in this study can play a significant role in altering the virulence of these virus strains on their infected hosts.

5.3.3   Evolution and Emergence of Lineage D EMCV

The novel EMCV strains identified during the 2013 investigation are highly similar to those cases from the 2001–2002 investigative study, forming new members of the currently Singapore-exclusive lineage D of the EMCV phylogeny. Yet, since lineage D strains of EMCV has not been reported from any other part of the world, this suggests that the EMCV strains that caused deaths of primates in 2013 outbreak were not imported but has been circulating in the Singapore Zoological Gardens for more than a decade.

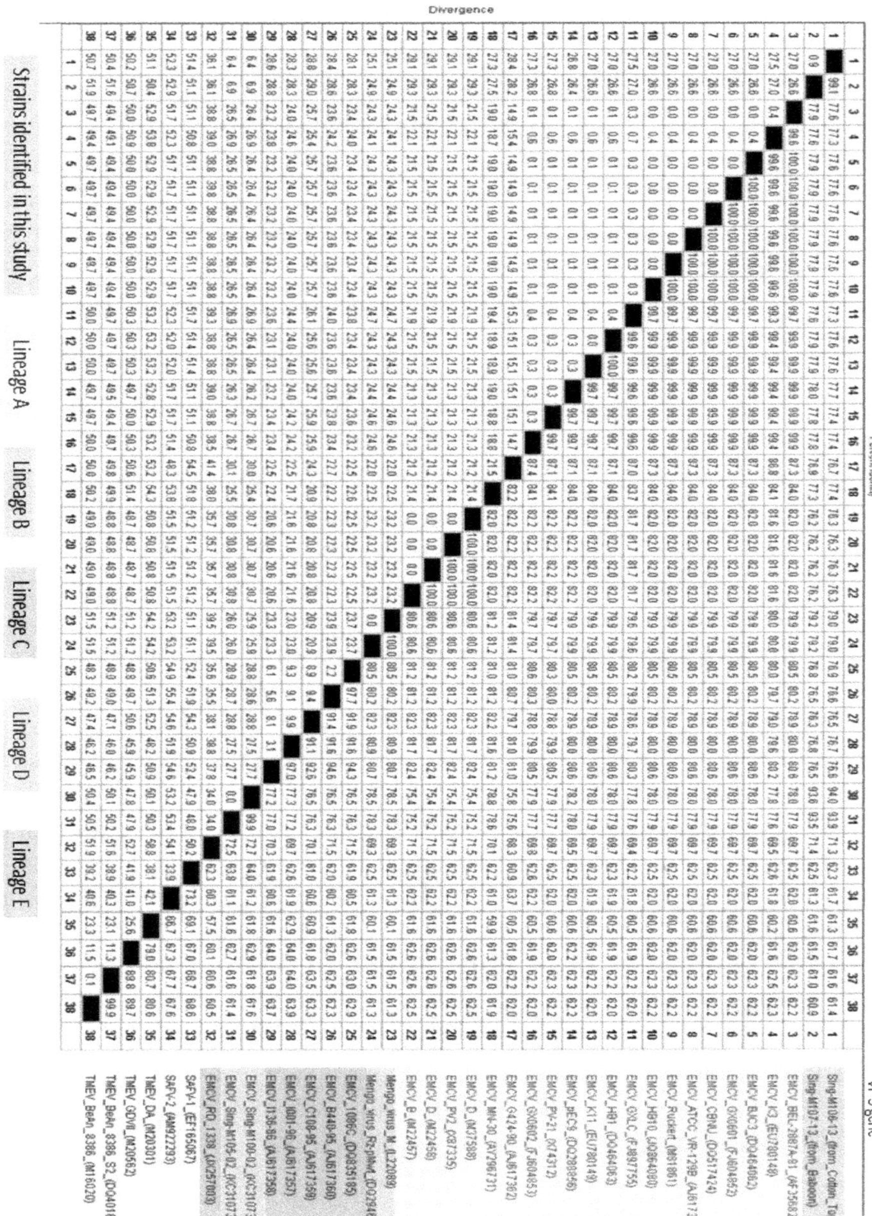

Figure 8: Chart for percentage divergence and identity of the VP3 gene for Encephalomyocarditis viruses (EMCV) and Theiloviruses based on nucleotide sequences. TMEV refers to Theiler's murine encephalomyelitis virus. SAFV refers to Saffold virus. Isolate names are followed by their NCBI GenBank accession number. EMCV strains are colour coded to highlight their lineages, except for the strains identified in this study, highlighted blue. Data was analysed by the DNASTAR program (U.S.A.).

The infected cotton-top tamarin and the infected hamadryas baboon were housed in isolated units, approximately 100 metres apart. That these animals were infected by highly similar strains, suggesting that there is an intermediate carrier of the virus. The two new strains identified in this study are also similar to the EMCV strains that infected the orang utans more than a decade prior. The orang utan habitat unit is approximately 200 metres away from the habitat units of both the cotton-top tamarin and the hamadryas baboon. These considerations further the probability that the wild rats are the vectors responsible for maintaining viral circulation in the zoo. The wild rats would have access to many animals in the zoo. Although EMCV was not detected in the squirrel monkey and pygmy marmoset investigated in the 2013 study, it does not eliminate the possibility that EMCV is indeed the etiological pathogen for these deaths. Thus far, EMCV of lineage D has only been identified in deaths of primates, specifically the orang utan, the cotton-top tamarin and the hamadryas baboon. It remains to be seen if these Singapore strains can be identified in other animal types succumbing to myocarditis.

6   Research on Potential Therapeutic Strategies

A good strategy in the prevention of future EMCV outbreaks would be the use of an effective vaccine. While there have been reports on the use of commercial vaccines on pigs and primates, these are no longer in production at the point when this chapter is prepared (Jeoung et al., 2012; Huneke et al., 1998; Carlson et al., 1993). However, these commercial vaccines may not offer complete protection on the Singapore primates as the Singapore strains of lineage D differ very much in terms of sequence identity from the rest of the EMCV. Several strategies for vaccine development have been reported, such as the use of inactivated virus, live attenuated virus, virus-like particles, and DNA vaccine (Jeoung et al., 2011; Jeoung et al., 2010; Suh et al., 2001; Backues et al., 1999; Hunter et al., 1998; Huneke et al., 1998; Sin et al., 1997; Osorio et al., 1996). In this study we report our preliminary results in developing an EMCV subunit vaccine for lineage D by cloning and expressing the two largest and most antigenic capsid proteins, VP1 (30.50 kDa) and VP2 (28.6 k Da), of the Sing-M105-02 strain.

6.1   Cloning of VP1 and VP2 Capsid Proteins of Sing-M105-02

The viral RNA of the strain Sing-M105-02 was extracted using the viral RNA minikit (Qiagen, Germany) and first strand cDNA synthesis carried out using Superscript® III First-Strand Synthesis for RT-PCR (Invitrogen). The cDNA of entire VP1and VP2 genes were PCR-amplified using the primers described in Table 3.

As shown in Figure 9, the respective amplicons were purified from agarose gel, linearized with EcoRI (New England Biolabs, U.S.A.), cloned into EcoRI-digested pDrive cloning vector (Qiagen, Netherlands) and transformed into Qiagen EZ competent cells (Qiagen, Netherlands).

Gene	Primer	Sequence (5' to 3')
VP1	Forward primer	GCC CCA TGG GGC GGA ATA GAA AAT GCA GAA
	Reverse primer	CCG GAA TTC CGG CTA CTC GAG CAT CAG AAC ACC
VP2	Forward primer	GCC CCA TGG GGC GAC CAA AAT ACA GAA GAA
	Reverse primer	CCG GAA TTC CGG CTA CTG TGT CTG GAG AGT TTC

Table 3: Details of primers designed for amplification and cloning of entire VP1 and VP2 genes of the Encephalomyocarditis virus strain Sing-M105-02.

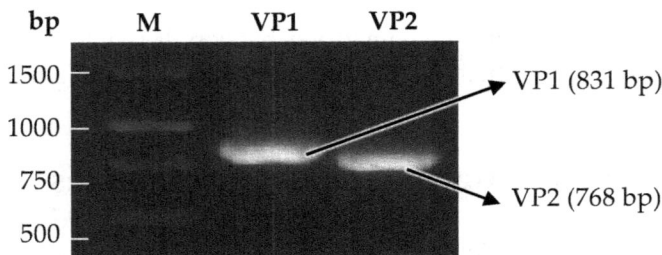

Figure 9: Agarose gel electrophoresis analysis showing the PCR-amplifed VP1 and VP2 capsid genes from EMCV strain Sing-M105-02. Lanes M represent the 1 kb DNA marker in bp (base pairs), VP1 and VP2 represent the respective gene inserts as highlighted by black arrows on the right.

6.2   Expression of VP1 and VP2 Capsid Proteins in Bacterial Expression System

The VP1 or VP2 gene inserts were next subcloned into the appropriate sites of pRSET C cloning vectors (Life Technologies, U.S.A.) by double-digestion with *Kpn*1 (New England Biolabs, U.S.A.) and *Hind*III (New England Biolabs, U.S.A.), and transformed into One Shot® BL21(DE3)pLysS competent cells (Invitrogen, Life Technologies, U.S.A.). Protein expression was induced with IPTG, the induced transformants were lysed and the recombinant VP1 and VP2 proteins purified using TALON® Metal Affinity Resin (Clontech, Takara Bio Inc, Japan). The recombinant proteins were separated by SDS-PAGE, transferred onto PVDF membrane (Immobilion-P, Millipore, USA) and protein bands visualized with anti-His tag antibody (see Fig 10). In the SDA-PAGE analysis, VP1 and VP2 capsid proteins were observed in the pellet fraction, indicating that these proteins are insoluble. As shown in Figure 10A and 10B, the protein species corresponding approximately to 37.5 kDa and 35.6 kDa represent the correct sizes for the respective recombinant VP1 and VP2 proteins, suggesting that the bacterial expression for both proteins were successful. Furthermore the visibly strong bands of these proteins, as seen on Figure 10A, indicate that expression of these recombinant proteins was robust by our method.

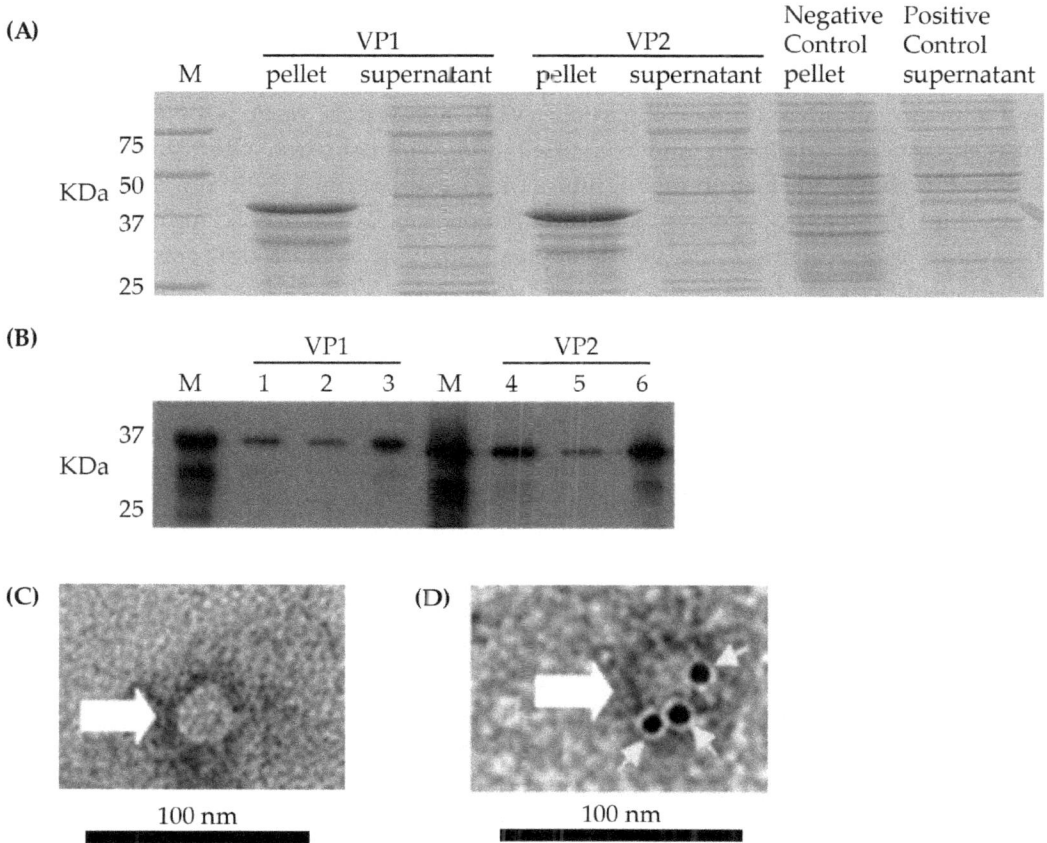

Figure 10: Recombinant VP1 and VP2 proteins expressed in bacteria. (A) Coomassie stained SDS-PAGE gel of the pellet and supernatant fractions of VP1 and VP2 transformed BL21(DE3)pLysS cells after cell lysis. Lane M represents the marker (Biorad, USA) in kilodaltons (kDa). The right end side indicates the positions of VP1 and VP2, at 37.5kDa and 35.5kDa respectively. Robust expression of VP1 and VP2 are observed in the pellet fractions. (B) Western blot for VP1 and VP2 proteins generated from expression of cloned bacteria. Bacterial lysate containing the pRSET C plasmids with VP1 and VP2 gene inserts were induced with IPTG and the expressed his-tagged proteins purified via nickel resin and eluted using 8M urea in 200 mM imidazole. Lanes 1 and 2 represent eluted VP1 protein from the nickel resin, and lane 3 represents the VP1 protein bound to the resin; lanes 4 and 5 represent eluted VP2 protein from the nickel resin, and lane 6 represents the VP2 protein bound to the resin. Lane M represents the marker (Biorad, USA) in kilodaltons (kDa). (C) An electron micrograph showing a recombinant virus-like-particle (white arrow) assembled from the bacterial expression of VP1 capsid protein. (D) An electron micrograph showing another recombinant virus-like-particle (white arrow) assembled from the bacterial expression of VP1 capsid protein reacting with gold particles (yellow arrows) conjugated to anti-His antibodies.

6.3   Expression of Virus-like Particles

The recombinant VP1 and VP2 capsid proteins were allowed to spontaneously assemble and the formation of virus-like particle (VLP) allowed to react with immunogold-labelled anti-His antibodies and examined under transmission electron microscope. Figure 10B shows an electron micrograph of a VLP approximately 30 nm formed by recombinant VP1 before reaction with immunogold-labelled anti-His antibodies. Figure 10C shows VLP reacting to the gold particles visualized as black dots conjugated with anti-His antibodies, when these were introduced. These VLPs formed with the recombinant VP1 protein were readily observed and resembled the same size and morphology as the true virus particles shown in Figure 3. No VLPs were observed with either the recombinant VP2 proteins nor with the bacterial lysate containing the pRSET C vector in the absence of any gene insert. The data indicated that the bacterial expressed VP1 can successfully form VLPs, and that the antigenicity of the recombinant VLPs can be investigated in order to determine its use as a potential vaccine candidate.

7   Possible future directions

The recurrent fatal myocarditis in an assortment of animals at the Singapore Zoological Gardens has prompted an investigation on the presence of EMCV in the Zoo. Our data suggests that the wild rodents may be the reservoir for the virus. Although control measures to eliminate the wild rodents are in place, wild rats continue to have free access to most habitats in the area of EMCV outbreaks. These localized outbreaks can spread to other areas in the Zoo, suggesting that an alternative strategy to control the EMCV infection needs to be urgently explored. The most effective way to prevent future outbreaks is to have a vaccine strategy in place, and as shown from our data above, a potential vaccine candidate is the recombinant VLP formed from bacterial VP1 expression.

Further study on of EMCV lineage D pertaining to its degree of virulence on non-human primates, as well as linking of our virological findings to histopathology, requires adherence to Koch's postulates using suitable non-human primate models. Since the zoo animals are commodities, these cannot be used as test subjects. Such considerations are equally applicable to the efficacy testing of our vaccine candidate. While vaccine safety dosage tests may be derived from small rodent subjects, vaccine efficacy tests require the use of suitable non-human primate models. These resources are currently not ready at our disposal, and work is in progress.

Acknowledgement

We would like to thank Eng-Eong Ooi and Hwee-Cheng Tan for work done for Table 1. In addition, we would like to thank Chin-Wen Jasper Liaw and Ai-Sim Elizabeth Lim for their technical contributions during the 2001–2002 investigation.

Appendix

VP 1 sequence for Sing-106-13 (831 nucleotides)

GGAATAGAAAATGCAGAAAAAGGTGTGACTGAAAATACAGATGCTACTG-
CAGATTTTGTAGCTCAGCCTGTCTACCTGCCTGAAAAC-
CAGACTAAGGTAAACTTCTTCTACGATCGATACAG-
TCCGATTGGTGCTTTTTCTGTAAAAAATGGAGCCATGGAGGGTGCTTTT-
GCGCCCTTTGCAAGTGATTTCTGTCCAAATTCGGTTATCTTGACACCAGGAC-
CACAGTATGACCCCAATAACCCCCAGGCACGACCCCAACGGCTCAC-
TGAAATTTGGGGAAATGGCAATGAAGACACTAGTAG-
TGTCTTCCCTCTCAAAACAAAACAGGACTACTCGTTTTGTCTCTTTTCCCCCTTT-
GTATATTATAAGTGTGATCTTGAAGTGACGATCAGCCCACATACATCTGG-
CAATCATGGCTTAGCTGTACGTTGGGCTCCAACAGGAACACCAACAAA-
GCCGACCACACAAGTGCTGCATGCTGTCGGTTCACTTTCTGAGGGAC-
GTACTCCCAAAATGTACAGTGCTGGGCCCGGAACTTCAAACCATATATCATTT-
GTTGTACCATACAACTCACCTCTGTCAGTCTTGCCCGCTGTCTGG-
TATAATGGACACAAGAAATTTGATAATACAGGCAGTTTGGG-
CATAGCCCCAAATTCAGACTTCGGTACTTTGTTCTTTGCTGGGACCAA-
GCCCGATGTGAAATTTACAGTGTACCTGAGATACAAGAACATGAAGGTTTTTT-
GTCCGAGACCCACTGTTTTCTTCCCTTGGCCCTCTGTTGGGGATAAGGTG-
GACATGACCCCCCGAGCTGGTGTCTTGATGCTCGAG

VP 3 sequence for Sing-106-13 (693 nucleotides)

TCCCCCATTCCGGTGACTATCCGTGAGCATGCTGGCACCTGGTATTCTACAC-
TTCCTGATACAACTGTCCCCATATATGGTAAAACTCCCGTTGCACCCTCTAAC-
TATATGGTAGGAGAATACACAGATTTCTTGGAGATTGCCCAGATAC-
CAACATTCATAGGAAACAAAACACCTAATGCGGTACCGTACATTGAGGCCAC-
GAACACAGTAGTGAAAACAAATCCACTTGCTACTTATCAAGTAACATT-
GTCATGTACATGTCTAGCCAACACTTTCCTGGCTGCAC-
TATCCAGAAATTTTTCCCAGTACAGAGGCTCAATGGTCTATACCTTT-
GTCTTCACTGGTACCGCGATGATGAAAGGAAAATTCCTGATTGCCTACACAC-
CTCCCGGCGCTGGAAAGCCCACTACTAGGGATCAGGCTATGCAA-
GCAACTTATGCTATCTGGGATTTGGGTTTAAATTCTAC-
CTACTCTTTTACTGTGCCCTTTATATCTCCCACACACTTTAGAATGGTT-
GGAACAGATCAAGTCAACATCACAAATGTTGATGGATGGGTCACAGTTTGG-
CAACTAACACCTCTGACGTACCCACCTGGCTGTCCGAACACTGCGAAAA-
TACTCACCATGGTTAGTGCCGGGAAAGACTTCACTGTTAAAATGCC-
TATTTCTCCTGCCCCATGGAGTCCACAG

VP 1 sequence for Sing-107-13 (831 nucleotides)

GGAATAGAAAATGCAGAAAAAGGTGTGACTGAAAATACAGATGCTACTG-

CAGATTTTGTAGCTCAGCCTGTCTACCTGCCTGAAAAC-
CAGACTAAGGTAAACTTCTTCTACGATCGATACAG-
TCCGATTGGTGCTTTTTCTGTAAAAAATGGAGCCATGGAGGGTGCTTTT-
GCGCCCTTTGCAAGTGATTTCTGTCCAAATTCGGTTATCTTGACACCAGGAC-
CACAGTATGACCCCAATAACCCCCAGGCACGACCCCAACGGCTCAC-
TGAAATTTGGGGAAATGGCAATGAAGACACTAGTAG-
TGTCTTCCCTCTCAAAACAAAACAGGACTACTCGTTTTGTCTCTTTTCCCCCTTT-
GTATATTATAAGTGTGATCTTGAAGTGACGATCAGCCCCCATACATCTGG-
CAATCATGGCTTAGCTGTACGTTGGGCTCCAACAGGAACACCAACAAA-
GCCGACCACACAAGTGCTGCATGCTGTGGGTTCACTTTCTGAGGGAC-
GTACTCCCAAAATGTACAGTGCTGGGCCCGGAACTTCAAACCATATATCATTT-
GTTGTACCATACAACTCACCTCTGTCAGTCTTGCCCGCTGTCTGG-
TATAATGGACACAAGAAATTTGATAATACAGGTAGTTTGGG-
CATAGCCCCAAATTCAGACTTCGGTACTTTGTTCTTTGCTGGGACCAA-
GCCCGATGTGAAATTTACAGTGTACCTGAGATACAAGAACATGAAGGTTTTTT-
GTCCGAGACCCACTGTTTTCTTCCCTTGGCCCTCTGTTGGGGATAAGGTG-
GACATGACCCCCCGAGCTGGTGTCTTGATGCTCGAG

VP 3 sequence for Sing-107-13 (693 nucleotides)

TCCCCCATTCCGGTGACTATCCGTGAGCATGCTGGCACCTGGTATTCTACAC-
TTCCTGATACAACTGTCCCCATATATGGTAAAACTCCCGTTGCACCCTCTAAC-
TATATGGTAGGAGAATACACAGATTTTTTGGAGATCGCCCAGATAC-
CAACATTCATAGGAAACAAAATACCTAATGCGGTACCGTACATTGAGGCCAC-
GAACACAGTAGTGAAAACAAATCCACTTGCTACTTATCAAGTAACATT-
GTCATGTACATGTCTAGCCAACACTTTCCTGGCTGCAC-
TATCCAGAAATTTTTCCCAGTACAGAGGCTCAATGGTCTATACCTTT-
GTCTTCACTGGTACCGCGATGATGAAAGGAAAATTCCTGATTGCCTACACAC-
CTCCCGGCGCTGGAAAGCCCACTACTAGAGATCAGGCCATGCAA-
GCAACTTATGCTATCTGGGATTTGGGTTTAAATTCTACAT-
ACTCTTTTACTGTGCCCTTTATATCTCCCACACACTTTAGAATGGTT-
GGAACAGATCAAGTCAACATCACAAATGTTGATGGATGGGTCACAGTTTGG-
CAACTAACACCTCTGACGTACCCACCTGGCTGTCCGAACACTGCGAAAA-
TACTCACCATGGTTAGTGCCGGGAAAGACTTCACTGTTAAAATGCC-
TATTTCTCCTGCCCCATGGAGTCCACAG

References

Backues, K. A., Hill, M., Palmenberg, A. C., Miller, C., Soike, K. F., & Aguilar, R. (1999). Genetically engineered Mengo virus vaccination of multiple captive wildlife species. Journal of wildlife diseases, 35 (2), 384–387.

Boege, U., Kobasa, D., Onodera, S., Parks, G. D., Palmenberg, A. C., & Scraba, D. G. (1991). Characterization of Mengo virus neutralization epitopes. Virology, 181 (1), 1–13.

Brown, B. A., Oberste, M. S., Alexander, J. P., Kennett, M. L., & Pallansch, M. A. (1999). Molecular epidemiology and evolution of enterovirus 71 strains isolated from 1970 to 1998. Journal of virology, 73 (12), 9969–9975.

Canelli, E., Luppi, A., Lavazza, A., Lelli, D., Sozzi, E., Martin, A. M., Gelmetti, D., Pascotto, E., Sandri, C., Magnone, W., & Cordioli, P. (2010). Encephalomyocarditis virus infection in an Italian zoo. Virol J, 7 (6), 4.

Carlson, J. H., & Joo, H. S. (1993). U.S. Patent No. 5,213,795. Washington, DC: U.S. Patent and Trademark Office.

Carocci, M., & Bakkali-Kassimi, L. (2012). The encephalomyocarditis virus. Virulence, 3 (4), 351–367.

Citino, S. B., Homer, B. L., Gaskin, J. M., & Wickham, D. J. (1988). Fatal encephalomyocarditis virus infection in a Sumatran orangutan (Pongo pygmaeus abelii). The Journal of Zoo Animal Medicine, 214–218.

Costa-Mattioli, M., Cristina, J., Romero, H., Perez-Bercof, R., Casane, D., Colina, R., ... & Ferré, V. (2002). Molecular evolution of hepatitis A virus: a new classification based on the complete VP1 protein. Journal of virology, 76 (18), 9516–9525.

Denis, P., Liebig, H. D., Nowotny, N., Billinis, C., Papadopoulos, O., O'Hara, R. S., Knowles, N. J., & Koenen, F. (2006). Genetic variability of encephalomyocarditis virus (EMCV) isolates. Veterinary microbiology, 113 (1), 1–12.

Dick, G. W., Haddow, A. J., Best, A. M., & Smithburn, K. C. (1948). Mengo encephalomyelitis: a hitherto unknown virus affecting man. The Lancet, 252 (6521), 286–289.

Doi, K. (2011). Experimental encephalomyocarditis virus infection in small laboratory rodents. Journal of comparative pathology, 144 (1), 25–40.

Domingo, E. (2000). Viruses at the edge of adaptation. Virology, 270 (2), 251–253.

Domingo, E. J. J. H., & Holland, J. J. (1997). RNA virus mutations and fitness for survival. Annual Reviews in Microbiology, 51 (1), 151–178.

Gajdusek, D. C. (1955). Encephalomyocarditis virus infection in childhood. Pediatrics, 16 (6), 902–906.

Gelmetti, D., Meroni, A., Brocchi, E., Koenen, F., & Cammarata, G. (2006). Pathogenesis of encephalomyocarditis experimental infection in young piglets: a potential animal model to study viral myocarditis. Veterinary research, 37 (1), 15–23.

Grobler, D. G., Raath, J. P., Braack, L. E. O., Keet, D. F., Gerdes, G. H., Barnard, B. J. H., Kriek, N. P. J., Jardine, J., & Swanepoel, R. (1995). An outbreak of encephalomyocarditis-virus infection in free-ranging African elephants in the Kruger National Park. Onderstepoort Journal of Veterinary Research, 62, 97–108

Haydon, D. T., Bastos, A. D., Knowles, N. J., & Samuel, A. R. (2001). Evidence for positive selection in foot-and-mouth disease virus capsid genes from field isolates. Genetics, 157 (1), 7–15.

Hu, D. G., Chan, C. H., Shieh, W. Y., & Chang, C. S. (1993). Epidemiological studies of swine Encephalomyocarditis virus infection. Research report—animal industry research institute, Taiwan Sugar Corporation. 1993: 149–154.

Hubbard, G. B., Soike, K. F., Butler, T. M., Carey, K. D., Davis, H., Butcher, W. I., & Gauntt, C. J. (1992). An encephalomyocarditis virus epizootic in a baboon colony. Laboratory animal science, 42 (3), 233–239.

Huneke, R. B., Michaels, M. G., Kaufman, C. L. & Ildstad, S. T. (1998). Antibody response in baboons

(Papio cynocephalus anubis) to a commercially available encephalomyocarditis virus vaccine. Comparative Medicine, 48 (5), 526–528.

Hunter, P., Swanepoel, S. P., Esterhuysen, J. J., Raath, J. P., Bengis, R. G., & Van der Lugt, J. J. (1998). The efficacy of an experimental oil-adjuvanted encephalomyocarditis vaccine in elephants, mice and pigs. Vaccine, 16 (1), 55–61.

Jeoung, H. Y., Lee, W. H., Jeong, W., Ko, Y. J., Choi, C. U., & An, D. J. (2010). Immune responses and expression of the virus-like particle antigen of the porcine encephalomyocarditis virus. Research in veterinary science, 89 (2), 295–300.

Jeoung, H. Y., Lee, W. H., Jeong, W., Shin, B. H., Choi, H. W., Lee, H. S., & An, D. J. (2011). Immunogenicity and safety of virus-like particle of the porcine encephalomyocarditis virus in pig. Virol J, 8 (1), 170.

Jeoung, H. Y., Shin, B. H., Jeong, W., Lee, M. H., Lee, W. H., & An, D. J. (2012). A novel vaccine combined with an alum adjuvant for porcine encephalomyocarditis virus (EMCV)-induced reproductive failure in pregnant sows. Research in veterinary science, 93 (3), 1508–1511.

Jones, P., Cordonnier, N., Mahamba, C., Burt, F. J., Rakotovao, F., Swanepoel, R., ... & Bakkali Kassimi, L. (2011). Encephalomyocarditis virus mortality in semi-wild bonobos (Pan panicus). Journal of medical primatology, 40 (3), 157–163.

Joo, H. S. (1992). Encephalomyocarditis virus. Diseases of swine, 257–262. Wolfe Publishing.

Kassimi, L. B., Boutrouille, A., Gonzague, M., Mbanda, A. L., & Cruciere, C. (2002). Nucleotide sequence and construction of an infectious cDNA clone of an EMCV strain isolated from aborted swine fetus. Virus research, 83 (1), 71–87.

Kim, H. S., Christianson, W. T., & Joo, H. S. (1989). Pathogenic properties of encephalomyocarditis virus isolates in swine fetuses. Archives of virology, 109 (1–2), 51–57.

Knowles, N. J., Dickinson, N. D., Wilsden, G., Carra, E., Brocchi, E., & De Simone, F. (1998). Molecular analysis of encephalomyocarditis viruses isolated from pigs and rodents in Italy. Virus research, 57 (1), 53–62.

Knowles, N. J., Hovi, T., Hyypiä, T., King, A. M. Q., Lindberg, A. M., Pallansch, M. A., Palmenberg, A. C., Simmonds, P., Skern, T., Stanway, G., Yamashita, T., & Zell, R. (2011). Picornaviridae, p 855–880. Virus taxonomy: classification and nomenclature of viruses. Ninth report of the International Committee on Taxonomy of Viruses. Elsevier, San Diego, CA.

Kobasa, D., Mulvey, M., Lee, J. S., & Scraba, D. G. (1995). Characterization of Mengo Virus Neutralization Epitopes II. Infection of Mice with an Attenuated Virus. Virology, 214 (1), 118–127.

Koenen, F., Vanderhallen, H., Dickinson, N. D., & Knowles, N. J. (1999). Phylogenetic analysis of European encephalomyocarditis viruses: comparison of two genomic regions. Archives of virology, 144 (5), 893–903.

Koenen, F., Vanderhallen, H., Papadopoulos, O., Billinis, C., Paschaleri-Papadopoulou, E., Brocchi, E., De Simone, F., Carra, E., & Knowles, N. J. (1997). Comparison of the pathogenic, antigenic and molecular characteristics of two encephalomyocarditis virus (EMCV) isolates from Belgium and Greece. Research in veterinary science, 62 (3), 239–244.

Koonin, E. V. (1991). The phylogeny of RNA-dependent RNA polymerases of positive-strand RNA viruses. J. Gen. Virol, 72 (Pt 9), 2197–2206.

Krishnaswamy, S., & Rossmann, M. G. (1990). Structural refinement and analysis of Mengo virus. Journal of molecular biology, 211 (4), 803–844.

Krylova, R. I., & Dzhikidze, E. K. (2005). Encephalomyocarditis in monkeys. Bulletin of experimental biology and medicine, 139 (3), 355–359.

LaRue, R., Myers, S., Brewer, L., Shaw, D. P , Brown, C., Seal, B. S., & Njenga, M. K. (2003). A wild-type porcine encephalomyocarditis virus containing a short poly (C) tract is pathogenic to mice, pigs, and cynomolgus macaques. Journal of virology, 77 (17), 9136–9146.

Lauring, A. S., & Andino, R. (2010). Quasispecies theory and the behavior of RNA viruses. PLoS pathogens, 6 (7), e1001005.

Lin, W., Liu, Y., Cui, S., & Liu, H. (2012). Isolation, molecular characterization, and phylogenetic analysis of porcine encephalomyocarditis virus strain HB10 in China. Infection, Genetics and Evolution, 12 (6), 1324–1327.

Lipton, H. L., Kumar, A. M., & Hertzler, S. (2005). Cardioviruses: Encephalomyocarditis Virus and Theiler's Murine Encephalomyelitis Virus. The Mouse in Biomedical Research: Diseases, 2, 311.

Lipton, H. L., Kumar, A. S. M., Hertzler, S. (2007) Chapter 12 – Cardioviruses: Encephalomyocarditis Virus and Theiler's Murine Encephalomyelitis Virus The Mouse in Biomedical Research (Second Edition), pp. 311–323

Liu, H., Yan, Q., Zhao, B., Luo, J., Wang, C., Du, Y., Yan, J., & He, H. (2013). Isolation, molecular characterization, and phylogenetic analysis of encephalomyocarditis virus from South China tigers in China. Infection, Genetics and Evolution, 19, 240–243.

Luo, M., Vriend, G., Kamer, G., Minor, I., Arnold, E., Rossmann, M. G, Boege, U., Scraba, D. G., Duke, G. M., & Palmenberg, A. C. (1987). The atomic structure of Mengo virus at 3.0 A resolution. Science, 235 (4785), 182–191.

Masek-Hammerman, K., Miller, A. D., Lin. K. C., MacKey, J., Weissenböck, H., Gierbolini, L., Perez, B. H., & Mansfield, K. G. (2012). Epizootic myocarditis associated with Encephalomyocarditis virus in a group of rhesus macaques (macaca mulatta). Veterinary Pathology Online, 49 (2), 386–392.

Maurice, H., Nielen, M., Brocchi, E., Nowotny, N., Bakkali Kassimi, L., Billinis, C., Loukaides, P., O'Hara, R. S., & Koenen, F. (2005). The occurrence of encephalomyocarditis virus (EMCV) in European pigs from 1990 to 2001. Epidemiology and infection, 133 (03), 547–557.

Maurice, H., Nielen, M., Vyt, P., Frankena, K., & Koenen, F. (2007). Factors related to the incidence of clinical encephalomyocarditis virus (EMCV) infection on Belgian pig farms. Preventive veterinary medicine, 78 (1), 24–34.

McMinn, P., Lindsay, K., Perera, D., Chan, H. M., Chan, K. P., & Cardosa, M. J. (2001). Phylogenetic analysis of enterovirus 71 strains isolated during linked epidemics in Malaysia, Singapore, and Western Australia. Journal of virology, 75 (16), 7732–7738.

Miyagi, J., Tsuhako, K., Kinjo, T., Iwamasa, T., Kamada, Y., Kinju, T., & Koyanagi, Y. (1999). Coxsackievirus B4 myocarditis in an orangutan. Veterinary Pathology Online, 36 (5), 452–456.

Mulders, M. N., Salminen, M., Kalkkinen, N., & Hovi, T. (2000). Molecular epidemiology of coxsackievirus B4 and disclosure of the correct VP1/2Apro cleavage site: evidence for high genomic diversity and long-term endemicity of distinct genotypes. Journal of General Virology, 81 (3), 803–812.

Nelsen-Salz, B., Zimmermann, A., Wickert, S., Arnold, G., Botta, A., Eggers, H. J., & Kruppenbacher, J. P. (1996). Analysis of sequence and pathogenic properties of two variants of encephalomyocarditis virus differing in a single amino acid in VP1. Virus research, 41 (2), 109–122.

Nielsen, S. C. A., Mourier, T., Baandrup, U., Søland, T. M., Bertelsen, M. F., Gilbert, M. T. P., & Nielsen,

L. P. (2012). *Probable transmission of coxsackie B3 virus from human to chimpanzee, Denmark. Emerging infectious diseases, 18 (7), 1163.*

Norder, H., Bjerregaard, L., & Magnius, L. O. (2001). *Homotypic echoviruses share aminoterminal VP1 sequence homology applicable for typing. Journal of medical virology, 63 (1), 35–44.*

Oberste, M. S., Gotuzzo, E., Blair, P., Nix, W. A., Ksiazek, T. G., Comer, J. A., Rollin, P., Goldsmith, C. S., Olson, J., & Kochel, T. J. (2009). *Human febrile illness caused by encephalomyocarditis virus infection, Peru. Emerging infectious diseases, 15 (4), 640.*

Oberste, M. S., Maher, K., Flemister, M. R., Marchetti, G., Kilpatrick, D. R., & Pallansch, M. A. (2000). *Comparison of classic and molecular approaches for the identification of untypeable enteroviruses. Journal of clinical microbiology, 38 (3), 1170–1174.*

Oberste, M. S., Maher, K., Kilpatrick, D. R., & Pallansch, M. A. (1999). *Molecular evolution of the human enteroviruses: correlation of serotype with VP1 sequence and application to picornavirus classification. Journal of virology, 73 (3), 1941–1948.*

Oberste, M. S., Schnurr, D., Maher, K., al-Busaidy, S., & Pallansch, M. A. (2001). *Molecular identification of new picornaviruses and characterization of a proposed enterovirus 73 serotype. Journal of General Virology, 82 (2), 409–416.*

Osorio, J. E., Hubbard, G. B., Soike, K. F., Girard, M., van der Werf, S., Moulin, J. C., & Palmenberg, A. C. (1996). *Protection of non-murine mammals against encephalomyocarditis virus using a genetically engineered Mengo virus. Vaccine, 14 (2), 155–161.*

Palmenberg, A. C., Kirby, E. M., Janda, M. R., Drake, N. L., Duke, G. M., Potratz, K. F., & Collett, M. S. (1984). *The nucleotide and deduced amino acid sequences of the encephalomyocarditis viral polyprotein coding region. Nucleic acids research, 12 (6), 2969–2985.*

Papaioannou, N., Billinis, C., Psychas, V., Papadopoulos, O., & Vlemmas, I. (2003). *Pathogenesis of encephalomyocarditis virus (EMCV) infection in piglets during the viraemia phase: a histopathological, immunohistochemical and virological study. Journal of comparative pathology, 129 (2), 161–168.*

Park, N. Y., Ri, C. Y., Chung, C. Y., Kee, H. Y., & Bae, S. Y. (1992). *Pathological findings on Encephalomyocarditis virus infections of swine in Korea. Korean Journal of Veterinary Research (Korea Republic). 32, 99–109.*

Paschaleri-Papadopoulou, E., Axiotis, I., & Laspidis, C. (1990). *Encephalomyocarditis of swine in Greece. Veterinary Record, 126 (15), 364–365.*

Philipps, A., Dauber, M., Groth, M., Schirrmeier, H., Platzer, M., Krumbholz, A., Wutzler, P , & Zell, R. (2012). *Isolation and molecular characterization of a second serotype of the encephalomyocarditis virus. Veterinary microbiology, 161 (1), 49–57.*

Porter, F. W., Bochkov, Y. A., Albee, A. J., Wiese, C., & Palmenberg, A. C. (2006). *A picornavirus protein interacts with Ran-GTPase and disrupts nucleocytoplasmic transport. Proceedings of the National Academy of Sciences, 103 (33), 12417–12422.*

Reddacliff, L. A., Kirkland, P. D., Hartley, W. J., & Reece, R. L. (1997). *Encephalomyocarditis virus infections in an Australian zoo. Journal of Zoo and Wildlife Medicine, 153–157.*

Rodrigo, M. J., & Dopazo, J. (1995). *Evolutionary analysis of the picornavirus family. Journal of molecular evolution, 40 (4), 362–371.*

Santti, J., Harvala, H., Kinnunen, L., & Hyypiä, T. (2000). *Molecular epidemiology and evolution of coxsackievirus A9. Journal of General Virology, 81 (5), 1361–1372.*

Scraba, Douglas G. *Functional aspects of the capsid structure of Mengo virus*. Journal of structural biology 104, no. 1 (1990): 52–62.

Sidoli, L., Barigazzi, G., Foni, E., Marcato, P. S., & Barbieri, G. (1989). *Encephalomyocarditis (EMC) due to Cardiovirus in Po Valley swines: preliminary observations, clinical aspects, virus isolation, characterization and experimental transmission*. Selozoine Vet, 30, 249–260.

Simpson, C. F., Lewis, A. L., & Gaskin, J. M. (1977). *Encephalomyocarditis virus infection of captive elephants*. Journal of the American Veterinary Medical Association, 171 (9), 902–905.

Sin, J. I., Sung, J. H., Suh, Y. S., Lee, A. H., Chung, J. H., & Sung, Y. C. (1997). *Protective immunity against heterologous challenge with encephalomyocarditis virus by VP1 DNA vaccination: effect of coinjection with a granulocyte-macrophage colony stimulating factor gene*. Vaccine, 15 (17), 1827–1833.

Speir, R. W. (1962). *pH and thermal stability of Mengo virus*. Virology, 17 (4), 588–592.

Suh, Y. S., Ha, S. J., Lee, C. H., Sin, J. I., & Sung, Y. C. (2001). *Enhancement of VP1-specific immune responses and protection against EMCV-K challenge by co-delivery of IL-12 DNA with VP1 DNA vaccine*. Vaccine, 19 (15), 1891–1898.

Swiss Institute of Bioinformatics, 2008, http://viralzone.expasy.org/all_by_species/33.html

van Sandwyk, J. H., Bennett, N. C., Swanepoel, R., & Bastos, A. D. (2013). *Retrospective genetic characterisation of Encephalomyocarditis viruses from African elephant and swine recovers two distinct lineages in South Africa*. Veterinary microbiology, 162 (1), 23–31.

Vanderhallen, H., & Koenen, F. (1997). *Rapid diagnosis of encephalomyocarditis virus infections in pigs using a reverse transcription-polymerase chain reaction*. Journal of virological methods, 66 (1), 83–89.

Vanderhallen, H., & Koenen, F. (1998). *Identification of encephalomyocarditis virus in clinical samples by reverse transcription-PCR followed by genetic typing using sequence analysis*. Journal of clinical microbiology, 36 (12), 3463–3467.

Villaverde, A., Martínez-Salas, E., & Domingo, E. (1988). *3D gene of foot-and-mouth disease virus: Conservation by convergence of average sequences*. Journal of molecular biology, 204 (3), 771–776.

Wells, Susan K., Andrew E. Gutter, Kenneth F. Szike, and Gary B. Baskin. *Encephalomyocarditis virus: epizootic in a zoological collection*. Journal of Zoo and Wildlife Medicine (1989): 291–296.

Yeo, D. S. Y., Lian, J. E., Fernandez, C. J., Lin, Y. N., Liaw, J. C. W., Soh, M. L., Lim, E. A. S., Chan, K. P., Ng, M. L., Tan, H. C., Oh, S., Ooi, E. E., & Tan, B. H. (2013). *A highly divergent Encephalomyocarditis virus isolated from nonhuman primates in Singapore*. Virology journal, 10(1), 248.

Zhang, G. Q., Ge, X. N., Guo, X., & Yang, H. C. (2007). *Genomic analysis of two porcine encephalomyocarditis virus strains isolated in China*. Archives of virology, 152 (6), 1209–1213.

Zimmerman, J. J. (1994). *Encephalomyocarditis*. CRC Handbook Series in Zoonoses. Section B: Viral, 2nd Edition. CRC Press, Boca Raton, FL, 423–435.

Chapter 2

The Physiology and Pathology of Synaptic Cell Adhesion Molecules

Chen Zhang[1], Xiaofei Yang[2]

1   Introduction

The brain was characterized by an enormous degree of complexity and diversity of neural networks, making it one of the most complicated organs. This complexity and diversity came from the vast numbers of neurons, but also from the variety of synapses where neurons pass electrical or chemical signals to other cells. In the brain, neurons recognized each other and form stable synaptic connections through synaptic cell adhesion molecules (CAMs). Synaptic CAMs served as the "glue" that connects the pre- and post-synaptic neurons. These CAMs played important roles in 1) the initial target recognition between pre- and post-synaptic neurons during synapse formation (Sanes & Yamagata, 2009; Williams et al., 2010) and 2) enrichment of synaptic components at pre- and post-synaptic terminals in the early stages of synapse development (Dalva et al., 2007; Chavis & Westbrook, 2001). During the later stages of synapse development and in mature synapses, CAMs also regulated synaptic structure and function. Alterations in CAMs led to changes in synaptic morphology and function, leading to dysfunction of neural circuits, whose function was highly reliant on precisely controlled cell-cell adhesions. Thus, it was not surprising that many CAMs were associated with many neuropsychiatric disorders including autism, Alzheimer's desease (AD) and schizophrenia. For example, mutations in

[1] State Key Laboratory of Membrane Biology, McGovern Institute for Brain Research, Peking University, Beijing, China.

[2] Key Laboratory of Cognitive Science, Hubei Key Laboratory of Medical Information Analysis and Tumor Diagnosis & Treatment, Laboratory of Membrane Ion Channels and Medicine, College of Biomedical Engineering, South-Central University for Nationalities, Wuhan, China.

neurexins (Nrxs) and neuroligins (NLs) were found in patients with autism spectrum disorder (ASD) (Südhof, 2008) and Eph receptor alterations were highly related to AD (Chen et al., 2012).

Here we would like to summarize some of the known CAMs, their physiology, and their roles in brain pathologies involving protein-protein interactions at synapses.

2 CAMs between pre- & post- synapses

2.1 Neurexin and Neuroligin

2.1.1 Physiology

Nrxs, discovered as receptors for α-latrotoxin (Südhof, 2008), were type-I transmembrane proteins localized presynaptically (Berninghausen et al., 2007). There were three different genes coding for Nrxs (Nrx1, Nrx2, Nrx3) in mammals, expressing three α-Nrxs (long form) and three β-Nrxs (short form) due to two different promoters (Baudouin & Scheiffele, 2010). NLs were also type-I proteins found on the postsynaptic membrane. At least four (in mice and rats) or five (in humans) NL isoforms had been identified (Lisé and El-Husseini, 2006; Jamain et al., 2008). Nrxs and NLs interacted with each other with high affinity via their extracellular regions (Scheiffele et al., 2000; Comoletti et al., 2006). The crystal structures of Nrxs and NLs indicated that these extracellular parts formed a trans-synaptic complex in the synaptic cleft (Araç et al., 2007). The binding of Nrxs and NLs was dependent on the extracellular Ca^{2+} (Boucard et al., 2005; Chen et al., 2008; Ichtchenko et al., 1995; Nguyen and Südhof, 1997) and splicing sites on both proteins. Splicing sites 4 (SS4) on Nrxs and splice site B on NLs controlled the binding affinity between these two proteins (Boucard et al., 2005; Chih et al., 2006; Reissner et al., 2013; Ichtchenko et al., 1995). The α-Nrxs and β-Nrxs both bound to NL1, which lacked splice site B, and were independent of SS4 in Nrxs. In the presence of splice site B, NL1 bound only to β-Nrxs, but did not bind to α-Nrxs, without SS4 (Boucard et al., 2005). This apparent splice insert dependency of Nrx/NL interaction raised a splice-code hypothesis that specific pairings of Nrx/NL complex according to their roles at different location (Nam & Chen, 2005; Boucard et al., 2005; Ichtchenko et al., 1995; Chih et al., 2006).

The C-terminal of Nrxs and NLs interacted with intracellular scaffolding proteins to mediate pre- and post-synaptic differentiation and function. Nrxs bound CASK (Ca^{2+}/calmodulin-activated Ser-Thr kinase), while CASK bound Velis/MALs proteins and Mints/X11 proteins in the presynaptic terminal (Butz et al., 1998; Borg et al., 1999). At postsynaptic sites, the NLs/Nrxs interaction caused an increase in PSD-95 clustering and the recruitment of postsynaptic NMDA (N-methyl-D-aspartate) and AMPA (α-amino-3-hydroxy-5-methyl-4-isoxazolepropionic acid) receptors (Nam & Chen, 2005; Heine et al., 2008; Chih et al., 2005; Barrow et al., 2009). Thus, the binding of Nrxs and NLs to their partners helped to align the presynaptic release machinery and postsynaptic receptors.

How exactly did the Nrx/NL complex function at synapses? *In vitro* studies suggested that Nrx/NL interactions promoted synapse formation. Expression of NLs in non-neuronal cells induced presynaptic differentiation at the contacting axons of cultured neurons, whereas expressing β-Nrx in non-neuronal cells induced postsynaptic differentiation at the contacting dendrites of neurons (Gokce & Südhof, 2013). Overexpression of NLs in cultured neurons increased synapse numbers in a synapse-type and NL-isoform-dependent manner (Chih et al., 2004, Chih et al., 2005; Varoqueaux et al., 2004; Levinson et al., 2005). Suppression of NLs expression by RNA interference (RNAi) or disruption of Nrx/NL interaction consistently reduced the number of synapses (Chih et al., 2005; Levinson et al., 2005).

In vivo analysis from knockout (KO) mice showed that NLs and Nrxs were essential for synaptic maturation and function (Varoqueaux et al., 2006; Missler et al., 2003; Chubykin et al., 2007). The α-Nrx KO mice showed reduced neurotransmitter release (Missler et al., 2003). The KO of NL1 in mice reduced the synaptic strength at excitatory synapses, whereas the neurons lacking NL2 showed synaptic dysfunction at inhibitory synapses. The NL1-3 triple KO mice were neonatal lethal, and massive synaptic impairments had been observed from both in vitro and in situ analysis of these mice (Varoqueaux et al., 2006). In addition, Nrxs and NLs also contributed to the long-term plasticity of synapses via an activity-dependent mechanism (Varoqueaux et al., 2004; Jedlicka et al., 2013). Constitutive inclusion of an alternative SS4 in Nrx-3 impaired the recruitment of the postsynaptic AMPA receptor (AMPAR) in mice during NMDA receptor (NMDAR)-dependent LTP (Aoto et al., 2013).

2.1.2   Pathology

Nrxs and NLs had been genetically associated with ASDs. ASDs were characterized by impairments in social interaction and communication, and were stereotypic or repetitive behaviors (Südhof, 2008). ASDs altered the connection and organization of nerve cells and their synapses in the brain. Five ultra-rare structural variants, including a predicted splicing mutation, had been found in the α-Nrx1 gene from 116 Caucasian patients with autism but only one ultra-rare structural variant occurred in controls (Yan et al., 2008). The β-Nrx1 gene had two putative missense structural variants that were detected in four Caucasian patients with autism and not in healthy controls (Feng et al., 2006). More recently, Nrx2 disruption had also been implicated to the pathogenesis of ASD (Gauthier et al., 2011). In 2012, rare Nrx3 deletions in ASD had been reported (Vaags et al., 2012). Two base pair deletions in NL4 had been found in male autistic patients, resulting in altered interactions with β-Nrxs (Laumonnier et al., 2004). The R451C and R87W substitutions in the NL3 and NL4 genes, respectively, had been associated with autistic patients (Comoletti et al., 2004; Zhang et al., 2009). This R451C mutation impaired NL3 trafficking, resulting in lower cell surface expression of NL3 and largely reducing β-Nrx1 binding activity. The R451C knock-in (KI) mice showed increased spatial learning and impairments in social interactions, accompanied by specific increases in inhibitory synaptic transmission (Tabuchi et al., 2007). Unlike the R451C knock-in mice, a loss-of-function mutation in the mouse NL4 impaired reciprocal social interactions and communication (Jamain et al., 2008).

The interactions of Nrxs and NLs not only controlled the balance between excitatory and inhibitory neurotransmitter release, but they also functioned in β-amyloid metabolism which was a key process in AD pathogenesis (Sindi et al., 2014). A genome-wide association study compared 1256 SNPs in Nrx1, Nrx2, Nrx3, and NL1 genes among 3009 AD patients and 3006 controls respectively, and identified AD susceptibility may increase by Nrx3 in males (Martinez-Mir et al., 2013). The NLs had been implicated a role in Aβ accumulation in AD (Scholl & Scheiffele, 2003). Recently, NL1 but not NL2 was reported to display a high affinity interaction with oligomeric forms of Aβ via its extracellular domain (Dinamarca et al., 2011; Dinamarca et al., 2012), thus indicating that NL1 stabilized oligomeric assemblies of Aβ in the glutamatergic synapse postsynaptically. Processing of Nrx3β was altered by the introduction of several PS1 mutations that caused early-onset familial AD (Bot et al., 2011). In hippocampal neurons, accumulation of Nrx C-terminal fragments was associated with the inhibition of presenilin/γ-secretase (Saura et al., 2011).

Nrxs and NLs had also been associated with schizophrenia. A whole-genome analysis identified a deletion in two affected siblings that disrupted Nrx1 (Kirov et al., 2008). Nrx1α exonic deletions had since been found in three patients with paranoid-type schizophrenia (Vrijenhoek et al., 2008). A later study of 2977 schizophrenia patients and 33746 controls examined Nrx1 for copy number variants (CNVs) and identified 66 deletions and 5 duplications in NRXN1 from the patients, confirming that Nrx1 was a risk gene for schizophrenia (Rujescu et al., 2009). Nrx3 was also shown to contribute to the degree of nicotine dependence in patients with schizophrenia (Novak et al., 2009). A loss-of-function mutation R215H in NL2 was associated with GABAergic synapse formation (Sun et al., 2011). Systematic screening had also confirmed the key role of NL4 in schizophrenia (Sand et al., 2006).

Mutations in Nrxs and NLs had been found in epilepsy. Biallelic Nrx1 deletions resulted in a severe recessive mental retardation syndrome and early onset epilepsy (Harrison et al., 2011). Furthermore, a screen in 1569 patients with idiopathic generalized epilepsy (IGE) and 6201 controls had revealed that exon-disrupting deletions of Nrx1 increased the risk of IGE syndromes (Møller et al., 2013). Furthermore, the Nrx2 expression level was elevated in the dentate gyrus in kainate- and pentylenetetrazole-induced seizures, whereas Nrx1 and 3 expression were observed no specific changes (Górecki et al., 1999). Postsynaptically, a partial NL1 deletion was found by genomic microarray in a child with seizure disorder (Millson et al., 2012). Moreover, mutations in NL4 have been associated with seizures because of its function in development of synaptic structures (Laumonnier et al., 2004).

2.2   N-cadherin/β-catenin

2.2.1   Physiology

Cadherins were transmembrane proteins containing an extracellular domain with a repeated "cadherin motif" or "cadherin repeat" sequence (Takeichi, 1988). There were more than 100 members in humans, grouping into classic cadherins and protocadherins. N-cadherin was the most abundant cadherin in excitatory synapses with a highly conserved cytoplasmic domain binding β-catenin and p120-catenin (Takeichi, 1988; Takeichi, 2007).

N-cadherin mediated Ca^{2+}-dependent homophilic protein interactions (Hirano and Takeichi, 2012). During synaptic maturation, the location of N-cadherin shifted from the cleft to the outer rims of the active zone (Uchida et al., 1996; Fannon & Colman, 1996). Classical cadherins bound to β-catenin at its central armadillo repeat domain, and β-catenin interacted with the actin cytoskeleton through α-catenin. Cultured neurons lacking N-cadherin or β-catenin showed reduced spine number, more filopodia-like spines, thinner spines, or spines with smaller heads (Mendez et al., 2010; Saglietti et al., 2007; Okuda et al., 2007). Suppression of β-catenin expression decreased the amplitude but not the frequency of spontaneous excitatory synaptic currents in cultures. Similar treatment impaired synaptic scaling induced by a two-day blockade of neural activity with tetrodotoxin or bicuculline (Okuda et al., 2007). Conditional KO mice showed reductions in the stability of coordinated spine enlargement and LTP in the CA1 region (Bozdagi et al., 2010). The LTP-induced long-term stabilization of synapses was also impaired in expression mutants or knockdown of N-cadherin (Mendez et al., 2010). Cooperation between NL1 and N-cadherin had recently been revealed that promotes the formation of glutamatergic synapses and controls vesicle clustering at nascent synapses (Aiga et al., 2011; Stan et al., 2010).

Beyond the postsynaptic functions, N-cadherin and β-catenin were also involved in regulating transmitter release. Overexpression of the extracellular domain of N-cadherin increased the frequency of miniature excitatory postsynaptic currents (mEPSCs) (Saglietti et al., 2007). The absence of N-cadherin dramatically impaired short-term plasticity from facilitation to depression at glutamatergic synapses (Jüngling et al., 2006). Mice deficient in β-catenin showed a reduction in the number of reserved pool vesicles and impairment in their response to prolonged repetitive stimulation (Bamji et al., 2003). Axonal knockdown β-catenin had been shown to affect the dynamics of vesicle release (Taylor et al., 2013). Therefore, N-cadherin and β-catenin were structurally and functionally linked in the processes of synapse stabilization as well as in the processes of synaptic transmission from both sides of the synapses.

2.2.2   Pathology

Many cadherin genes were found to be genetically associated with ASD. A genome-wide recurrent *de novo* analysis included the CDH13 gene in rare copy-number variations in autism families (Sanders et al., 2011). A scan for the IQ discrepancy in ASD patients revealed a unique truncated cadherin, cadherin 13 (CDH13) (Chapman et al., 2011). The cadherin 15 (CDH15) gene had been found in a sporadic patient with autism (Willemsen et al., 2010). Cadherin 8 (CDH8), which presents in the developing human cortex, was reported as an autism susceptibility gene in other recent research (Pagnamenta et al., 2011). Moreover, variants of cadherin 11 (CDH11), cadherin 10 (CDH10) and cadherin 9 (CDH9) had been identified in ASD (Wang et al., 2009; Crepel et al., 2014). Protocadherin 10 (PCDH10), which regulates neuronal activity and controls axon outgrowth, was one potential candidate gene for autism (Morrow et al., 2008; Uemura et al., 2007). Protocadherin 19 (PCDH19) mutations had also been associated with ASD recently (van Harssel et al., 2013).

PCDH11 had been implicated to associate with hominid speciation, language acquisition and the sexual dimorphism of brain asymmetry, thereby functioning in schizophrenia as predicted (Crow 2002). Another study was observed an increase of PCDH17 expression in schizophrenia patients in Brodmann's area 46 (Dean et al., 2007). Furthermore, a deletion between CDH12 and CDH18 genes on 5p14 had been identified in a monozygotic twin pair discordant for schizophrenia (Singh et al., 2010). Disrupted in schizophrenia 1 (DISC1), a promising gene in schizophrenia, had been reported to regulate N-cadherin expression at the cell membrane in primary neurons, thus indicating the linkage between cadherin and schizophrenia (Hattori et al., 2010).

The contribution of cadherins in epilepsy had also been reported. In 2008, PCDH19 was first implicated in epilepsy or mental retardation (Dibbens et al., 2008). Later on, in two unrelated girls with seizures, larger genomic deletions comprising PCDH19 had been identified (Vincent et al., 2012). *De novo* PCDH19 mutations in epilepsy female restricted mental retardation syndrome had implicated that PCDH19 was a major gene for epilepsy (Jamal et al., 2010). Furthermore, the gonadal mosaicism of a PCDH19 mutation in a parent could be an important mechanism as reported (Dibbens et al., 2011).

2.3   Ephrins and Eph Receptors

2.3.1   Physiology

Eph receptors (EphA and B) was a family of receptor tyrosine kinases, containing an intracellular tyrosine kinase domain and a PDZ-binding motif (Kullander & Klein, 2002; Himanen, 2012). EphA receptors bound to glycosylphosphatidylinositol(GPI)-anchored proteins ephrinA, while EphB receptors bound to transmembrane ephrinB ligands. Eph–ephrin interaction also could mediate signal transductions between the receptor-expressing cell and the ligand-expressing cell in a bidirectional manner (Daar, 2012). Eph and ephrin expressions were found at both the pre- and postsynaptic membranes, and also, at least some isoforms, on astrocytes (Klein. 2009). Eph and ephrin signaling was involved in many regulation processes, including axon guidance and cell migration (Davy and Soriano, 2005; Xu and Henkemeyer, 2012; Egea & Klein, 2007). The activation of cyclin-dependent kinase 5 (Cdk5) and ephexin1 by ephrin-A1 promoted EphA4-dependent spine retraction, followed by a scaling-down of excitatory synaptic strength (Fu et al., 2007; Peng et al., 2013). EphA4 inhibited integrin signaling pathways (Bourgin et al., 2007), and EphA4 activation by ephrin-A3 reduced tyrosine phosphorylation of the scaffolding protein Crk-associated substrate (Cas), the tyrosine kinase focal adhesion kinase (FAK), and proline-rich tyrosine kinase 2 (Pyk2) while down-regulating the association of Cas with the Src family kinase Fyn and the adaptor Crk. The EphA4 receptor linked with spine-associated RapGAP (SPAR), which was activated by GTPase, regulated the activities of the Rap GTPase, and therefore neuronal morphology (Richter et al., 2007, Clifford et al., 2011). EphA–ephrinA signaling played important roles in the synaptic strength and plasticity in addition to regulating cell morphology (Hruska and Dalva, 2012). The activation of EphA4 decreased synaptic and surface GluR1, and attenuates mEPSCs amplitude (Fu et al., 2011). The Eph4-deficient hippocampal CA1 region showed altered dendritic spine maturation (Murai et al., 2003), impaired LTP and long-term depression (LTD) (Grunwald et al., 2004). Postsynaptic expression of EphA4 and its ligand ephrin-A3 in astrocytes mediated neuron-glia interactions, which were also required for LTP expression at CA3-CA1 synapses in the hippocampus (Filosa et al., 2009).

EphB–ephrinB signaling promoted excitatory synaptogenesis. EphrinB binding to the EphB receptor elevated excitatory synapse formation via degradation of Ephexin5, a RhoA guanine nucleotide exchange factor (Margolis et al., 2010). Suppression of the expression of the EphB receptor reduced excitatory synapses and the clustering of NMDARs and AMPARs, and altered dendritic spine formation as well (Henkemeyer et al., 2003). The PDZ domain of EphB2 also controlled localization of the AMPA-type glutamate receptor, while the ephrin binding domain of EphB2 initiated presynaptic differentiation (Kayser et al., 2006). EphBs were thought to control synaptogenesis by associating the motility of filopodia and the binding ability of ephrin (Kayser et al., 2008). The Rho-GEF kalirin, Rac1, and its effector PAK were involved in the ephrinB-EphB signaling pathway during spine development (Penzes et al., 2003). Suppression of EphB2 expression by siRNA in the postsynaptic neuron reduced mEPSCs frequency in cultured cortical neurons (Kayser et al., 2006). EphB2 deficient mice showed reduced NMDA-mediated synaptic responses and impaired LTP (Henderson et al., 2001), which could be rescued by expressing C-terminal truncated EphB2 (Grunwald et al., 2001). The tyrosine phosphorylation sites in ephrinB2 were necessary for maintaining LTP but not LTD, whereas the C-terminal PDZ interaction site was required for both (Bouzioukh et al., 2007). EphrinB3-deficient mice showed reduced amplitude of mEPSCs, but increased NMDA/AMPA ratios in CA1 neurons (Antion et al., 2010). Blocking the interaction between EphRs and the PDZ protein GRIP or extracellular application of soluble forms of B-ephrins (presynaptic ligands for the EphB receptors) reduced mossy fiber LTPs in the CA3 region, suggesting a requirement for trans-synaptic interactions between EphB receptors and B-ephrins (Contractor et al., 2002). Replacement of the cytoplasmic C-terminal signaling domain of the ephrinB3 with β-galactosidase selectively blocked mossy fiber LTPs (Armstrong et al., 2006). Therefore, trans-synaptic ephrin–Eph adhesion regulated synaptic maturation and plasticity in a bidirectional way in both developing and adult brains.

2.3.2   Pathology

Copy number variations in ephrinA5 were associated with schizophrenia in 2006 (Wilson et al., 2006). EphrinB2 was suggested to be a schizophrenia susceptibility gene on chromosome 13q33 in the Han Chinese population (Zhang et al., 2010). Loss of function of ephrinBs blocked the phosphorylation of Dab1 by Reelin, which was associated with epilepsy, schizophrenia and AD (Sentürk et al., 2011). Morphological abnormalities of spines were closely associated with mental retardation and schizophrenia (Wong & Guo, 2013), where ephrin-Eph receptor signaling was indicated in these processes via the regulation of Rho GTPase (Irie & Yamaguchi, 2004). The up-regulation of EphA10 and ephrinA4 were observed after status epilepticus (SE), suggesting their involvement in the pilocarpine-induced epileptogenesis (Xia et al., 2013). Moreover, receptor EphA5 and ligand ephrin-A3 functionally retarded the development of behavioral seizures induced by perforant path stimulation (Xu et al., 2003).

Dysfunctions in Ephs and ephrins signaling pathways had been found to be involved in the pathogenesis of AD (Chen et al., 2012). In AD model mice, abnormal expression of EphA4 and EphB2 were detected much earlier than the decrease in synaptic proteins and the onset of cognitive decline (Simón et al., 2009), indicating that Eph receptors may act as early stage markers of AD. EphA4 had been reported to be one of γ-secretase's substrates (Inoue et al., 2009), the key enzyme that cleaved amyloid precursor protein (APP) to generate Aβ. However, familial mutations in PS1 in AD patients slowed down this process of EphA4, resulting in a reduced formation of dendritic spines. The amount of Rac1 decreased dramatically corresponding with the level of EphA4-ICD in AD patients (Matsui et al., 2012). The processing of the EphB2 receptor was also regulated by γ-secretase and inhibited by familial AD mutations of PS1 (Litterst et al., 2007). The Aβ peptide bound to the extracellular domain of EphB2 and triggers EphB2 degradation in the proteasome, leading to a decrease in surface and total EphB2 in neurons. A lack of EphB2 expression caused neuronal dysfunction and memory impairments through the NMDAR dependent pathway (Cissé et al., 2011). More interestingly, increasing EphB2 level could reverse these impairments.

With limited research results, Eph and ephrin were also considered as potential risking genes in ASD. Decreased expression levels of EphrinB3 were identified in the autistic group than in the controls by real-time reverse-transcriptase PCR (Suda et al., 2011). EphB/Ephexin5 signaling during the development of synapses affected cognitive function in ASD in another study (Margolis et al., 2010). However, the association still remained to be confirmed.

2.4   NCAM

2.4.1   Physiology

The neural cell adhesion molecule (NCAM) was a glycoprotein expressed in both the pre- and postsynaptic membranes. The extracellular part of NCAM had five Ig domains that bound to NCAM, and two fibronectin type III (FNIII) domains related to neurite outgrowth. At least 27 alternatively spliced NCAM mRNAs were present in rat brains (Reyes et al., 1991). Numerous studies had shown that NCAM regulated synapse formation, maturation, and function through homo- and heterophilic interactions (Bukalo and Dityatev, 2012). The ablation of NCAM reduced the number of synapses (Dityatev et al., 2000). NCAM associated with the postsynaptic spectrin-based scaffold to form a complex that was responsible for recruiting NMDARs and Ca^{2+}/calmodulin-dependent protein kinase II alpha (CaMKIIalpha) to synapses, and was important for NMDAR-dependent LTP and LTD (Sytnyk et al., 2006; Bukalo et al., 2004; Muller et al., 1996). NCAM also had presynaptic functions (Rafuse et al., 2000; Polo-Parada et al., 2001). Deleting NCAM at the neuromuscular junction (NMJ) led to smaller NMJs with impaired accumulation of presynaptic proteins, reduced number of docked vesicles, and altered paired-pulse facilitation

(PPF). The C-terminal of NCAM played a key role in maintaining effective transmission via a pathway involving myosin light chain kinase (MLCK) and probably MLC and myosin II (Polo-Parada et al., 2005). Chromaffin cells showed impairment of catecholamine granule trafficking in the absence of NCAM, resulting in a reduced rate of granule fusion under physiological stimulation. These findings suggested that NCAM was involved in vesicle recycling in both neuronal and endocrine cells (Chan et al., 2005).

2.4.2   Pathology

NCAM had long been implicated in various neurological disorders. Embryonic NCAM dysfunction was linked with schizophrenia more than 20 years ago (Conrad & Scheibel, 1987). Unlike the case of ASD patients (Plioplys et al., 1990), NCAM levels in serum and cerebrospinal fluid (CSF) increased in schizophrenic patients (Lyons et al., 1988; Poltorak et al., 1996). Interestingly, the hippocampus of schizophrenic patients showed a reduction of polysialylated NCAM (PSA-NCAM) (Barbeau et al., 1995). An increase in the cytosolic isoform of NCAM had also been observed in the hippocampus of schizophrenia patients (Vawter et al., 1998b). An increase in the cytosolic NCAM/synaptophysin ratio was demonstrated in the hippocampus of schizophrenia patients (Vawter et al., 1999). Similarly, the cingulate cortex of schizophrenics also showed elevated NCAM/synaptophysin ratios (Honer et al., 1997). In another study, ChAT/NCAM ratios were reduced in the frontal and temporal cortexes of AD patients as compared to controls (Aisa et al., 2010). Besides schizophrenia, the levels of NCAM serum fragment had also been found significant decreased in autistic patients compared with age-matched controls (Plioplys et al., 1990).

The cytosolic NCAM isoform (cN-CAM) underwent a tremendous reduction in BP disorder (-140%) in hippocampal tissue (Vawter, 2000). Quantitative western blot analysis had revealed that cytosolic NCAM protein and mRNA levels increased in the hippocampus and prefrontal cortex in patients (Vawter et al., 1998b). Interestingly, NCAM infusion reduced astrocyte division, while BP disorder decreased glia numbers (Krushel et al., 1995; Ongür et al., 1998). Recently, novel variants of ST8SIA2, a BP disorder related gene, in its region of interaction with NCAM1 had been described in 48 Caucasian cases with BP disorder (Shaw et al., 2014).

Interestingly, reduced CSF-NCAM-1 concentration was found in either epileptic group compared to the control group or in the drug-refractory epilepsy group compared to the drug-effective epilepsy group, therefore indicating CSF-NCAM-1 as a potential biomarker for epilepsy (Wang et al., 2012). Approximately 10 years ago, a largely increased number of highly PSA-NCAM positive cells in the bilateral dentate gyrus were observed in rats with repeated exposure to amygdaloid kindled generalized seizures (Sato et al., 2003). Later, degeneration of CA3 neurons and dentate gyrus granule cells in the epileptic focus and early onset of focal seizures were induced by the inactivation of PSA-NCAM by endoneuraminidase (EndoN) administration into the contralateral ventricle of kainic acid-treated mice, suggesting that PSA-NCAM mediated GDNF signaling to transport neuroprotective signals into the lesioned hippocampus (Duveau & Fritschy, 2010). Plannexin, a NCAM-derived peptide that mimicked trans-homophilic NCAM interaction, represented protective roles for immature neurons *in vivo* after status epilepticus (Zellinger et al., 2011).

2.5 L1-CAMs

2.5.1 Physiology

L1-CAMs was a family of transmembrane proteins, with at least four members in vertebrates: L1CAM, close homolog of L1 (CHL1), NgCAM-related cell adhesion molecule (NrCAM), and neurofascin. The L1-CAMs were involved in many neuronal functions, including axonal guidance, neurite outgrowth and fasciculation, and cell migration (Chang et al., 1987; Lindner et al., 1983; Fischer et al., 1986; Maness & Schachner, 2007). L1-deficient mice showed a significant reduction in frequency of miniature inhibitory postsynaptic currents (mIPSCs) and a reduction in the amplitude of putative unitary IPSCs (Saghatelyan et al., 2004). However, the conditional inactivation of L1 in the adult brain increased the basal excitatory synaptic transmission and decreases anxiety in the open field, which differed from the response seen in L1 constitutive KO mice (Law et al., 2003). The ankyrin-mediated localization of L1CAMs was implicated in the organization of GABAergic synapses in Purkinje neurons (Ango et al., 2004). Loss of the L1/ankyrin interaction impaired branching of GABAergic interneurons and specifically reduced the number of perisomatic synapses (Guan & Maness, 2010).

CHL1 was implicated in synaptogenesis of inhibitory interneurons, although it functioned differently from L1. The hippocampal CA1 region in juvenile CHL1 mutant mice showed an increase in IPSCs and a decrease in LTP at CA3-CA1 synapses. The length and linear density of active zones and the numbers of perisomatic puncta containing inhibitory axonal markers were also increased (Nikonenko et al., 2006). CHL1 also maintained inhibitory synapses between stellate axons and Purkinje dendrites, indicating a role in connecting glia and neuron (Ango et al., 2008). CHL1-deficient mice showed enhancement of basal synaptic transmission in the lateral and medial perforant path projections to the dentate gyrus, while reactivity to environmental stimuli and social behaviors were altered (Morellini et al., 2007).

2.5.2 Pathology

L1-CAMs was largely increased in the CSF of AD patients, independent of age and gender (Strekalova et al., 2006). CHL1 was detected to co-localize with β-site APP-cleaving enzyme (BACE1) in the terminals of hippocampal mossy fibers, olfactory sensory neuron axons and growth cones of primary hippocampal neurons (Hitt et al., 2012) Moreover, L1-CAMs and CHL1 were cleaved by BACE1 physiologically (Zhou et al., 2012). After four months of L1-CAMs injection into adult AD model mice, Aβ plaque load, levels of Aβ42, Aβ42/40 ratio, and astrogliosis were reduced and densities of inhibitory synapses on pyramidal cells in the hippocampus were increased as compared to control, implying L1-CAMs as a candidate to ameliorate the pathology of AD (Djogo et al., 2013)

In 2002, three novel L1-CAM variations were determined in exon 18, intron 11, and intron 25 from Japanese schizophrenic patients (Kurumaji et al., 2001). A missense poly-morphism of CHL1 in the signal peptide region was observed in 24 Japanese patients with schizophrenia in another study (Sakurai et al., 2002). This positive association be-tween CHL1 gene and schizophrenia was confirmed by further analyzing SNPs in the gene in the Han Chinese population (Chen et al., 2005). L1-CAM was also suggested to regulate schizophrenia with NCAM. Increased N-CAM and decreased L1-CAM antigen in CSF of schizophrenia patients were reported (Poltorak et al., 1997). The correlation be-tween expression levels of L1-CAM and NCAM had been impaired in schizophrenia pa-tients (Vawter et al., 1998a).

2.6   Nectins

2.6.1   Physiology

Nectins (Nectin 1-4) were Ca^{2+}-independent Ig-CAMs (Takai et al., 2003). Nectins form homo-*cis* dimers followed by *trans*-interaction in an either heterophilic or homophilic manner through their extracellular domains (Mizoguchi et al., 2002). Nectins interacted with actin-binding protein afadin, an α-catenin interact protein, through the C-terminal PDZ binding domain (Giagtzoglou et al., 2009). Similar to N-cadherin, Nectin-1 mainly located at matured excitatory synapses (Lim et al., 2008). The CA3 area of the adult hip-pocampus showed an asymmetric localization of Nectin-1 and -3 at the pre- and postsyn-aptic sides. Reduction in nectin-based adhesion led to a decrease in synapse size and an accompanying increase in synapse number, suggesting a role of the nectin-afadin system in synaptogenesis (Mizoguchi et al., 2002). Mice deficient in either Nectin-1 or Nectin-3 showed a reduced number of puncta adherentia junctions (PAJs) and abnormal mossy fiber trajectory (Honda et al., 2006). Conversely, conditional inactivation of afadin re-duced the signal of nectins, N-cadherin, β-catenin and disrupts PAJs, whereas it increased the numbers of perforated synapses. Thus, the nectin-afadin interaction appeared to par-ticipate in synaptic remodeling by regulating the stability of synaptic junctions (Majima et al., 2009).

The nectin-afadin complex also interacted with many synaptic proteins that func-tion at synapses. The synaptic scaffolding molecule (S-SCAM) had been reported to co-localize with nectins via the PDZ-binding domain of the latter (Yamada et al., 2003). S-SCAM was involved in the presynaptic vesicle clustering mediated by N-cadherin and NL-1 cooperation (Stan et al., 2010). Thus, several CAMs could function either separately or synergistically in synapse maturation (Sakisaka et al., 2007).

2.6.2   Pathology

Nectin-1 and -3 served as substrates for PS/γ-secretase proteolytic activity (Kim et al., 2002; Kim et al., 2011). Recently, an association between reduced expression of Nectin-3 in the stratum lacunosum moleculare and the triggering of tauopathy had been suggested (Maurin et al., 2013). In AD, the excessive production of Aβ peptide could be prevent by

ADAM10-mediated α-secretase activity toward APP (Postina et al., 2004). Reduced expression of Nectin-1 had been revealed in ADAM10 conditional KO mice recently, suggesting the involvement of Nectin-1 in AD (Prox et al., 2013). However, more investigations would be necessary to uncover the mechanisms of nectins in diseases.

2.7   Contactins

2.7.1   Physiology

Contactins (CNTN) were a group of GPI-linked Ig-CAMs containing six N-terminal Ig-like domains and four fibronectin III-like domains. Six members were recognized in the CNTN family: CNTN-1, CNTN-2/TAG-1, CNTN-3/BIG-1, CNTN-4/BIG-2, CNTN-5/NB2, and CNTN-6/NB3. Both CNTN-1 and CNTN-2 were involved in axon growth and guidance (Buttiglione et al., 1996; Perrin et al., 2001). CNTNs may therefore function at both pre- and postsynaptic sites, although the mechanisms remain unclear. CNTN-6 was prominently expressed presynaptically in the developing nervous system. CNTN-6 deficient mice showed increased numbers of immature granule cells in the internal granule cell layer (IGL) (Sakurai et al., 2009) and a decreased density of excitatory but not inhibitory synapse density (Sakurai et al., 2010). CNTN 4 and 5 were also involved in synapse differentiation, especially at early stages (Mercati et al., 2013). Unlike the presynaptic localization of CNTN-6, CNTN-1 had been detected in PSD in CA1 pyramidal cells. Inactivation of CNTN-1 expression affected PPF and NMDA receptor-dependent LTD, without altering synaptic morphology (Murai et al., 2002). In adult mice, overexpression of contactin increased LTP as well as spatial and object recognition memory (Puzzo et al., 2013).

2.7.2   Pathology

CNTN was another family of CAMs heavily related to ASD. CNTN4, CNTN5, and CNTN6 were suggested as potential risking genes. For example, a deletion at the 5' end of the CNTN4 gene had been identified in an autism patient (Cottrell et al., 2011). Disruption of the CNTN4 gene caused 3p deletion syndrome and impairs normal CNS development (Fernandez et al., 2004). Rare copy number variations (CNVs) in CNTN4 had been reported to influence autism susceptibility in Asian populations (Guo et al., 2012). A loss of CNTN5 co-segregated with autism in one family, as well as one *de novo* CNV and one non-cosegregating inherited CNV in CNTN6, was found in a Utrecht cohort (van Daalen et al., 2011). Mice models based on clinic observations on CNTN had been generated (Momoi et al., 2009), and more investigations were needed to reveal the underlying mechanism between these molecules and ASD.

A homozygous mutation of CNTNAP2 in Old Order Amish children with focal epilepsy was reported (Strauss et al., 2006). The CNTNAP2 gene had emerged as a genetic risk in both autism and schizophrenia (Burbach & van der Zwaag, 2009). CNTN2, together with CNTN associated protein-like 2 (CNTNAP2) were required for maintaining voltage-gated potassium channels at the juxtaparanodal region, was reported to be associated with seizures as well (Stogmann et al., 2013).

A downstream of CNTN2 that was linked to three conserved SNPs in the 3'-UTR of CNTN2 was significant following random effects meta-analysis, thus suggesting CNTN2 as a new biomarker in AD (Medway et al., 2010). A recent study demonstrated CNTN2 levels were decreased in AD brain samples, whereas BACE1 levels increased in the same samples, therefore indicating CNTN2 as a physiological substrate for BACE1 and presenting the possibility that CNTN2 regulated AD via BACE1-mediated pathway (Gautam et al., 2014).

2.8   LRRTMs

2.8.1   Physiology

The LRRTM (LRRTM 1-4) proteins were a group of PSD-enriched type-I transmembrane proteins that contained extracellular leucine rich repeats and a short cytoplasmic tail (Laurén et al., 2003). Non-neuronal cells expressing LRRTMs induced presynaptic differentiation when cocultured with neurons (Linhoff et al., 2009). Knocking down LRRTM2 reduced, whereas overexpression of LRRTM2 increased, the number of excitatory synapses, but not inhibitory synapses in a cultured system (de Wit et al., 2009; Ko et al., 2009). The extracellular LRR domain of LRRTM2 mediated this excitatory presynaptic differentiation (Siddiqui et al., 2013). LRRTM4-Null dentate gyrus granule cells showed reduced numbers of excitatory synapses and impairments in both mEPSCs and action-potential-evoked EPSCs (Siddiqui et al., 2013). LRRTM2 bound Nrxs, and the LRRTM-Nrx interaction played a key role in regulating excitatory synapse formation (Ko et al., 2009). Single, double, or triple knockdowns of LRRTM1, LRRTM2 and NL-3 in cultured hippocampal neurons had no effect on synapse numbers, whereas triple knockdown (TKD) of two LRRTMs and NL-3 in cultured NL-1 KO neurons led to a ~40% reduction in excitatory synapses (Ko et al., 2011). Knockdown of LRRTM1 and LRRTM2 selectively reduced AMPA receptor-mediated synaptic currents, while knockdown of both LRRTMs, together with NL-3, reduced AMPAR and NMDAR-mediated currents in NL-1 deficiency mice in the synapses forming stage (Soler-Llavina et al., 2011), suggesting a functional redundancy between NLs and LRRTMs in developing excitatory synapses. In mature synapses, LRRTMs acted in a NLs-independent manner. For example, inactivation of LRRTM expression, starting from P21 to P35-40, had no effect on excitatory synaptic transmission, while KO of NL1 reduced the NMDAR/AMPAR ratio at similar ages (Soler-Llavina et al., 2011). LRRTM1-KO mice exhibited an increase in the size of presynaptic terminals in the hippocampal CA1 region, and an extraordinary phenotype where the animals showed avoidance of small enclosures, an increase in social interaction, and a decrease in nest building (Linhoff et al., 2009; Voikar et al., 2013). In acute hippocampal slices, double knockdown of LRRTM1 and LRRTM2 impaired LTP, which could be rescued by expression of the LRRTM2 extracellular domain (Soler-Llavina et al., 2013). These results indicated that LRRTMs not only played a key role in synapse development and maturation, but they were also directly involved in synaptic transmission and more complicated behaviors.

2.8.2   Pathology

LRRTMs had been implicated in several neurologic disorders by limited evidences. LRRTM1, considered the first potential genetic influence on human handedness and first putative genetic effect on variability in human brain asymmetry, was associated with schizophrenia (Francks et al., 2007). LRRTM3 was reported to promote APP processing by β-site APP-cleaving enzyme 1 (BACE1) (Majercak et al., 2006). LRRTM3 bound to pre-senilin-1 and is implicated in the clearance of Aβ deposition (Edwards et al., 2009). Moreover, a family-based association study implicated LRRTM3 in ASD susceptibility (Sousa et al., 2010).

2.9   SynCAM

2.9.1   Physiology

Synaptic cell adhesion molecules (SynCAM1-4) was a family of type-1 transmembrane proteins with three extracellular Ig-like domains (Thomas et al., 2008). All SynCAMs were highly enriched in the brain, and SynCAM 1 was also found in the lung and testis (Fogel et al., 2007). Like the NLs, SynCAM recruited synaptic proteins and promoted neuron differentiation presynaptically in co-culture assays (Sara et al., 2005). During synapse development, SynCAMs were located in both pre- and postsynaptic compartments and underwent homo- and heterophilic adhesive interactions. SynCAMs also bound many other proteins via the C-terminal domain. SynCAMs bound to the scaffold proteins syntenin and CASK via the C-terminal PDZ domain, and recruited CASK to the plasma membrane (Biederer et al., 2002). SynCAM1 also bound to protein 4.1B intracellularly, which, in turn, recruited NMDAR to the postsynaptic plasma membrane, resulting in an increase in the frequency of NMDAR-mediated mEPSCs in cultured hippocampal neurons (Hoy et al., 2009). *In vivo* studies had revealed a role for SynCAM 1 in the regulation of synapse numbers and plasticity. Mouse neurons formed fewer excitatory synapses in the absence of SynCAM 1 (Giza et al., 2013), while overexpression of SynCAM 1 resulted in an increase in excitatory synapse number. The LTD and spatial learning were also regulated by the expression of SynCAM 1 (Robbins et al., 2010).

2.9.2   Pathology

The involvement of SynCAM in diseases was still not well investigated. The intracellular domain of APP could form a complex with Mint1 and Cask and be replaced by SynCAM sequences, thus implicating a possible involvement of SynCAM in AD (Wang et al., 2009). In a culture system, more polysialylation of SynCAM 1 occured in the presence of ST8SIA2, a gene associated with schizophrenia, suggesting SynCAM may be involved in schizophrenia through an indirect manner (Rollenhagen et al., 2012). Thereby more investigations would be needed in this area.

2.10 SALMs

2.10.1   Physiology

Synaptic adhesion-like molecules (SALMs) were a newly discovered family of adhesion molecules with at least five members. SALMs 1-3 contained an extracellular region consisting of a leucine-rich repeat (LRR), a fibronectin type III domain, Ig-like domains, a transmembrane domain, and a C-terminal PDZ-binding motif that interacted with PSD-95. SALMs 4 and 5 lacked the PDZ-binding domain (Seabold et al., 2008). SALMs 1-3 bound to each other, while SALMs 4 and 5 formed homomeric complexes. Transfected heterologous cells showed that only SALMs 4 and 5 formed homomeric associations mediated by the extracellular N terminus (Seabold et al., 2008). SALMs bound to many synaptic proteins. SALM1 interacted with postsynaptic NMDA receptors, possibly through the extracellular or transmembrane regions, and with scaffold proteins PSD-95, SAP 97, and SAP 102 via the PDZ-binding domain. Immunostaining experiments showed that SALM1 recruited PSD-95 and NMDA receptors to postsynaptic sites (Wang et al., 2006; Seabold et al., 2012). SALM2 interacted with PSD-95 and other postsynaptic proteins, including guanylate kinase-associated protein (GKAP) and AMPA receptors (Ko et al., 2006). SALM3 and SALM5 recruited vesicular glutamate transporter (VGluT) and vesicular GABA transporter (VGAT), the presynaptic vesicle protein synaptophysin, and the presynaptic active zone protein Piccolo (Mah et al., 2010). Functional assays revealed that overexpression of SALMs promoted neurite outgrowth in cultured neurons (Wang et al., 2008a). Suppression of SALM2 expression decreased the number of excitatory synapses and dendritic spines, and selectively reduced the frequency but not the amplitude of mEPSCs (Ko et al., 2006). Knockdown of SALM5 reduced both spontaneous excitatory and inhibitory synaptic transmissions, affecting both frequency and amplitude (Mah et al., 2010). Thus, SALMs regulated excitatory and inhibitory synapse function through distinct mechanisms.

2.10.2   Pathology

The reports of SALMs involvement in neurologic disorders were also quite limited now. In a 19-year-old severely autistic and mentally retarded girl, SALM5 was observed to have a 10-fold decreased expression compared to control in fibroblasts (de Bruijn et al., 2010). In another study, SALM5 had been suggested in familial schizophrenia by using rare copy number variant and linkage scans (Xu et al., 2009).

2.11 NGLs

2.11.1   Physiology

NGL (netrin-G ligand) proteins were a family of LRR–containing CAMs with three members: NGL1-3. NGLs were mainly located postsynaptically at excitatory synapses. NGL-1 and -2 bound to netrin-G1 and netrin-G2 through their cytosolic tails in an isoform-specific manner (Kim et al., 2006). The LRR domain of NGL-3 interacted with presynaptic

LAR protein to induce synapse formation (Kwon et al., 2010). PTPσ interacted with NGL-3 to promote a bidirectional synapse formation, whereas PTPδ-NGL-3 interaction induced presynaptic differentiation in a unidirectional manner. Receptor tyrosine phosphatases LAR, the NGL-3 binding partner, was also required for maintaining the number of excitatory synapses and dendritic spines (Dunah et al., 2005). Overexpression NGL-2 in cultured neurons showed increased number of dendritic protrusions. Suppression or competitive inhibition of NGL-2 reduced the number of excitatory synapses (Kim et al., 2006) and decreased EPSCs (Kim et al., 2006; Woo et al., 2009). In the retina, loss of NGL-2 impaired branching of horizontal cell axons that stratified in the outer plexiform layer and reduced synapse formation between horizontal cell axons and rods (Soto et al., 2013). LAR knockdown reduced both the amplitude and frequency of mEPSCs (Dunah et al., 2005). Thus, like other cell adhesion molecules, NGLs were also involved in synaptic maturation and transmission.

2.11.2   Pathology

NGL-1 localized at chromosome 1p13, a risk region with schizophrenia reported previously (Ohtsuki et al., 2008). Decreased mRNA expression levels of NGL-1 and NGL-2 were observed in the brains of schizophrenia and BP disorder patients (Aoki-Suzuki et al., 2005). Moreover, NGL-1 had been reported to be phosphorylated via the interaction with cyclin-dependent kinase-like 5, and the phosphorylation of NGL-1 stabilized the association between NGL-1 and PSD95, thereby arguably suggesting a role for NGL-1 in disorders like autism and early-onset intractable epilepsy beyond its synaptic functions (Ricciardi et al., 2012).

2.12 IgLONs

2.12.1   Physiology

IgLONs were a group of GPI-anchored proteins with three extracellular C2 domains. Four genes were identified in this family: LAMP (limbic system-associated membrane protein), OBCAM (opioid-binding cell-adhesion molecule), NTM (neurotrimin), and Kilon. The LAMP, NTM, and OBCAM molecules interacted homophilically with themselves and heterophilically with each other (Lodge et al., 2000; Gil et al., 2002). The Ig-LONs were implicated in synaptogenesis. Overexpression of LAMP or OBCAM increased the synapse number in cultured hippocampal neurons (Hashimoto et al., 2009). Consistently, down regulation of OBCAM expression reduced the synapse number (Yamada et al., 2007). Overexpression of Kilon reduced the synapse number at early stages but increased the number of dendritic synapses in mature neurons with the alteration of lipid raft dependence (Hashimoto et al., 2008).

2.12.2   Pathology

IgLONs were implicated in the neuronal disorders with limited researches. Down-regulation of OBCAM was determined in the cerebral cortex, frontal lobe, and meninges, but not in cerebellum in most cases of brain tumors (Reed et al., 2007). Stronger expression of NTM was also identified in nervous tumors than that in normal brain tissues (Liu et al., 2004). Additionally, NTM and OBCAM had been suggested as having a role in developmental delay (Minhas et al., 2013).

2.13 LAR-RPTPs

2.13.1   Physiology

Leukocyte antigen-related receptor protein tyrosine phosphatases (LAR-RPTPs) were type-I transmembrane proteins with two intracellular PTP domains (Pulido et al., 1995). Three vertebrate members (LAR, PTPδ, and PTPσ) and a few invertebrate members had been identified (Chagnon et al., 2004). LAR and PTPσ were enriched in glutamatergic synapses, and LAR was associated with AMPARs (Wyszynski et al., 2002; Takahashi et al., 2011); whereas PTPδ was mainly localized in inhibitory synapses (Takahashi et al., 2012). LAR-RPTPs regulated synapse formation via various protein interactions. Overexpression of dominant-negative LAR impaired the normal function of β-catenin–cadherin complex that regulated synaptic differentiation (Brigidi & Bamji, 2011). EPSCs were dramatically impaired by overexpression of LAR dominant-negative constructs (Dunah et al., 2005). Loss of LAR-RPTPs reduced the amplitude and frequency of mEPSCs. Mice deficient in PTPδ showed increased PPF and LTP in the hippocampus (Uetani et al., 2000). Receptor protein tyrosine phosphatase σ (RPTPσ) null mice showed an increase in PPF and mEPSCs frequency, but reduced LTP (Horn et al., 2012). PTPσ and PTPδ were required for excitatory and inhibitory synaptic differentiation, respectively, via interactions with Slit- and Trk-like proteins (Slitrks), a family of proteins belonging to the LRR superfamily (Yim et al., 2013). Activation of LAR-RPTPs resulted in specific mAChR-LTD, but not mGluR-LTD (Dickinson et al., 2009). Mice lacking LAR phosphatase domains exhibited spatial learning impairment in Morris water maze, and were more active in exploration and nest-building (Kolkman et al., 2004). Similar learning impairment had been found in mice lacking PTPδ (Uetani et al., 2000). On the contrary, loss of RPTPσ in mice caused an enhancement in novel object recognition memory (Horn et al., 2012).

2.13.2   Pathology

With very few research results, LAR-RPTPs seem to play a role in neuropsychiatric disease. PS/γ-secretase sequentially cleaved LAR and controlled LAR-β-catenin interaction (Haapasalo et al., 2007). On the other hand, Slitrks, which interacted with PTPσ and PTPδ, were linked to schizophrenia and Tourette syndrome (Hayashi-Takagi & Sawa, 2010; Bloch et al., 2011). Moreover, the Slitrk5 mutant mice had caused a reduction in striatal volume and dendritic complexity of striatal medium spiny neurons and an increase in neuronal activity in orbito-frontal cortex, indicating its role in human obsessive-compulsive disorder (OCD) (Ting & Feng, 2011).

Mole.	Synaptic Location	Interaction	Functions	References
Nrxs	pre	α-latrotoxin, CASK, NLs, LRRTMs, GABA_A-receptor	α-latrotoxin receptor	Südhof, 2008
			Maintained presynaptic differentiation, the basal synaptic transmission and long-term plasticity of synapses	Levinson et al., 2005; Varoqueaux et al.,2004; Varoqueaux et al.,2006
			↑PSD-95, ↑NMDA and AMPA receptors	Barrow et al.,2009; Chih et al.,2005; Heine et al.,2008; Nam & chen,2005
			Related to ASD, AD, schizophrenia & epilepsy	Harrison et al., 2011; Reissner et al.,2013; Sindi et al., 2014; Südhof, 2008
			Induced postsynaptic differentiation (β-Nrx)	Gokce & Südhof,2013
			Impaired the recruitment of the postsynaptic AMPAR (Nrx3)	Aoto et al., 2013
NLs	post	Nrxs, PSD-95	Induced pre- and postsynaptic differentiation and function	Chih et al.,2005; Gokce & Südhof,2013
			Maintained the numbers of synapses, the basal synaptic transmission and long-term plasticity of synapses	Varoqueaux et al.,2004; Varoqueaux et al., 2006
			↑PSD-95, ↑NMDA and AMPA receptors	Barrow et al.,2009; Chih et al.,2005; Heine et al.,2008; Nam and chen,2005

Continued on next page….

Mole.	Synaptic Location	Interaction	Functions	References
			Related to ASD, AD, schizophrenia & epilepsy	Millson et al., 2012; Sand et al., 2006; Sindi et al., 2014; Südhof, 2008
			Maintained LTP and the synaptic strength at excitatory synapses (NL1)	Jedlicka et al., 2013
			↑ the inhibitory synapse numbers (NL2)	Levinson et al., 2005
			↑social interactions and communication (NL4)	Jamain et al., 2008
N cadherin	post	β-catenin, AMPAR subunit GluA2, NL1	Mediated Ca^{2+}-dependent homophilic protein interaction	Hirano & Takeichi,2012
			Regulated the development of postsynaptic spines and dendritic spine stabilization	Mendez et al.,2010; Okuda et al.,2007; Saglietti et al., 2007
			Maintained synaptic transmission, short-term plasticity, LTP, ↑mEPSCs	Bozdagi t al.,2010; Mendez et al.,2010; Saglietti et al., 2007
			Related to ASD, schizophrenia & epilepsy	Chapman et al., 2011; Crow 2002; Dibbens et al., 2008 Pagnamenta et al., 2011
β-catenin	post	N-cadherin, AChR	Maintained the development of postsynaptic spines and the number of reserved pool vesicles	Bamji et al.,2003; Okuda et al,2007
			Regulated excitatory synaptic currents	Okuda et al,2007
			↑vesicle recycling	Taylor et al., 2013

Continued on next page....

Mole.	Synaptic Location	Interaction	Functions	References
Eph Receptors	both	Ephrin, SPAR	Mediated axon guidance, cell migration, presynaptic differentiation and spine maturation	Clifford et al., 2011; Davy & Soriano, 2005; Egea & Klein, 2007; Murai et al., 2003; Xu & Henkemeyer, 2012
			Mediated neuron-glia interactions (EphA4)	Filosa et al., 2009
			↓mEPSCs, ↓LTP & LTD (EphA4)	Fu et al.,2011; Grunwald et al., 2004
			Maintained excitatory synapses and the clustering of NMDARs and AMPARs (EphB)	Henkemeyer et al., 2003
			↓mEPSCs (EphB2)	Kayser et al., 2006;
			Related to AD & ASD	Chen et al., 2012; Margulis et al., 2010; Simón et al., 2009
Ephrins	both	Cdk5, Eph	Mediated axon guidance, cell migration	Davy & Soriano, 2005; Egea & Klein, 2007; Xu & Henkemeyer, 2012
			Maintained NMDA-mediated current and LTP (ephrinB2)	Bouzioukh et al., 2007; Henderson et al., 2001
			↓mEPSCs, ↑NMDA/AMPA ratios, ↓mossy fiber LTPs(EphrinB3)	Antion et al.,2010; Armstrong et al.,2006; Contractor et al. 2002;
			Related to ASD, AD, schizophrenia & epilepsy	Chen et al., 2012; Sentürk et al., 2011; Suda et al., 2011

Continued on next page....

Mole.	Synaptic Location	Interaction	Functions	References
NCAM	both	homo- & heterophilic interactions	Maintained synapses number	Dityatev et al., 2000
			↑NMDA receptor, ↑CaMKIIalpha LTP, LTD	Bukalo et al., 2004; Muller et al., 1996; Sytnyk et al., 2006
			↑vesicle recycling	Chan et al.,2005; Polo-Parada et al., 2001; Polo-Parada et al., 2005; Rafuse et al., 2000
			Linked with schizophrenia, epilepsy & BP	Conrad & Scheibel, 1987; Vawter et al., 1998b; Wang et al., 2012
L1-CAMs	pre		Controlled axonal guidance, neurite outgrowth and fasciculation, and cell migration	Chang et al., 1987; Fischer et al., 1986; Lindner et al., 1983; Maness & Schachner, 2007
			↓ inhibitory synaptic response (L1)	Saghatelyan et al., 2004
			↑vesicle recycling (CHL1)	Ango et al., 2008; Morellini et al., 2007; Nikonenko et al.,2006
			Related to ASD & schizophrenia	Djogo et al., 2013; Sakurai et al., 2002; Strekalova et al., 2006

Continued on next page….

Mole.	Synaptic Location	Interaction	Functions	References
Nectins	both	afadin, N-cadherin-catenin complex, S-SCAM	Initial synapses formation	Giagtzoglou et al.,2009; Lim et al.,2008
			Regulated the stability of synaptic junctions	Majima et al., 2009
			Related to AD	Kim et al., 2002; Kim et al. 2011
Contactins	both		Mediated axon connections	Buttiglione et al., 1996; Perrin et al., 2001
			↑PPF, ↑LTD, ↑LTP & spatial and object recognition memory (CNTN-1)	Murai et al., 2002; Puzzo et al.,2013
			Extended the length of neurites (CNTN-4)	Mercati et al,2013
			↑root (CNTN-5)	Mercati et al,2013
			Postnatal glutamatergic synapse development (CNTN-6)	Sakurai et al.,2009 Sakurai ot al,2010
			Related to ASD, AD, schizophrenia & epilepsy	Burbach & van der Zwaag, 2009; Cottrell et al., 2011; Gautam et al., 2014; Strauss et al., 2006; van Daalen et al., 2011
LRRTMs	post	Nrxs	Induced presynaptic differentiation (LRRTM1)	Linhoff et al., 2009
			Maintained excitatory synapses numbers and synaptic transmission (LRRTM2 & 4)	de Wit et al., 2009; Ko et al., 2009; Siddiqui et al., 2013
			Related to ASD, AD & schizophrenia	Edwards et al., 2009; Francks et al., 2007; Sousa et al., 2010

Continued on next page…

Mole.	Synaptic Location	Interaction	Functions	References
SynCAM	both	CASK, protein 4.1B & NMDAR, heterophilic interactions	recruited synaptic proteins and promotes neuron differentiation	Sara et al., 2005
			Postsynaptic scaffolding, NMDAR trafficking, ↑NMDAR-mediated current, ↓LTD, not LTP in CA1 (SynCAM-1)	Biederer et al.,2002; Hoy et al., 2009
			↑Vesicle recycling, ↑number of presynaptic terminals, ↑excitatory synapse number & synaptic transmission (SynCAM-1 & 2)	Fogel et al., 2007; Robbins et al., 2010; Sara et al., 2005
			Related to AD & schizophrenia	Rollenhagen et al., 2012; Wang et al., 2009
SALMs	both	PSD-95, SAP 97, SAP 102, NMDAR, GKAP, AMPAR	Postsynaptic scaffolding, NMDAR trafficking (SALM-1)	Seabold et al.,2012; Wang et al.,2006
			↑frequency of mEPSCs Postsynaptic scaffolding (SALM-2)	Ko et al.,2006
			Postsynaptic scaffolding, recruit presynaptic proteins (SALM-3)	Mah et al.,2010
			↑frequency and amplitude of mEPSCs Postsynaptic scaffolding, recruit presynaptic proteins (SALM-5)	Mah et al.,2010
			Related to ASD & schizophrenia	de Bruijn et al., 2010; Xu et al., 2009
NGLs	post	netrin-G, LAR, PTPσ, PTPδ	Postsynaptic scaffolding	Dunah et al.,2005; Kwon et al.,2010
			Maintained excitatory synapses & synaptic currents	Kim et al., 2006;
			Induces branching of horizontal cell axons (NGL-2)	Soto et al., 2013
			Maintained excitatory synaptic currents (NGL-3)	Woo et al., 2009

Continued on next page...

Mole.	Synaptic Location	Interaction	Functions	References
			Related to schizophrenia & BP	Aoki-Suzuki et al., 2005 Ohtsuki et al., 2008
IgLONs	both	homo- and heterophilic interactions	Postsynaptic scaffolding	Hashimoto et al.,2008
			↑synapse number (LAMP, OBCAM)	Hashimoto et al., 2009
			↓synapse number at early stages, ↑increases number of dendritic synapses in mature neurons (Kilon)	Hashimoto et al., 2008
			Related to brain tumors	Reed et al., 2007
LAR-RPTPs	post	NGL-3, Slitrks	maintained excitatory synapses and dendritic spines, AMPAR trafficking, ↑AMPAR-mediated current (LAR)	Dunah et al., 2005
			excitatory synaptic differentiation ↑ PPF, mEPSCs frequency, ↓LTP (PTPσ)	Horn et al., 2012; Yim et al., 2013
			inhibitory synaptic differentiation ↑ PPF, LTP (PTPδ)	Uetani et al., 2000; Yim et al., 2013
			Related to AD & OCD	Haapasalo et al., 2007; Ting & Feng, 2011

Table1: Interactions and functions mediated by CAMs between pre & post synapses

pre: presynaptic; post: postsynaptic;   both: pre- & postsynaptic;
ND: non-determined;   ↑: increase;   ↓: decrease

3   CAMs between synapses & ECM or others

3.1   Integrins

3.1.1   Physiology

Integrins were transmembrane receptors forming heterodimers with two type-I trans-membrane chains, the α and β subunits. At least 19 α and 8 β subunits were known, re-sulting in 25 unique heterodimers in mammals (Humphries, 2000). Some integrin subu-nits were concentrated at synapses. For example, postsynaptic β3 integrin bound to the GluA2 subunit of AMPARs through their cytoplasmic tails (Cingolani et al., 2008; Pozo et al., 2012). Overexpression of β3 integrin in the postsynaptic neurons reduced the am-plitude of mEPSCs and altered the subunit composition of AMPAR, while inactivation of β3 integrin abolished the synaptic scaling induced by pharmacological silencing of neu-ronal activity (Harburger & Calderwood, 2009). Homeostatic synaptic scaling required β3 integrin, but the function of this protein in synaptic transmission was still not very clear. Excitatory synaptic currents in primary hippocampal pyramidal neurons were in-creased or decreased by overexpression of wild type or dominant-negative β3 integrin, respectively (Cingolani et al., 2008). However, expressing β3 integrin mutants, including wild-type, in constitutively inactive or constitutively active mutants had no differential effects in excitatory synaptic responses (Pozo et al., 2012). Deletion of β3 integrin also leaved LTP, LTD, and short-term plasticity unaltered (McGeachie et al., 2012). Therefore, more investigations were needed to determine the exact role of integrins in synaptic transmission.

3.1.2   Pathology

Integrins had been involved in AD. The α4 integrin and a fibronectin specific antibody were detected at the tau positive plaques in AD patients (Van Gool et al., 1994). High stained level of vitronectin and its receptor β3 integrin were found in senile plaques and neurofibrillary tangles in Alzheimer brain tissue (Akiyama et al., 1991). A recent study demonstrated that the inhibition of Aβ in LTP could be eliminated by α5 integrin in both the dentate gyrus *in vitro* and the CA1 *in vivo* (Wang et al., 2008b). Integrins had also shown their importance in the process that Aβ increases NMDA evoked neuronal activity (Uhász et al., 2010). In addition, APP was specifically colocalized with α1β1 and α5β1 integrins at the cell surface of rat hippocampal neurons and rat cortical astrocytes (Yama-zaki et al., 1997).

The contributions of integrins in epilepsy had been confirmed with numerous re-searches. Native low expression of β1 integrin could be strongly enhanced in hippocam-pal neurons and astroglial cells induced by seizure (Pinkstaff et al., 1998). Moreover, α2 integrin and laminin β1 were intensely increased in the anterior temporal neocortex tissue of patients with intractable epilepsy as compared with controls (Wu et al., 2011). In reac-tive astrocytes after pilocarpine-induced SE, immunoreactivity for α1, α2, α4, α5, β1, β3, and β4 integrin was intensely detected (Fasen et al., 2003). Similarly, an increase in α6 integrin was observed in both seizure-induced neurons and glia (Gall & Lynch, 2004). In schizophrenia studies, the potential importance of integrins had been announced. The localization of integrins in the hippccampus had been considered to be functionally correlated with their roles in neuronal epileptiform activities (Grooms & Jones, 1997). In 2002, an increase of α2b and β3a integrin expression was described in the platelet of patients with schizophrenia (Walsh et al., 2002). Genetic analysis showed variants of β3 integrin associated with age at onset of schizophrenia (Wang et al., 2013). Recently in another study, gender-specific altered α8 integrin was found in schizophrenia (Supriyanto et al., 2013). Furthermore, Reelin, a glycoprotein that bound to integrin receptors, was decreased in the prefrontal cortex of patients with schizophrenia (Guidotti et al., 2000).

Integrins had been involved in ASD. An association between β3 integrin and ASD was suggested (Napolioni et al., 2011). An association between α4 integrin and levels of a serum autoantibody directed to brain tissue was identified to relate α4 integrin to the etiology of autism (Correia et al., 2009). Similar with NL3 R451C KI mice, a significant reduction in total brain volume and a lack of preference for social novelty were detected in β3 integrin KO mice (Ellegood et al., 2012).

3.2   Telencephalin

3.2.1   Physiology

Telencephalin (TLCN), also known as intercellular adhesion molecule 5 (ICAM5), was a type I transmembrane glycoprotein expressed only in the soma and dendritic membrane in brain (Oka et al., 1990). This dendritic distribution was mainly decided by its C-terminal sequence (Mitsui et al., 2005). Neuronal surface expressed TLCN exhibited homophilic binding ability between neurons, and heterophilic binding ability between neurons and leukocytes (Tian et al., 2000). TLCN also interacted with multiple proteins. An interaction between TLCN and ERM (ezrin/radixin/moesin) family proteins indicated the linkage of actin cytoskeleton and membrane proteins (Furutani et al., 2007). TLCN was reported to interact with β(1) integrins and stimulate β(1) integrin-dependent phosphorylation of cofilin (Conant et al., 2011).

TLCN played a role in neuronal development. In cultured hippocampal neurons, TLCN promoted dendritic elongation and branching (Tian et al., 2000). Overexpression of TLCN increased the density of dendritic filopodia and decreased the density of spines simultaneously. Consistently, TLCN-deficient neurons showed decreased density of filopodia displayed (Matsuno et al., 2006). Furthermore, the neurons lacking TLCN retracted the growth of spine heads and spine numbers in contrast to WT neurons in response to NMDA stimulation (Tian et al., 2007). TLCN also functioned in the synaptic plasticity. In TLCN-deficient hippocampal neurons, LTP induced by tetanic stimulation had been largely enhanced, while the basal synaptic transmission was normal, suggesting a TLCN-regulation of synaptic plasticity by determining the dynamic range of synaptic efficacy (Nakamura et al., 2001).

3.2.2   Pathology

TLCN may play an important role in AD development by preventing the processing of APP by γ-secretase (Annaert et al., 2001). TLCN was revealed to functionally but not structurally bound with Presenilin 1 and 2 (PS1 and PS2) (Annaert et al., 2001). Interestingly, APP competed the same binding region of PS1 with TLCN. This binding region of PS1 was often mutated in AD patients. In the brain of AD patients, the immunoreactivity of TLCN was decreased dramatically (Hino et al., 1997).

Several observations also suggested a role of TLCN in epilepsy. The concentrations of sTLCN were reduced in epilepsy patient plasmas, concomitant with an increase of TARC (thymus and activation regulated chemokines, CCL17) concentrations. Therefore raising a hypothesis that the ratio of TARC/sICAM5 distinguished between patients and controls (Pollard et al., 2013). Furthermore, TLCN was found in response to temporal-lobe dysfunction as well. The concentration of soluble TLCN (sTLCN) in serum and cerebral spinal fluid increased in adult temporal lobe epilepsy patients (Rieckmann et al., 1998). In localization-related epilepsy and secondarily generalized seizures patients whose TLCN was detected, lower functional MRI activation in the frontotemporal region was found concomitantly, making TLCN a potential biomarker in localization-related epilepsy (Jansen et al., 2008).

3.3   MHC-1

3.3.1   Physiology

Major histocompatibility complex (MHC) proteins were first identified in immune systems that mediated interactions of leukocytes. Three subgroups of MHC proteins had been found: class I, class II, and class III. In these three classes of proteins, class I MHC (MHC-1) was expressed in neurons as well (Corriveau et al., 1998). In addition, both β2-microglobulin, a cosubunit of MHC-1, and CD3ζ, a component of a receptor complex for MHC-1, were expressed in neurons, indicating MHC-1 signaling may also be mediated in the neuronal system in addition to immune system. Later, MHC-1 was shown colocalization with PSD-95 at excitatory synapses postsynaptically (Goddard et al., 2007). MHC-1 was negative controlling glutamatergic and GABAergic synapse density (Glynn et al., 2011). Moreover, MHC-1 was reported to be necessary and sufficient for synapse elimination in the retinogeniculate system (Lee et al., 2014).

Functionally, MHC-1 was involved in regulating synaptic transmission and plasticity. Reducing the MHC-1 expression level resulted in a significant increase in mEPSC frequency, a modest enlargement of presynaptic buttons and an increase in vesicle numbers (Goddard et al., 2007). Neural homeostatic plasticity could also be mediated by MHC-1. Reduced MHC-1 expression led to a failure to induce the increase of mEPSC amplitude and frequency by TTX treatment (Goddard et al., 2007). These results thereby suggested that MHC-1 controlled presynaptic release properties and retrogradely translated a signal across the synapse. In MHC-1 deficient hippocampal neurons, the AMPA/NMDA ratio was decreased (Fourgeaud et al., 2010), NMDA-dependent LTP was increased and LTD was blocked (Huh et al., 2000). Furthermore, in Purkinje cells lacking

MHC-1, a lower threshold for induction of LTD was exhibited, correlating an alteration of motor learning (McConnell et al., 2009).

3.3.2   Pathology

MHC-1 (human leukocyte antigen, HLA) A2 allele, but not B alleles, was reported an increased frequency of inheritance for autistic children (Torres et al., 2006). Conversely, the expression of MHC-1 was decreased in the dorsolateral prefrontal cortex but not in the orbitofrontal cortex in nonsmoking schizophrenia patients (Kano et al., 2011). MHC-1 mRNA expression was largely increased in the dentate gyrus 9 hours after kainic acid injection, indicating its role in seizures (Corriveau et al., 1998).

4   Perspective

The most remarkable feature of the brain was the large scale neuron-connected network. To transfer the information flows from one to another in the network, neurons had to form synapses. The synapse was thus considered the key structure for conveying the neural signal. It had been found that the CAMs mediate protein-protein interactions in the synaptic cleft and were involved in the recognition and localization of pre- and postsynaptic sites, as well as trans-synaptic signaling. Alterations in CAMs led to changes in synaptic morphology and function, and were associated with many neurological disorders, including autism, AD, schizophrenia and so on. Current data clearly showed that multiple mutations in different CAMs could lead to a single disease (eg., ASD), but how these mutant proteins could synergistically affect the brain to present a common human behavior deficit seen in patients was still a mystery.

As was stated in this chapter, there was still no crystal-clear picture of how CAMs worked to initiate/regulate synapse formation, and how dysfunction of these molecules affected the function of brain circuit and behavior. In view of the large variety of synapses in the brain, the number of known synaptogenic molecules was surprisingly low and none of these mutants abolished the synapse formation either *in vitro* or *in vivo*. Thus, more efforts were expected to 1) study the precise function of the known CAMs in the synaptogenesis process, and 2) search and identify the new molecules in determining/regulating synapse formation by means of genome-wide screening, genetic engineering, and structural and functional analysis in animal models.

Acknowledgement

We sincerely apologize to the many authors whose works were not cited in this review due to space considerations. This work was supported by grants to Drs. Zhang Chen & Yang Xiaofei from National Basic Research Program of China (2011CB809102, 2014CB942804 and 2014BAI03B01), and National Science Foundation of China (31222025, 31171025 and 31300892), and National Science Foundation of Hubei (2014CFA027), and

Molecules	Synaptic location	Interaction	Functions	References
Integrins	both	cadherins, AMPAR	AMPAR trafficking ↓amplitude of mEPSCs altered the subunit composition of AMPAR ↑excitatory synaptic currents (Integrin-β3)	Cingolani et al., 2008; Harburger & Calderwood, 2009
			Related to ASD, AD, schizophrenia & epilepsy	Akiyama et al., 1991; Fasen et al., 2003; Napolioni et al., 2011; Walsh et al., 2002
Telencephalin	ND	ERM, β(1) integrins	slowed spine maturation LTP↓	Matsuno et al., 2006; Nakamura et al., 2001
			Relate to AD & epilepsy	Annaert et al., 2001; Jansen et al., 2008
MHC-1	post	β2-microglobulin, CD3ζ	negative controlling glutamatergic and GABAergic synapse density, synapse elimination mEPSC frequency ↓, AMPA/NMDA ratio ↓, LTP ↓	Glynn et al., 2011; Lee et al., 2014; Fourgeaud et al., 2010; Goddard et al., 2007; Huh et al., 2000
			Related to ASD, schizophrenia & epilepsy	Corriveau et al., 1998; Kano et al., 2011; Torres et al., 2006

pre: presynaptic; post: postsynaptic; both: pre- & postsynaptic;
ND: non-determined; ↑: increase; ↓: decrease

Table2: Interactions and functions mediated by CAMs between synapses & ECM or others.

Program for New Century Excellent Talents in University of Ministry of Education of China, and the Project Sponsored by the Scientific Research Foundation for the Returned Overseas Chinese Scholars, State Education Ministry.

References

Aiga, M., Levinson, JN., & Bamji, SX. (2011). N-cadherin and neuroligins cooperate to regulate synapse formation in hippocampal cultures. J Biol Chem, 286, 851–858.

Aisa, B., Gil-Bea, FJ., Solas, M., García-Alloza, M., Chen, CP., Lai, MK., Francis, PT., & Ramírez, MJ. (2010). Altered NCAM expression associated with the cholinergic system in Alzheimer's disease. J Alzheimers Dis, 20 (2), 659–668.

Akiyama, H., Kawamata, T., Dedhar, S., & McGeer, PL.(1991). Immunohistochemical localization of vitronectin, its receptor and beta-3 integrin in Alzheimer brain tissue. J Neuroimmunol, 32 (1), 19–28.

Ango, F., di Cristo, G., Higashiyama, H., Bennett. V., Wu, P., & Huang, ZJ. (2004). Ankyrin-based subcellular gradient of neurofascin, an immunoglobulin family protein, directs GABAergic innervation at purkinje axon initial segment. Cell, 119, 257–272.

Ango, F., Wu, C., Van der Want, JJ., Wu, P., Schachner, M., & Huang, ZJ. (2008). Bergmann glia and the recognition molecule CHL1 organize GABAergic axons and direct innervation of Purkinje cell dendrites. PLoS Biol, 6, e103.

Annaert, WG., Esselens, C., Baert, V., Boeve, C., Snellings, G., Cupers, P., Craessaerts, K., & De Strooper, B. (2001). Interaction with telencephalin and the amyloid precursor protein predicts a ring structure for presenilins. Neuron, 32 (4): 579–589.

Antion, MD., Christie, LA., Bond, AM., Dalva, MB., & Contractor, A. (2010). Ephrin-B3 regulates glutamate receptor signaling at hippocampal synapses. Mol Cell Neurosci, 45, 378–388.

Aoki-Suzuki, M., Yamada, K., Meerabux, J., Iwayama-Shigeno, Y., Ohba, H., Iwamoto, K., Takao, H., Toyota, T., Suto, Y., Nakatani, N., Dean, B., Nishimura, S., Seki, K., Kato, T., Itohara, S., Nishikawa, T., & Yoshikawa T. (2005). A family-based association study and gene expression analyses of netrin-G1 and -G2 genes in schizophrenia. Biol Psychiatry, 57 (4), 382–393.

Aoto, J., Martinelli, DC., Malenka, RC., Tabuchi. K., & Südhof, TC. (2013). Presynaptic neurexin-3 alternative splicing trans-synaptically controls postsynaptic AMPA receptor trafficking. Cell, 154, 75–88.

Araç, D., Boucard, AA., Ozkan, E., Strop, P., Newell, E., Südhof, TC., & Brunger, AT. (2007). Structures of neuroligin-1 and the neuroligin-1/neurexin-1 beta complex reveal specific protein-protein and protein-Ca2+ interactions. Neuron, 56, 992–1003.

Armstrong, JN., Saganich, MJ., Xu, NJ., Henkemeyer, M., Heinemann, SF., & Contractor, A. (2006). B-ephrin reverse signaling is required for NMDA-independent long-term potentiation of mossy fibers in the hippocampus. J Neurosci, 26, 3474–3481.

Bamji, SX., Shimazu, K., Kimes, N., Huelsken, J., Birchmeier, W., Lu, B., & Reichardt, LF. (2003). Role of beta-catenin in synaptic vesicle localization and presynaptic assembly. Neuron, 40, 719–731.

Barbeau, D., Liang, JJ., Robitalille, Y., Quirion, R., & Srivastava, LK. (1995). Decreased expression of the embryonic form of the neural cell adhesion molecule in schizophrenic brains. Proc Natl Acad Sci U S A, 92, 2785–2789.

Barrow, SL., Constable, JR., Clark, E., El-Sabeawy, F., McAllister, AK., & Washbourne, P. (2009). Neuroligin1: a cell adhesion molecule that recruits PSD-95 and NMDA receptors by distinct mechanisms during synaptogenesis. Neural Dev, 4, 17.

Baudouin, S., & Scheiffele, P. (2010). SnapShot: Neuroligin-neurexin complexes. Cell, 141, 908, 908.

Berninghausen, O., Rahman, MA., Silva, JP., Davletov, B., Hopkins, C., & Ushkaryov, YA. (2007). Neurexin Ibeta and neuroligin are localized on opposite membranes in mature central synapses. J Neurochem, 103, 1855–1863.

Biederer, T., Sara, Y., Mozhayeva, M., Atasoy, D., Liu, X., Kavalali, ET., & Südhof, TC. (2002). SynCAM, a synaptic adhesion molecule that drives synapse assembly. Science, 297, 1525–1531.

Bloch, M., State, M., & Pittenger, C. (2011). Recent advances in Tourette syndrome. Curr Opin Neurol, 24,119–125.

Borg, JP., Lõpez-Figueroa, MO., de Taddèo-Borg, M., Kroon, DE., Turner, RS., Watson, SJ., & Margolis, B. (1999). Molecular analysis of the X11-mLin-2/CASK complex in brain. J Neurosci, 19, 1307–1316.

Bot, N., Schweizer, C., Ben Halima, S., & Fraering, PC. (2011). Processing of the synaptic cell adhesion molecule neurexin-3beta by Alzheimer disease alpha- and gamma-secretases. J Biol Chem, 286, 2762–2773.

Boucard, AA., Chubykin, AA., Comoletti, D., Taylor, P., & Südhof, TC. (2005). A splice code for trans-synaptic cell adhesion mediated by binding of neuroligin 1 to alpha- and beta-neurexins. Neuron, 48, 229–236.

Bourgin, C., Murai, KK., Richter, M., & Pasquale, EB. (2007). The EphA4 receptor regulates dendritic spine remodeling by affecting beta1-integrin signaling pathways. J Cell Biol, 178, 1295–1307.

Bouzioukh, F., Wilkinson, GA., Adelmann, G.,Frotscher, M., Stein, V., & Klein, R. (2007). Tyrosine phosphorylation sites in ephrinB2 are required for hippocampal long-term potentiation but not long-term depression. J Neurosci, 7, 1279–1288.

Bozdagi, O., Wang, XB., Nikitczuk, JS., Anderson, TR., Bloss, EB., Radice, GL., Zhou, Q., Benson, DL., & Huntley, GW. (2010). Persistence of coordinated long-term potentiation and dendritic spine enlargement at mature hippocampal CA1 synapses requires N-cadherin. J Neurosci, 30, 9984–9989.

Brigidi, GS., & Bamji, SX. (2011). Cadherin-catenin adhesion complexes at the synapse. Curr Opin Neurobiol, 21, 208–214.

Bukalo, O., & Dityatev, A. (2012). Synaptic cell adhesion molecules. Adv Exp Med Biol, 970, 97–128.

Bukalo, O., Fentrop, N., Lee, AY., Salmen, B., Law, JW., Wotjak, CT., Schweizer, M., Dityatev, A., & Schachner, M. (2004). Conditional ablation of the neural cell adhesion molecule reduces precision of spatial learning, long-term potentiation, and depression in the CA1 subfield of mouse hippocampus. J Neurosci, 24, 1565–1577.

Burbach, JP., & van der Zwaag, B. (2009). Contact in the genetics of autism and schizophrenia. Trends Neurosci, 32 (2), 69–72.

Buttiglione, M., Revest, JM., Rougon, G., & Faivre-Sarrailh, C. (1996). F3 neuronal adhesion molecule controls outgrowth and fasciculation of cerebellar granule cell neurites: a cell-type-specific effect mediated by the Ig-like domains. Mol Cell Neurosci, 8, 53–69.

Butz, S., Okamoto, M., & Südhof, TC. (1998). A tripartite protein complex with the potential to couple synaptic vesicle exocytosis to cell adhesion in brain. Cell, 94, 773–782.

Chagnon, MJ., Uetani, N., & Tremblay, ML. (2004). Functional significance of the LAR receptor protein tyrosine phosphatase family in development and diseases. *Biochem Cell Biol*, 82, 664–675.

Chan, SA., Polo-Parada, L., Landmesser, LT., & Smith. C. (2005). Adrenal chromaffin cells exhibit impaired granule trafficking in NCAM knockout mice. *J Neurophysiol*, 94, 1037–1047.

Chang, S., Rathjen, FG., & Raper, JA. (1987). Extension of neurites on axons is impaired by antibodies against specific neural cell surface glycoproteins. *J Cell Biol*, 104, 355–662.

Chapman, NH., Estes, A., Munson, J., Bernier, R., Webb, SJ., Rothstein, JH., Minshew, NJ., Dawson, G., Schellenberg, GD., & Wijsman, EM. (2011). Genome-scan for IQ discrepancy in autism: evidence for loci on chromosomes 10 and 16. *Hum Genet*, 129, 59–70.

Chavis, P., & Westbrook, G. (2001). Integrins mediate functional pre- and postsynaptic maturation at a hippocampal synapse. *Nature*, 411, 317–321.

Chen, QY., Chen, Q., Feng, GY., Lindpaintner, K., Chen, Y., Sun, X., Chen, Z., Gao, Z., Tang, J., & He, L. (2005). Case-control association study of the close homologue of L1 (CHL1) gene and schizophrenia in the Chinese population. *Schizophr Res*, 73 (2–3), 269–274.

Chen, X., Liu, H., Shim, AH., Focia, PJ., & He, X. (2008). Structural basis for synaptic adhesion mediated by neuroligin-neurexin interactions. *Nat Struct Mol Biol*, 15, 50–56.

Chen, Y., Fu, AK., Ip, & NY. (2012). Eph receptors at synapses: implications in neurodegenerative diseases. *Cell Signal*, 24, 606–611.

Chih, B., Afridi, SK., Clark, L., & Scheiffele, P. (2004). Disorder-associated mutations lead to functional inactivation of neuroligins. *Hum Mol Genet*, 13, 1471–1477.

Chih, B., Engelman, H., & Scheiffele, P. (2005). Control of excitatory and inhibitory synapse formation by neuroligins. *Science*, 307, 1324–1328.

Chih, B., Gollan, L., & Scheiffele, P. (2006). Alternative splicing controls selective trans-synaptic interactions of the neuroligin-neurexin complex. *Neuron*, 51, 171–178.

Chubykin, AA., Atasoy, D., Etherton, MR., Brose, N., Kavalali, ET., Gibson, JR., & Südhof, TC. (2007). Activity-dependent validation of excitatory versus inhibitory synapses by neuroligin-1 versus neuroligin-2. *Neuron*, 54, 919–931.

Cingolani, LA., Thalhammer, A., Yu, LM., Catalano, M., Ramos, T., Colicos, MA., & Goda, Y. (2008). Activity-dependent regulation of synaptic AMPA receptor composition and abundance by beta3 integrins. *Neuron*, 58, 749–762.

Cissé, M., Halabisky, B., Harris, J., Devidze, N., Dubal, DB., Sun, B., Orr, A., Lotz, G., Kim, DH., Hamto, P., Ho, K., Yu, GQ., & Mucke, L. (2011). Reversing EphB2 depletion rescues cognitive functions in Alzheimer model. *Nature*, 469, 47–52.

Clifford, MA., Kanwal, JK., Dzakpasu, R., & Donoghue, MJ. (2011). EphA4 expression promotes network activity and spine maturation in cortical neuronal cultures. *Neural Dev*, 6, 21.

Comoletti, D., De Jaco, A., Jennings, LL., Flynn, RE., Gaietta, G., Tsigelny, I., Ellisman, MH., & Taylor, P. (2004). The Arg451Cys-neuroligin-3 mutation associated with autism reveals a defect in protein processing. *J Neurosci*, 24, 4889–4893.

Comoletti, D., Flynn, RE., Boucard, AA., Demeler, B., Schirf, V., Shi, J., Jennings, LL., Newlin, HR., Südhof, TC., & Taylor, P. (2006). Gene selection, alternative splicing, and post-translational processing regulate neuroligin selectivity for beta-neurexins. *Biochemistry*, 45, 12816–12827.

Conant, K., Lonskaya, I., Szklarczyk, A., Krall, C., Steiner, J., Maguire-Zeiss, K., & Lim, ST. (2011). Methamphetamine-associated cleavage of the synaptic adhesion molecule intercellular adhesion *molecule-5. J Neurochem, 118 (4), 521–532.*

Conrad, AJ., & Scheibel, AB. (1987). Schizophrenia and the hippocampus: the embryological hypothesis extended. Schizophr Bull, 13, 577–587.

Contractor, A., Rogers, C., Maron, C., Henkemeyer, M., Swanson, GT., & Heinemann, SF. (2002). Trans-synaptic Eph receptor-ephrin signaling in hippocampal mossy fiber LTP. Science, 296, 1864–1869.

Corriveau, RA., Huh, GS., & Shatz, CJ. (1998). Regulation of class I MHC gene expression in the developing and mature CNS by neural activity. Neuron, 21 (3), 505–520.

Cottrell, CE., Bir, N., Varga, E., Alvarez, CE., Bouyain, S., Zernzach, R., Thrush, DL., Evans, J., Trimarchi, M., Butter, EM., Cunningham, D., Gastier-Foster, JM., McBride, KL., & Herman, GE. (2011). Contactin 4 as an autism susceptibility locus. Autism Res, 4, 189–199.

Crepel, A., De Wolf, V., Brison, N., Ceulemans, B., Walleghem, D., Peuteman, G., Lambrechts, D., Steyaert, J., Noens, I., Devriendt, K., & Peeters, H. (2014). Association of CDH11 with non-syndromic ASD. Am J Med Genet B Neuropsychiatr Genet, 165B (5), 391–398.

Crow, TJ. (2002). Handedness, language lateralisation and anatomical asymmetry: relevance of protocadherin XY to hominidspeciation and the aetiology of psychosis. Point of view. Br J Psychiatry, 181, 295–297.

Daar, IO. (2012). Non-SH2/PDZ reverse signaling by ephrins. Semin Cell Dev Biol, 23, 65–74.

Dalva, MB., McClelland, AC., & Kayser, MS. (2007). Cell adhesion molecules: signalling functions at the synapse. Nat Rev Neurosci, 8, 206–220.

Davy, A., & Soriano, P. (2005). Ephrin signaling in vivo: look both ways. Dev Dyn, 232, 1–10.

de Bruijn, DR., van Dijk, AH., Pfundt, R., Hoischen, A., Merkx, GF., Gradek, GA., Lybæk, H., Stray-Pedersen, A., Brunner, HG., & Houge, G. (2010). Severe Progressive Autism Associated with Two de novo Changes: A 2.6-Mb 2q31.1 Deletion and a Balanced t (14; 21)(q21.1; p11.2) Translocation with Long-Range Epigenetic Silencing of LRFN5 Expression. Mol Syndromol, 1 (1), 46–57.

de Wit, J., Sylwestrak, E., O'Sullivan, ML., Otto, S., Tiglio, K., Savas, JN., Yates, JR 3rd., Comoletti, D., Taylor, P., & Ghosh, A. (2009). LRRTM2 interacts with Neurexin1 and regulates excitatory synapse formation. Neuron, 64, 799–806.

Dean, B., Keriakous, D., Scarr, E., & Thomas, EA. (2007). Gene expression profiling in Brodmann's area 46 from subjects with schizophrenia. Aust N Z J Psychiatry, 41 (4), 308–320.

Dibbens, LM., Kneen, R., Bayly, MA., Heron, SE., Arsov, T., Damiano, JA., Desai, T., Gibbs, J., McKenzie, F., Mulley, JC., Ronan, A., & Scheffer, IE. (2011). Recurrence risk of epilepsy and mental retardation in females due to parental mosaicism of PCDH19 mutations. Neurology, 76 (17), 1514–1519.

Dibbens, LM., Tarpey, PS., Hynes, K., Bayly, MA., Scheffer, IE., Smith, R., Bomar, J., Sutton, E., Vandeleur, L., Shoubridge, C., Edkins, S., Turner, SJ., Stevens, C., O'Meara, S., Tofts, C., Barthorpe, S., Buck, G., Cole, J., Halliday, K., Jones, D., Lee, R., Madison, M., et al. (2008). X-linked protocadherin 19 mutations cause female-limited epilepsy and cognitive impairment. Nat Genet, 40 (6), 776–781.

Dickinson, BA., Jo, J., Seok, H., Son, GH., Whitcomb, DJ., Davies, CH., Sheng, M., Collingridge, GL., & Cho, K. (2009). A novel mechanism of hippocampal LTD involving muscarinic receptor-triggered interactions between AMPARs, GRIP and liprin-alpha. Mol Brain, 2, 18.

Dinamarca, MC., Ríos, JA., & Inestrosa, NC. (2012). Postsynaptic Receptors for Amyloid-β Oligomers as Mediators of Neuronal Damage in Alzheimer's Disease. Front Physiol, 3, 464.

Dinamarca, MC., Weinstein, D., Monasterio, O., & Inestrosa, NC. (2011). The synaptic protein neuroligin-

1 interacts with the amyloid β-peptide. Is there a role in Alzheimer's disease? Biochemistry, 50 (38), 8127–8137.

Dityatev, A., Dityateva, G., & Schachner, M. (2000). Synaptic strength as a function of post- versus presynaptic expression of the neural cell adhesion molecule NCAM. Neuron, 26, 207–217.

Djogo, N., Jakovcevski, I., Müller, C., Lee, HJ., Xu, JC., Jakovcevski, M., Kügler, S., Loers, G., & Schachner, M. (2013). Adhesion molecule L1 binds to amyloid beta and reduces Alzheimer's disease pathology in mice. Neurobiol Dis, 56, 104–115.

Dosemeci, A., Tao-Cheng, JH., Vinade, L., & Jaffe, H. (2006). Preparation of postsynaptic density fraction from hippocampal slices and proteomic analysis. Biochem Biophys Res Commun, 339, 687–694.

Dunah, AW., Hueske, E., Wyszynski, M., Hoogenraad, CC., Jaworski, J., Pak, DT., Simonetta, A., Liu, G., & Sheng, M. (2005). LAR receptor protein tyrosine phosphatases in the development and maintenance of excitatory synapses. Nat Neurosci, 8, 458–467.

Duveau, V., & Fritschy, JM. (2010). PSA-NCAM-dependent GDNF signaling limits neurodegeneration and epileptogenesis in temporal lobe epilepsy. Eur J Neurosci, 32 (1), 89–98.

Edwards, TL., Pericak-Vance, M., Gilbert, JR., Haines, JL., Martin, ER., & Ritchie, MD. (2009). An association analysis of Alzheimer disease candidate genes detects an ancestral risk haplotype clade in ACE and putative multilocus association between ACE, A2M, and LRRTM3. Am J Med Genet B Neuropsychiatr Genet, 150B (5), 721–735.

Egea, J., & Klein, R. (2007). Bidirectional Eph-ephrin signaling during axon guidance. Trends Cell Biol, 17, 230–238.

Ellegood, J., Henkelman, RM., & Lerch, JP. (2012). Neuroanatomical Assessment of the Integrin β3 Mouse Model Related to Autism and the Serotonin System Using High Resolution MRI. Front Psychiatry, 3, 37.

Fannon, AM., & Colman, DR. (1996). A model for central synaptic junctional complex formation based on the differential adhesive specificities of the cadherins. Neuron, 17, 423–434.

Fasen, K., Elger, CE., & Lie, AA. (2003). Distribution of alpha and beta integrin subunits in the adult rat hippocampus after pilocarpine induced neuronal cell loss, axonal reorganization and reactive astrogliosis. Acta Neuropathol, 106(4), 319–322.

Feng, J., Schroer, R., Yan, J., Song, W., Yang, C., Bockholt, A., Cook EH, Jr., Skinner, C., Schwartz, CE., & Sommer, SS. (2006). High frequency of neurexin 1beta signal peptide structural variants in patients with autism. Neurosci Lett, 409, 10–13.

Fernandez, T., Morgan, T., Davis, N., Klin, A., Morris, A., Farhi, A., Lifton, RP., & State, MW. (2004). Disruption of contactin 4 (CNTN4) results in developmental delay and other features of 3p deletion syndrome. Am J Hum Genet, 74, 1286–1293.

Filosa, A., Paixão, S., Honsek, SD., Carmona, MA., Becker, L., Feddersen, B., Gaitanos, L., Rudhard, Y., Schoepfer, R., Klopstock, T., Kullander, K., Rose, CR., Pasquale, EB., & Klein, R. (2009). Neuron-glia communication via EphA4/ephrin-A3 modulates LTP through glial glutamate transport. Nat Neurosci, 12, 1285–1292.

Fischer, G., Künemund, V., & Schachner, M. (1986). Neurite outgrowth patterns in cerebellar microexplant cultures are affected by antibodies to the cell surface glycoprotein L1. J Neurosci, 6, 605–612.

Fogel, AI., Akins, MR., Krupp, AJ., Stagi, M., Stein, V., & Biederer, T. (2007). SynCAMs organize synapses through heterophilic adhesion. J Neurosci, 27, 12516–12530.

Fourgeaud, L., Davenport, CM., Tyler, CM., Cheng, TT., Spencer, MB., & Boulanger, LM. (2010). MHC class I modulates NMDA receptor function and AMPA receptor trafficking. Proc Natl Acad Sci U S A, 107 (51), 22278–22283.

Francks, C., Maegawa, S., Laurén, J., Abrahams, BS., Velayos-Baeza, A., Medland, SE., Colella, S., Groszer, M., McAuley, EZ., Caffrey, TM., Timmusk, T., Pruunsild, P., Koppel, I., Lind, PA., Matsumoto-Itaba, N., Nicod, J., Xiong, L., Joober, R., Enard, W., et al. (2007). LRRTM1 on chromosome 2p12 is a maternally suppressed gene that is associated paternally with handedness and schizophrenia. Mol Psychiatry, 12 (12), 1129–1139, 1057

Fu, AK., Hung, KW., Fu, WY., Shen, C., Chen, Y., Xia, J., Lai, KO., & Ip, NY. (2011). APC(Cdh1) mediates EphA4-dependent downregulation of AMPA receptors in homeostatic plasticity. Nat Neurosci, 14, 181–189.

Fu, WY., Chen, Y., Sahin, M., Zhao, XS., Shi, L., Bikoff, JB., Lai, KO., Yung, WH., Fu, AK., Greenberg, ME., & Ip, NY. (2007). Cdk5 regulates EphA4-mediated dendritic spine retraction through an ephexin1-dependent mechanism. Nat Neurosci, 10, 67–76.

Furutani, Y., Matsuno, H., Kawasaki, M., Sasaki, T., Mori, K., & Yoshihara, Y. (2007). Interaction between telencephalin and ERM family proteins mediates dendritic filopodia formation. J Neurosci, 27 (33), 8866–8876.

Gall, CM., & Lynch, G. (2004). Integrins, synaptic plasticity and epileptogenesis. Adv Exp Med Biol, 548, 12–33.

Gautam, V., D'Avanzo, C., Hebisch, M., Kovacs, DM., & Kim, DY. (2014). BACE1 activity regulates cell surface contactin-2 levels. Mol Neurodegener, 9, 4.

Gauthier, J., Siddiqui, TJ., Huashan, P., Yokomaku, D., Hamdan, FF., Champagne, N., Lapointe, M., Spiegelman, D., Noreau, A., Lafrenière, RG., Fathalli, F., Joober, R., Krebs, MO., DeLisi, LE., Mottron, L., Fombonne, E., Michaud, JL., Drapeau, P., Carbonetto, S., Craig, AM., & Rouleau, GA. (2011). Truncating mutations in NRXN2 and NRXN1 in autism spectrum disorders and schizophrenia. Hum Genet, 130 (4), 563–573.

Giagtzoglou, N., Ly, CV., & Bellen, HJ. (2009). Cell adhesion, the backbone of the synapse: "vertebrate" and "invertebrate" perspectives. Cold Spring Harb Perspect Biol, 1, a003079.

Gil, OD., Zhang, L., Chen, S., Ren, YQ., Pimenta, A., Zanazzi, G., Hillman, D., Levitt, P., & Salzer, JL. (2002). Complementary expression and heterophilic interactions between IgLON family members neurotrimin and LAMP. J Neurobiol, 51, 190–204.

Giza, JI., Jung, Y., Jeffrey, RA., Neugebauer, NM., Picciotto, MR., & Biederer, T. (2013). The synaptic adhesion molecule SynCAM 1 contributes to cocaine effects on synapse structure and psychostimulant behavior. Neuropsychopharmacology, 38, 628–638.

Glynn, MW., Elmer, BM., Garay, PA., Liu, XB., Needleman, LA., El-Sabeawy, F., & McAllister, AK. (2011). MHCI negatively regulates synapse density during the establishment of cortical connections. Nat Neurosci, 14 (4), 442–451.

Goddard, CA., Butts, DA., & Shatz, CJ. (2007). Regulation of CNS synapses by neuronal MHC class I. Proc Natl Acad Sci U S A, 104 (16), 6828–6833.

Gokce, O., & Südhof, TC. (2013). Membrane-tethered monomeric neurexin LNS-domain triggers synapse formation. J Neurosci, 33, 14617–14628.

Górecki, DC., Szklarczyk, A., Lukasiuk, K., Kaczmarek, L., & Simons, JP. (1999). Differential seizure-induced and developmental changes of neurexin expression. Mol Cell Neurosci, 13 (3), 218–227.

Correia, C., Coutinho, AM., Almeida, J., Lontro, R., Lobo, C., Miguel, TS., Martins, M., Gallagher, L., Conroy, J., Gill, M., Oliveira, G., & Vicente, AM. (2009). Association of the alpha4 integrin subunit gene (ITGA4) with autism. Am J Med Genet B Neuropsychiatr Genet, 150B (8), 1147–1151.

Grooms, SY., & Jones, LS. (1997). RGDS tetrapeptide and hippocampal in vitro kindling in rats: evidence for integrin-mediated physiological stability. Neurosci Lett, 231 (3), 139–142.

Grunwald, IC., Korte, M., Adelmann, G., Plueck, A., Kullander, K., Adams, RH., Frotscher, M., Bonhoeffer, T., & Klein, R. (2004). Hippocampal plasticity requires postsynaptic ephrinBs. Nat Neurosci, 7, 33–40.

Grunwald, IC., Korte, M., Wolfer, D., Wilkinson, GA., Unsicker, K., Lipp, HP., Bonhoeffer, T., & Klein, R. (2001). Kinase-independent requirement of EphB2 receptors in hippocampal synaptic plasticity. Neuron, 32, 1027–1040.

Guan, H., & Maness, PF. (2010). Perisomatic GABAergic innervation in prefrontal cortex is regulated by ankyrin interaction with the L1 cell adhesion molecule. Cereb Cortex, 20, 2684–2693.

Guidotti, A., Auta, J., Davis, JM., Di-Giorgi-Gerevini, V., Dwivedi, Y., Grayson, DR., Impagnatiello, F., Pandey, G., Pesold, C., Sharma, R., Uzunov, D., & Costa, E. (2000). Decrease in reelin and glutamic acid decarboxylase67 (GAD67) expression in schizophrenia and bipolar disorder: a postmortem brain study. Arch Gen Psychiatry, 57 (11), 1061–1069.

Guo, H., Xun, G., Peng, Y., Xiang, X., Xiong, Z., Zhang, L., He, Y., Xu, X., Liu, Y., Lu, L., Long, Z., Pan, Q., Hu, Z., Zhao, J., & Xia, K. (2012). Disruption of Contactin 4 in two subjects with autism in Chinese population. Gene, 505, 201–205.

Haapasalo, A., Kim, DY., Carey, BW., Turunen, MK., Pettingell, WH., & Kovacs, DM. (2007). Presenilin/gamma-secretase-mediated cleavage regulates association of leukocyte-common antigen-related (LAR) receptor tyrosine phosphatase with beta-catenin. J Biol Chem, 282 (12), 9063–9072.

Harburger, DS., & Calderwood, DA. (2009). Integrin signalling at a glance. J Cell Sci, 122, 159–163.

Harrison, V., Connell, L., Hayesmoore, J., McParland, J., Pike, MG., & Blair, E. (2011). Compound heterozygous deletion of NRXN1 causing severe developmental delay with early onset epilepsy in two sisters. Am J Med Genet A, 155A (11), 2826–2831.

Hashimoto, T., Maekawa, S., & Miyata, S. (2009). IgLON cell adhesion molecules regulate synaptogenesis in hippocampal neurons. Cell Biochem Funct, 27, 496–498.

Hashimoto, T., Yamada, M., Maekawa, S., Nakashima, T., & Miyata, S. (2008). IgLON cell adhesion molecule Kilon is a crucial modulator for synapse number in hippocampal neurons. Brain Res, 1224, 1–11.

Hattori, T., Shimizu, S., Koyama, Y., Yamada, K., Kuwahara, R., Kumamoto, N., Matsuzaki, S., Ito, A., Katayama, T., & Tohyama, M. (2010). DISC1 regulates cell-cell adhesion, cell-matrix adhesion and neurite outgrowth. Mol Psychiatry, 15 (8), 775, 798–809.

Hayashi-Takagi, A., & Sawa, A. (2010). Disturbed synaptic connectivity in schizophrenia: convergence of genetic risk factors during neurodevelopment. Brain Res Bull, 83, 140–146.

Heine, M., Thoumine, O., Mondin, M., Tessier, B., Giannone, G., & Choquet, D. (2008). Activity-independent and subunit-specific recruitment of functional AMPA receptors at neurexin/neuroligin contacts. Proc Natl Acad Sci U S A, 105, 20947–20952.

Henderson, JT., Georgiou, J., Jia, Z., Robertson, J., Elowe, S., Roder, JC., & Pawson, T. (2001). The receptor tyrosine kinase EphB2 regulates NMDA-dependent synaptic function. Neuron, 32, 1041–1056.

Henkemeyer, M., Itkis, OS., Ngo, M., Hickmott, PW., & Ethell, IM. (2003). Multiple EphB receptor tyrosine *kinases shape dendritic spines in the hippocampus. J Cell Biol, 163, 1313–1326.*

Himanen, JP. (2012). Ectodomain structures of Eph receptors. Semin Cell Dev Biol, 23, 35–42.

Hino, H., Mori, K., Yoshihara, Y., Iseki, E., Akiyama, H., Nishimura, T., Ikeda, K., & Kosaka, K. (1997). Reduction of telencephalin immunoreactivity in the brain of patients with Alzheimer's disease. Brain Res, 753 (2), 353–357.

Hirano, S., & Takeichi, M. (2012). Cadherins in brain morphogenesis and wiring. Physiol Rev, 92, 597–634.

Hitt, B., Riordan, SM., Kukreja, L., Eimer, WA., Rajapaksha, TW., & Vassar, R. (2012). β-Site amyloid precursor protein (APP)-cleaving enzyme 1 (BACE1)-deficient mice exhibit a close homolog of L1(CHL1) loss-of-function phenotype involving axon guidance defects. J Biol Chem, 287 (46), 38408–38425.

Honda, T., Sakisaka, T., Yamada, T., Kumazawa, N., Hoshino, T., Kajita, M., Kayahara, T., Ishizaki, H., Tanaka-Okamoto, M., Mizoguchi, A., Manabe, T., Miyoshi, J., & Takai, Y. (2006). Involvement of nectins in the formation of puncta adherentia junctions and the mossy fiber trajectory in the mouse hippocampus. Mol Cell Neurosci, 31, 315–325.

Honer, WG., Falkai, P., Young, C., Wang, T., Xie, J., Bonner, J., Hu, L., Boulianne, GL., Luo, Z., & Trimble, WS. (1997). Cingulate cortex synaptic terminal proteins and neural cell adhesion molecule in schizophrenia. Neuroscience, 78, 99–110.

Horn, KE., Xu, B., Gobert, D., Hamam, BN., Thompson, KM., Wu, CL., Bouchard, JF., Uetani, N., Racine, RJ., Tremblay, ML., Ruthazer, ES., Chapman, CA., & Kennedy, TE. (2012). Receptor protein tyrosine phosphatase sigma regulates synapse structure, function and plasticity. J Neurochem, 122, 147–161.

Hoy, JL., Constable, JR., Vicini, S., Fu, Z., & Washbourne, P. (2009). SynCAM1 recruits NMDA receptors via protein 4.1B. Mol Cell Neurosci, 42, 466–483.

Hruska, M., & Dalva, MB. (2012). Ephrin regulation of synapse formation, function and plasticity. Mol Cell Neurosci, 50, 35–44.

Huh, GS., Boulanger, LM., Du, H., Riquelme, PA., Brotz, TM., & Shatz, CJ. (2000). Functional requirement for class I MHC in CNS development and plasticity. Science, 290 (5499), 2155–2159.

Humphries, MJ. (2000). Integrin structure. Biochem. Soc. Trans, 28 (4), 311–339.

Ichtchenko, K., Hata, Y., Nguyen, T., Ullrich, B., Missler, M., Moomaw, C., & Südhof, TC. (1995). Neuroligin 1: a splice site-specific ligand for beta-neurexins. Cell, 81, 435–443.

Inoue, E., Deguchi-Tawarada, M., Togawa, A., Matsui, C., Arita, K., Katahira-Tayama, S., Sato, T., Yamauchi, E., Oda, Y., & Takai, Y. (2009). Synaptic activity prompts gamma-secretase-mediated cleavage of EphA4 and dendritic spine formation. J Cell Biol, 185, 551–564.

Irie, F., & Yamaguchi, Y. (2004). EPHB receptor signaling in dendritic spine development. Front Biosci, 9, 1365–1373.

Jamain, S., Radyushkin, K., Hammerschmidt, K., Granon, S., Boretius, S., Varoqueaux, F., Ramanantsoa, N., Gallego, J., Ronnenberg, A., Winter, D., Frahm, J., Fischer, J., Bourgeron, T., Ehrenreich, H., & Brose, N. (2008). Reduced social interaction and ultrasonic communication in a mouse model of monogenic heritable autism. Proc Natl Acad Sci U S A, 105, 1710–1715.

Jamal, SM., Basran, RK., Newton, S., Wang, Z., & Milunsky, JM. (2010). Novel de novo PCDH19 mutations in three unrelated females with epilepsy female restricted mental retardation syndrome. Am J Med Genet A, 152A(10), 2475–2481.

Jansen, JF., Vlooswijk, MC., de Baets, MH., de Krom, MC., Rieckmann, P., Backes, WH., Aldenkamp, AP.;

& SEGAED Study Group. (2008). Cognitive fMRI and soluble telencephalin assessment in patients with localization-related epilepsy. Acta Neurol Scand, 118 (4), 232–239.

Jedlicka, P., Vnencak, M., Krueger, DD., Jungenitz, T., Brose, N., & Schwarzacher, SW. (2013). Neuroligin-1 regulates excitatory synaptic transmission, LTP and EPSP-spike coupling in the dentate gyrus in vivo. Brain Struct Funct.

Jüngling, K., Eulenburg, V., Moore, R., Kemler, R., Lessmann, V., & Gottmann, K. (2006). N-cadherin transsynaptically regulates short-term plasticity at glutamatergic synapses in embryonic stem cell-derived neurons. J Neurosci, 26, 6968–6978.

Kano, S., Nwulia, E., Niwa, M., Chen, Y., Sawa, A., & Cascella, N. (2011). Altered MHC class I expression in dorsolateral prefrontal cortex of nonsmoker patients with schizophrenia. Neurosci Res, 71 (3), 289–293.

Kayser, MS., McClelland, AC., Hughes, EG., & Dalva, MB. (2006). Intracellular and trans-synaptic regulation of glutamatergic synaptogenesis by EphB receptors. J Neurosci, 26, 12152–12164.

Kayser, MS., Nolt, MJ., & Dalva, MB. (2008). EphB receptors couple dendritic filopodia motility to synapse formation. Neuron, 59, 56–69.

Kim, DY., Ingano, LA., & Kovacs, DM. (2002). Nectin-1alpha, an immunoglobulin-like receptor involved in the formation of synapses, is a substrate for presenilin/gamma-secretase-like cleavage. J Biol Chem, 277, 49976–49981.

Kim, J., Chang, A., Dudak, A., Federoff, HJ., & Lim, ST. (2011). Characterization of nectin processing mediated by presenilin-dependent γ-secretase. J Neurochem, 119, 945–956.

Kim, S., Burette, A., Chung, HS., Kwon, SK., Woo, J., Lee, HW., Kim, K., Kim, H., Weinberg, RJ., & Kim, E. (2006). NGL family PSD-95-interacting adhesion molecules regulate excitatory synapse formation. Nat Neurosci, 9, 1294–1301.

Kirov, G., Gumus, D., Chen, W., Norton, N., Georgieva, L., Sari, M., O'Donovan, MC., Erdogan, F., Owen, MJ., Ropers, HH., & Ullmann, R. (2008). Comparative genome hybridization suggests a role for NRXN1 and APBA2 in schizophrenia. Hum Mol Genet, 17, 458–465.

Klein, R. (2009). Bidirectional modulation of synaptic functions by Eph/ephrin signaling. Nat Neurosci, 12, 15–20.

Ko, J., Fuccillo, MV., Malenka, RC., & Südhof, TC. (2009). LRRTM2 functions as a neurexin ligand in promoting excitatory synapse formation. Neuron, 64, 791–798.

Ko, J., Kim, S., Chung, HS., Kim, K., Han, K., Kim, H., Jun, H., Kaang, BK., & Kim, E. (2006). SALM synaptic cell adhesion-like molecules regulate the differentiation of excitatory synapses. Neuron, 50, 233–245.

Ko, J., Soler-Llavina, GJ., Fuccillo, MV., Malenka, RC., & Südhof, TC. (2011). Neuroligins/LRRTMs prevent activity- and Ca2+/calmodulin-dependent synapse elimination in cultured neurons. J Cell Biol, 194, 323–334.

Kolkman, MJ., Streijger, F., Linkels, M., Bloemer, M., Heeren, DJ., Hendriks, WJ., & Van der Zee, CE. (2004). Mice lacking leukocyte common antigen-related (LAR) protein tyrosine phosphatase domains demonstrate spatial learning impairment in the two-trial water maze and hyperactivity in multiple behavioural tests. Behav Brain Res, 154, 171–182.

Krushel, LA., Sporns, O., Cunningham, BA., Crossin, KL., & Edelman, GM. (1995). Neural cell adhesion molecule (N-CAM) inhibits astrocyte proliferation after injury to different regions of the adult rat brain. Proc Natl Acad Sci U S A, 92, 4323–4327.

Kullander, K., & Klein, R. (2002). Mechanisms and functions of Eph and ephrin signalling. Nat Rev Mol Cell Biol, 3, 475–486.

Kwon, SK., Woo, J., Kim, SY., Kim, H., & Kim, E. (2010). Trans-synaptic adhesions between netrin-G ligand-3 (NGL-3) and receptor tyrosine phosphatases LAR, protein-tyrosine phosphatase delta (PTPdelta), and PTPsigma via specific domains regulate excitatory synapse formation. J Biol Chem, 285, 13966–13978.

Kurumaji, A., Nomoto, H., Okano, T., & Toru, M. (2001). An association study between polymorphism of L1CAM gene and schizophrenia in a Japanese sample. Am J Med Genet, 105 (1), 99–104.

Laumonnier, F., Bonnet-Brilhault, F., Gomot, M., Blanc, R., David, A., Moizard, MP., Raynaud, M., Ronce, N., Lemonnier, E., Calvas, P., Laudier, B., Chelly, J., Fryns, JP., Ropers, HH., Hamel, BC., Andres, C., Barthélémy, C., Moraine, C., & Briault, S. (2004). X-linked mental retardation and autism are associated with a mutation in the NLGN4 gene, a member of the neuroligin family. Am J Hum Genet, 74, 552–557.

Laurén, J., Airaksinen, MS., Saarma, M., & Timmusk, T. (2003). A novel gene family encoding leucine-rich repeat transmembrane proteins differentially expressed in the nervous system. Genomics, 81, 411–421.

Law, JW., Lee, AY., Sun, M., Nikonenko, AG., Chung, SK., Dityatev, A., Schachner, M., & Morellini, F. (2003). Decreased anxiety, altered place learning, and increased CA1 basal excitatory synaptic transmission in mice with conditional ablation of the neural cell adhesion molecule L1. J Neurosci, 23, 10419–10432.

Lee, H., Brott, BK., Kirkby, LA., Adelson, JD., Cheng, S., Feller, MB., Datwani, A., & Shatz, CJ. (2014). Synapse elimination and learning rules co-regulated by MHC class I H2-Db. Nature, 509 (7499), 195–200.

Levinson, JN., Chéry, N., Huang, K., Wong, TP., Gerrow, K., Kang, R., Prange, O., Wang, YT., & El-Husseini, A. (2005). Neuroligins mediate excitatory and inhibitory synapse formation: involvement of PSD-95 and neurexin-1beta in neuroligin-induced synaptic specificity. J Biol Chem, 280, 17312–17319.

Lim, ST., Lim, KC., Giuliano, RE., & Federoff, HJ. (2008). Temporal and spatial localization of nectin-1 and l-afadin during synaptogenesis in hippocampal neurons. J Comp Neurol, 507, 1228–1244.

Lindner, J., Rathjen, FG., & Schachner, M. (1983). L1 mono- and polyclonal antibodies modify cell migration in early postnatal mouse cerebellum. Nature, 305, 427–430.

Linhoff, MW., Laurén, J., Cassidy, RM., Dobie, FA., Takahashi, H., Nygaard, HB., Airaksinen, MS., Strittmatter, SM., & Craig, AM. (2009). An unbiased expression screen for synaptogenic proteins identifies the LRRTM protein family as synaptic organizers. Neuron, 61, 734–749.

Lisé, MF., & El-Husseini, A. (2006). The neuroligin and neurexin families: from structure to function at the synapse. Cell Mol Life Sci, 63, 1833–1849.

Litterst, C., Georgakopoulos, A., Shioi, J., Ghersi, E., Wisniewski, T., Wang, R., Ludwig, A., & Robakis, NK. (2007). Ligand binding and calcium influx induce distinct ectodomain/gamma-secretase-processing pathways of EphB2 receptor. J Biol Chem, 282, 16155–16163.

Liu, J., Li, G., Peng, X., Liu, B., Yin, B., Tan, X., Fan, M., Fan, W., Qiang, B., & Yuan, J. (2004). The cloning and preliminarily functional analysis of the human neurotrimin gene. Sci China C Life Sci, 47(2), 158–164.

Lodge, AP., Howard, MR., McNamee, CJ., & Moss, DJ. (2000). Co-localisation, heterophilic interactions and regulated expression of IgLON family proteins in the chick nervous system. Brain Res Mol Brain Res, 82, 84–94.

Lyons, F., Martin, ML., Maguire, C., Jackson, A., Regan, CM., & Shelley, RK. (1988). *The expression of an N-CAM serum fragment is positively correlated with severity of negative features in type II schizophrenia. Biol Psychiatry, 23, 769–775.*

Mah, W., Ko, J., Nam, J., Han, K., Chung, WS., & Kim, E. (2010). *Selected SALM (synaptic adhesion-like molecule) family proteins regulate synapse formation. J Neurosci, 30, 5559–5568.*

Majercak, J., Ray, WJ., Espeseth, A., Simon, A., Shi, XP., Wolffe, C., Getty, K., Marine, S., Stec, E., Ferrer, M., Strulovici, B., Bartz, S., Gates, A., Xu, M., Huang, Q., Ma, L., Shughrue, P., Burchard, J., Colussi, D., Pietrak, B., Kahana, J., Beher, D., et al. (2006). *LRRTM3 promotes processing of amyloid-precursor protein by BACE1 and is a positional candidate gene for late-onset Alzheimer's disease. Proc Natl Acad Sci U S A, 103 (47), 17967–17972.*

Majima, T., Ogita, H., Yamada, T., Amano, H., Togashi, H., Sakisaka, T., Tanaka-Okamoto, M., Ishizaki, H., Miyoshi, J., & Takai, Y. (2009). *Involvement of afadin in the formation and remodeling of synapses in the hippocampus. Biochem Biophys Res Commun, 385, 539–544.*

Maness, PF., & Schachner, M. (2007). *Neural recognition molecules of the immunoglobulin superfamily: signaling transducers of axon guidance and neuronal migration. Nat Neurosci, 10, 19–26.*

Margolis, SS., Salogiannis, J., Lipton, DM., Mandel-Brehm, C., Wills, ZP., Mardinly, AR., Hu, L., Greer, PL., Bikoff, JB., Ho, HY., Soskis, MJ., Sahin, M., & Greenberg, ME. (2010). *EphB-mediated degradation of the RhoA GEF Ephexin5 relieves a developmental brake on excitatory synapse formation. Cell, 143, 442–455.*

Martinez-Mir, A., González-Pérez, A., Gayán, J., Antúnez, C., Marín, J., Boada, M., Lopez-Arrieta, JM., Fernández, E., Ramírez-Lorca, R., Sáez, ME., Ruiz, A., Scholl, FG., & Real, LM. (2013). *Genetic study of neurexin and neuroligin genes in Alzheimer's disease. J Alzheimers Dis, 35 (2), 403–412.*

Matsui, C., Inoue, E., Kakita, A., Arita, K., Deguchi-Tawarada, M., Togawa, A., Yamada, A., Takai, Y., & Takahashi, H. (2012). *Involvement of the γ-secretase-mediated EphA4 signaling pathway in synaptic pathogenesis of Alzheimer's disease. Brain Pathol, 22, 776–787.*

Matsuno, H., Okabe, S., Mishina, M., Yanagida, T., Mori, K., & Yoshihara, Y. (2006). *Telencephalin slows spine maturation. J Neurosci, 26 (6), 1776–1786.*

Maurin, H., Seymour, CM., Lechat, B., Borghgraef, P., Devijver, H., Jaworski, T., Schmidt, MV., Kuegler, S., & Van Leuven, F. (2013). *Tauopathy differentially affects cell adhesion molecules in mouse brain: early down-regulation of nectin-3 in stratum lacunosum moleculare. PLoS One, 8 (5), e63589.*

McConnell, MJ., Huang, YH., Datwani, A., & Shatz, CJ. (2009). *H2-K(b) and H2-D(b) regulate cerebellar long-term depression and limit motor learning. Proc Natl Acad Sci U S A, 106 (16), 6784–6789.*

McGeachie, AB., Skrzypiec, AE., Cingolani, LA., Letellier, M., Pawlak, R., & Goda, Y. (2012). *β3 integrin is dispensable for conditioned fear and hebbian forms of plasticity in the hippocampus. Eur J Neurosci, 36, 2461–2469.*

Medway, C., Shi, H., Bullock, J., Black, H., Brown, K., Vafadar-Isfahani, B., Matharoo-Ball, B., Ball, G., Rees, R., Kalsheker, N., & Morgan, K. (2010). *Using In silico LD clumping and meta-analysis of genome-wide datasets as a complementary tool to investigate and validate new candidate biomarkers in Alzheimer's disease. Int J Mol Epidemiol Genet, 1(2), 134–144.*

Mendez, P., De Roo, M., Poglia, L., Klauser, P., & Muller, D. (2010). *N-cadherin mediates plasticity-induced long-term spine stabilization. J Cell Biol, 189, 589–600.*

Mercati, O., Danckaert, A., André-Leroux, G., Bellinzoni, M., Gouder, L., Watanabe, K., Shimoda, Y., Grailhe, R., De Chaumont, F., Bourgeron, T., & Cloëz-Tayarani, I. (2013). *Contactin 4, -5 and -6 differentially regulate neuritogenesis while they display identical PTPRG binding sites. Biol Open, 2, 324–334.*

Millson, A., Lagrave, D., Willis, MJ., Rowe, LR., Lyon, E., & South, ST. (2012). *Chromosomal loss of 3q26.3-3q26.32, involving a partial neuroligin 1 deletion, identified by genomic microarray in a child with microcephaly, seizure disorder, and severe intellectual disability. Am J Med Genet A, 158A (1), 159–165.*

Minhas, HM., Pescosolido, MF., Schwede, M., Piasecka, J., Gaitanis, J., Tantravahi, U., & Morrow, EM. (2013). *An unbalanced translocation involving loss of 10q26.2 and gain of 11q25 in a pedigree with autism spectrum disorder and cerebellar juvenile pilocytic astrocytoma. Am J Med Genet A, 161A (4), 787–791.*

Missler, M., Zhang, W., Rohlmann, A., Kattenstroth, G., Hammer, RE., Gottmann, K., & Südhof, TC. (2003). *Alpha-neurexins couple Ca2+ channels to synaptic vesicle exocytosis. Nature, 423, 939–948.*

Mitsui, S., Saito, M., Hayashi, K., Mori, K., & Yoshihara, Y. (2005). *A novel phenylalanine-based targeting signal directs telencephalin to neuronal dendrites. J Neurosci, 25(5), 1122–1131.*

Mizoguchi, A., Nakanishi, H., Kimura, K., Matsubara, K., Ozaki-Kuroda, K., Katata, T., Honda, T., Kiyohara, Y., Heo, K., Higashi, M., Tsutsumi, T., Sonoda, S., Ide, C., & Takai, Y. (2002). *Nectin: an adhesion molecule involved in formation of synapses. J Cell Biol, 156, 555–565.*

Møller, RS., Weber, YG., Klitten, LL., Trucks, H., Muhle, H., Kunz, WS., Mefford, HC., Franke, A., Kautza, M., Wolf, P., Dennig, D., Schreiber, S., Rückert, IM., Wichmann, HE., Ernst, JP., Schurmann, C., Grabe, HJ., Tommerup, N., Stephani, U., Lerche, H., Hjalgrim, H., Helbig, I., Sander, T; & EPICURE Consortium. (2013). *Exon-disrupting deletions of NRXN1 in idiopathic generalized epilepsy. Epilepsia, 54 (2), 256–264.*

Momoi, T., Fujita, E., Senoo, H., & Momoi, M. (2009). *Genetic factors and epigenetic factors for autism: endoplasmic reticulum stress and impaired synaptic function. Cell Biol Int, 34 (1),13–19.*

Morellini, F., Lepsveridze, E., Kähler, B., Dityatev, A., & Schachner, M. (2007). *Reduced reactivity to novelty, impaired social behavior, and enhanced basal synaptic excitatory activity in perforant path projections to the dentate gyrus in young adult mice deficient in the neural cell adhesion molecule CHL1. Mol Cell Neurosci, 34, 121–136.*

Morrow, EM., Yoo, SY., Flavell, SW., Kim, TK., Lin, Y., Hill, RS., Mukaddes, NM., Balkhy, S., Gascon, G., Hashmi, A., Al-Saad, S., Ware, J., Joseph, RM., Greenblatt, R., Gleason, D., Ertelt, JA., Apse, KA., Bodell, A., Partlow, JN., Barry, B., Yao, H., Markianos, K., Ferland, RJ., Greenberg, ME., & Walsh, CA. (2008). *Identifying autism loci and genes by tracing recent shared ancestry. Science, 321, 218–223.*

Muller, D., Wang, C., Skibo, G., Toni, N., Cremer, H., Calaora, V., Rougon, G., & Kiss, JZ. (1996). *PSA-NCAM is required for activity-induced synaptic plasticity. Neuron, 17, 413–422.*

Murai, KK., Misner, D., & Ranscht, B. (2002). *Contactin supports synaptic plasticity associated with hippocampal long-term depression but not potentiation. Curr Biol, 12, 181–190.*

Murai, KK., Nguyen, LN., Koolpe, M., McLennan, R., Krull, CE., & Pasquale, EB. (2003). *Targeting the EphA4 receptor in the nervous system with biologically active peptides. Mol Cell Neurosci, 24, 1000–1011.*

Nakamura, K., Manabe, T., Watanabe, M., Mamiya, T., Ichikawa, R., Kiyama, Y., Sanbo, M., Yagi, T., Inoue, Y., Nabeshima, T., Mori, H., & Mishina, M. (2001). *Enhancement of hippocampal LTP, reference memory and sensorimotor gating in mutant mice lacking a telencephalon-specific cell adhesion molecule. Eur J Neurosci, 13 (1), 179–189.*

Nam, CI., & Chen, L. (2005). Postsynaptic assembly induced by neurexin-neuroligin interaction and neurotransmitter. Proc Natl Acad Sci U S A, 102, 6137–6142.

Napolioni, V., Lombardi, F., Sacco, R., Curatolo, P., Manzi, B., Alessandrelli, R., Militerni, R., Bravaccio, C., Lenti, C., Saccani, M., Schneider, C., Melmed, R., Pascucci, T., Puglisi-Allegra, S., Reichelt, KL., Rousseau, F., Lewin, P., & Persico, AM. (2011). Family-based association study of ITGB3 in autism spectrum disorder and its endophenotypes. Eur J Hum Genet, 19 (3), 353–359.

Nguyen, T., & Südhof, TC. (1997). Binding properties of neuroligin 1 and neurexin 1beta reveal function as heterophilic cell adhesion molecules. J Biol Chem, 272, 26032–26039.

Nikonenko, AG., Sun, M., Lepsveridze, E., Apostolova, I., Petrova, I., Irintchev, A., Dityatev, A., & Schachner, M. (2006). Enhanced perisomatic inhibition and impaired long-term potentiation in the CA1 region of juvenile CHL1-deficient mice. Eur J Neurosci, 23, 1839–1852.

Novak, G., Boukhadra, J., Shaikh, SA., Kennedy, JL., & Le Foll, B. (2009). Association of a polymorphism in the NRXN3 gene with the degree of smoking in schizophrenia: a preliminary study. World J Biol Psychiatry, 10 (4 Pt 3), 929–935.

Ohtsuki, T., Horiuchi, Y., Koga, M., Ishiguro, H., Inada, T., Iwata, N., Ozaki, N., Ujike, H., Watanabe, Y., Someya, T., & Arinami, T. (2008). Association of polymorphisms in the haplotype block spanning the alternatively spliced exons of the NTNG1 gene at 1p13.3 with schizophrenia in Japanese populations. Neurosci Lett, 435 (3), 194–197.

Oka, S., Mori, K., & Watanabe, Y. (1990). Mammalian telencephalic neurons express a segment-specific membrane glycoprotein, telencephalin. Neuroscience, 35 (1), 93–103.

Okuda, T., Yu, LM., Cingolani, LA., Kemler, R., & Goda, Y. (2007). beta-Catenin regulates excitatory postsynaptic strength at hippocampal synapses. Proc Natl Acad Sci U S A, 104, 13479–13484.

Ongür, D., Drevets, WC., & Price, JL. (1998). Glial reduction in the subgenual prefrontal cortex in mood disorders. Proc Natl Acad Sci U S A, 95, 13290–13295.

Pagnamenta, AT., Khan, H., Walker, S., Gerrelli, D., Wing, K., Bonaglia, MC., Giorda, R., Berney, T., Mani, E., Molteni, M., Pinto, D., Le Couteur, A., Hallmayer, J., Sutcliffe, JS., Szatmari, P., Paterson, AD., Scherer, SW., Vieland, VJ., & Monaco, AP. (2011). Rare familial 16q21 microdeletions under a linkage peak implicate cadherin 8 (CDH8) in susceptibility to autism and learning disability. J Med Genet, 48, 48–54.

Peng, YR., Hou, ZH., & Yu, X. (2013). The kinase activity of EphA4 mediates homeostatic scaling-down of synaptic strength via activation of Cdk5. Neuropharmacology, 65, 232–243.

Penzes, P., Beeser, A., Chernoff, J., Schiller, MR., Eipper, BA., Mains, RE., & Huganir, RL. (2003). Rapid induction of dendritic spine morphogenesis by trans-synaptic ephrinB-EphB receptor activation of the Rho-GEF kalirin. Neuron, 37, 263–274.

Perrin, FE., Rathjen, FG., & Stoeckli, ET. (2001). Distinct subpopulations of sensory afferents require F11 or axonin-1 for growth to their target layers within the spinal cord of the chick. Neuron, 30, 707–723.

Pinkstaff, JK., Lynch, G., & Gall, CM. (1998). Localization and seizure-regulation of integrin beta 1 mRNA in adult rat brain. Brain Res Mol Brain Res, 55, 265–276.

Plioplys, AV., Hemmens, SE., & Regan, CM. (1990). Expression of a neural cell adhesion molecule serum fragment is depressed in autism. J Neuropsychiatry Clin Neurosci, 2, 413–417.

Pollard, JR., Eidelman, O., Mueller, GP., Dalgard, CL., Crino, PB., Anderson, CT., Brand, EJ., Burakgazi, E., Ivaturi, SK., & Pollard, HB. (2013). The TARC/sICAM5 Ratio in Patient Plasma is a Candidate Biomarker for Drug Resistant Epilepsy. Front Neurol, 3, 181.

Polo-Parada, L., Bose, CM., & Landmesser, LT. (2001). Alterations in transmission, vesicle dynamics, and transmitter release machinery at NCAM-deficient neuromuscular junctions. Neuron, 32, 815–828.

Polo-Parada, L., Plattner, F., Bose, C., & Landmesser, LT. (2005). NCAM 180 acting via a conserved C-terminal domain and MLCK is essential for effective transmission with repetitive stimulation. Neuron, 46, 917–931.

Poltorak, M., Frye, MA., Wright, R., Hemperly, JJ., George, MS., Pazzaglia, PJ., Jerrels, SA., Post, RM., & Freed, WJ. (1996). Increased neural cell adhesion molecule in the CSF of patients with mood disorder. J Neurochem, 66, 1532–1538.

Poltorak, M., Wright, R., Hemperly, JJ., Torrey, EF., Issa, F., Wyatt, RJ., & Freed, WJ. (1997). Monozygotic twins discordant for schizophrenia are discordant for N-CAM and L1 in CSF. Brain Res, 751 (1), 152–154.

Postina, R., Schroeder, A., Dewachter, I., Bohl, J., Schmitt, U., Kojro, E., Prinzen, C., Endres, K., Hiemke, C., Blessing, M., Flamez, P., Dequenne, A., Godaux, E., van Leuven, F., & Fahrenholz, F. (2004). A disintegrin-metalloproteinase prevents amyloid plaque formation and hippocampal defects in an Alzheimer disease mouse model. J Clin Invest, 113 (10), 1456–1464.

Pozo, K., Cingolani, LA., Bassani, S., Laurent, F., Passafaro, M., & Goda, Y. (2012). β3 integrin interacts directly with GluA2 AMPA receptor subunit and regulates AMPA receptor expression in hippocampal neurons. Proc Natl Acad Sci U S A, 109, 1323–1328.

Prox, J., Bernreuther, C., Altmeppen, H., Grendel, J., Glatzel, M., D'Hooge, R., Stroobants, S., Ahmed, T., Balschun, D., Willem, M., Lammich, S., Isbrandt, D., Schweizer, M., Horré, K., De Strooper, B., & Saftig, P. (2013). Postnatal disruption of the disintegrin/metalloproteinase ADAM10 in brain causes epileptic seizures, learning deficits, altered spine morphology, and defective synaptic functions. J Neurosci, 33 (32), 12915–12928,

Pulido, R., Serra-Pagès, C., Tang, M., & Streuli, M. (1995). The LAR/PTP delta/PTP sigma subfamily of transmembrane protein-tyrosine-phosphatases: multiple human LAR, PTP delta, and PTP sigma isoforms are expressed in a tissue-specific manner and associate with the LAR-interacting protein LIP.1. Proc Natl Acad Sci U S A, 92, 11686–11690.

Puzzo, D., Bizzoca, A., Privitera, L., Furnari, D., Giunta, S., Girolamo, F., Pinto, M., Gennarini, G., & Palmeri, A. (2013). F3/Contactin promotes hippocampal neurogenesis, synaptic plasticity, and memory in adult mice. Hippocampus, 23, 1367–1382.

Rafuse, VF., Polo-Parada, L., & Landmesser, LT. (2000). Structural and functional alterations of neuromuscular junctions in NCAM-deficient mice. J Neurosci, 20, 6529–6539.

Reed, JE., Dunn, JR., du Plessis, DG., Shaw, EJ., Reeves, P., Gee, AL., Warnke, PC., Sellar, GC., Moss, DJ., & Walker, C. (2007). Expression of cellular adhesion molecule 'OPCML' is down-regulated in gliomas and other brain tumours. Neuropathol Appl Neurobiol, 33(1), 77–85.

Reissner, C., Runkel, F., & Missler, M. (2013). Neurexins. Genome Biol, 14, 213–227.

Reyes, AA., Small, SJ., & Akeson, R. (1991). At least 27 alternatively spliced forms of the neural cell adhesion molecule mRNA are expressed during rat heart development. Mol Cell Biol, 11, 1654–1661.

Ricciardi, S., Ungaro, F., Hambrock, M., Rademacher, N., Stefanelli, G., Brambilla, D., Sessa, A., Magagnotti, C., Bachi, A., Giarda, E., Verpelli, C., Kilstrup-Nielsen, C., Sala, C., Kalscheuer, VM., & Broccoli, V. (2012). CDKL5 ensures excitatory synapse stability by reinforcing NGL-1-PSD95 interaction in the postsynaptic compartment and is impaired in patient iPSC-derived neurons. Nat Cell Biol, 14 (9), 911–923.

Richter, M., Murai, KK., Bourgin, C., Pak, DT., & Pasquale, EB. (2007). The EphA4 receptor regulates neuronal morphology through SPAR-mediated inactivation of Rap GTPases. J Neurosci, 27, 14205–14215.

Rieckmann, P., Turner, T., Kligannon, P., & Steinhoff. BJ. (1998). Telencephalin as an indicator for temporal-lobe dysfunction. Lancet, 352 (9125), 370–371.

Robbins, EM., Krupp, AJ., Perez de Arce, K., Ghosh, AK., Fogel, AI., Boucard, A., Südhof, TC., Stein, V., & Biederer, T. (2010). SynCAM 1 adhesion dynamically regulates synapse number and impacts plasticity and learning. Neuron, 68, 894–906.

Rollenhagen, M., Kuckuck, S., Ulm, C., Hartmann, M., Galuska, SP., Geyer, R., Geyer, H., & Mühlenhoff, M. (2012). Polysialylation of the synaptic cell adhesion molecule 1 (SynCAM 1) depends exclusively on the polysialyltransferase ST8SiaII in vivo. J Biol Chem, 287 (42), 35170–35180.

Rujescu, D., Ingason, A., Cichon, S., Pietiläinen, OP., Barnes, MR., Toulopoulou, T., Picchioni, M., Vassos, E., Ettinger, U., Bramon, E., Murray, R., Ruggeri, M., Tosato, S., Bonetto, C., Steinberg, S., Sigurdsson, E., Sigmundsson, T., Petursson, H., Gylfason, A., Olason, PI., et al. (2009). Disruption of the neurexin 1 gene is associated with schizophrenia. Hum Mol Genet, 18, 988–996.

Saghatelyan, AK., Nikonenko, AG., Sun, M., Rolf, B., Putthoff, P., Kutsche, M., Bartsch, U., Dityatev, A., Schachner, M. (2004). Reduced GABAergic transmission and number of hippocampal perisomatic inhibitory synapses in juvenile mice deficient in the neural cell adhesion molecule L1. Mol Cell Neurosci, 26, 191–203.

Saglietti, L., Dequidt, C., Kamieniarz, K., Rousset, MC., Valnegri, P., Thoumine, O., Beretta, F., Fagni, L., Choquet, D., Sala, C., Sheng, M., & Passafaro, M. (2007). Extracellular interactions between GluR2 and N-cadherin in spine regulation. Neuron, 54, 461–477.

Sakisaka, T., Ikeda, W., Ogita, H., Fujita, N., & Takai, Y. (2007). The roles of nectins in cell adhesions: cooperation with other cell adhesion molecules and growth factor receptors. Curr Opin Cell Biol, 19, 593–602.

Sakurai, K., Toyoshima, M., Takeda, Y., Shimoda, Y., & Watanabe, K. (2010). Synaptic formation in subsets of glutamatergic terminals in the mouse hippocampal formation is affected by a deficiency in the neural cell recognition molecule NB-3. Neurosci Lett, 473, 102–106.

Sakurai, K., Toyoshima, M., Ueda, H., Matsubara, K., Takeda, Y., Karagogeos, D., Shimoda, Y., & Watanabe, K. (2009). Contribution of the neural cell recognition molecule NB-3 to synapse formation between parallel fibers and Purkinje cells in mouse. Dev Neurobiol, 69, 811–824.

Sakurai, K., Migita, O., Toru, M., & Arinami, T. (2002). An association between a missense polymorphism in the close homologue of L1 (CHL1, CALL) gene and schizophrenia. Mol Psychiatry, 7 (4), 412–415.

Sand, P., Langguth, B., Hajak, G., Perna, M., Prikryl, R., Kucerova, H., Ceskova, E., Kick, C., Stoertebecker, P., & Eichhammer, P. (2006). Screening for Neuroligin 4 (NLGN4) truncating and transmembrane domain mutations in schizophrenia. Schizophr Res, 82 (2–3), 277–278.

Sanders, SJ., Ercan-Sencicek, AG., Hus, V., Luo, R., Murtha, MT., Moreno-De-Luca, D., Chu, SH., Moreau, MP., Gupta, AR., Thomson, SA., Mason, CE. Bilguvar, K., Celestino-Soper, PB., Choi, M., Crawford, EL., Davis, L., Wright, NR., Dhodapkar, RM., DiCola, M., DiLullo, NM., et al. (2011). Multiple recurrent de novo CNVs, including duplications of the 7q11.23 Williams syndrome region, are strongly associated with autism. Neuron, 70, 863–885.

Sanes, JR., & Yamagata, M. (2009). Many paths to synaptic specificity. Annu Rev Cell Dev Biol, 25, 161–195.

Sara, Y., Biederer, T., Atasoy, D., Chubykin, A., Mozhayeva, MG., Südhof, TC., & Kavalali, ET. (2005). Selective capability of SynCAM and neuroligin for functional synapse assembly. J Neurosci, 25, 260–270.

Sato, K., Iwai, M., Zhang, WR., Kamada, H., Ohta, K., Omori, N., Nagano, I., Shoji, M., & Abe, K. (2003). Highly polysialylated neural cell adhesion molecule (PSA-NCAM) positive cells are increased and change localization in rat hippocampus by exposure to repeated kindled seizures. Acta Neurochir Suppl, 86, 575–579.

Saura, CA., Servián-Morilla, E., & Scholl, FG. (2011). Presenilin/γ-secretase regulates neurexin processing at synapses. PLoS One, 6, e19430.

Scheiffele, P., Fan, J., Choih, J., Fetter, R., & Serafini, T. (2000). Neuroligin expressed in nonneuronal cells triggers presynaptic development in contacting axons. Cell, 101, 657–669.

Scholl, FG., & Scheiffele, P. (2003). Making connections: cholinesterase-domain proteins in the CNS. Trends Neurosci, 26(11), 618–624.

Seabold, GK., Wang, PY., Chang, K., Wang, CY., Wang, YX., Petralia, RS., & Wenthold, RJ. (2008). The SALM family of adhesion-like molecules forms heteromeric and homomeric complexes. J Biol Chem, 283, 8395–8405.

Seabold, GK., Wang, PY., Petralia, RS., Chang, K., Zhou, A., McDermott, MI., Wang, YX., Milgram, SL., & Wenthold, RJ. (2012). Dileucine and PDZ-binding motifs mediate synaptic adhesion-like molecule 1 (SALM1) trafficking in hippocampal neurons. J Biol Chem, 287, 4470–4484.

Sentürk, A., Pfennig, S., Weiss, A., Burk, K., & Acker-Palmer, A. (2011). Ephrin Bs are essential components of the Reelin pathway to regulate neuronal migration. Nature, 472 (7343), 356–360.

Shaw, AD., Tiwari, Y., Kaplan, W., Heath, A., Mitchell, PB., Schofield, PR., & Fullerton, JM. (2014). Characterisation of genetic variation in ST8SIA2 and its interaction region in NCAM1 in patients with bipolar disorder. PLoS One, 9(3), e92556.

Siddiqui, TJ., Tari, PK., Connor, SA., Zhang, P., Dobie, FA., She, K., Kawabe, H., Wang, YT., Brose, N., & Craig, AM. (2013). An LRRTM4-HSPG complex mediates excitatory synapse development on dentate gyrus granule cells. Neuron, 79, 680–695.

Simón, AM., de Maturana, RL., Ricobaraza, A., Escribano, L., Schiapparelli, L., Cuadrado-Tejedor, M., Pérez-Mediavilla, A., Avila, J., Del Río, J., & Frechilla, D. (2009). Early changes in hippocampal Eph receptors precede the onset of memory decline in mouse models of Alzheimer's disease. J Alzheimers Dis, 17, 773–786.

Sindi, IA., Tannenberg, RK., & Dodd, PR. (2014). A role for the neurexin-neuroligin complex in Alzheimer's disease. Neurobiol Aging, 35, 746–56.

Singh, SM., Castellani, C., & O'Reilly, R. (2010). Autism meets schizophrenia via cadherin pathway. Schizophr Res, 116 (2–3), 293–294.

Soler-Llavina, GJ., Arstikaitis, P., Morishita, W., Ahmad, M., Südhof, TC., & Malenka, RC. (2013). Leucine-rich repeat transmembrane proteins are essential for maintenance of long-term potentiation. Neuron, 79, 439–446.

Soler-Llavina, GJ., Fuccillo, MV., Ko, J., Südhof, TC., & Malenka, RC. (2011). The neurexin ligands, neuroligins and leucine-rich repeat transmembrane proteins, perform convergent and divergent synaptic functions in vivo. Proc Natl Acad Sci U S A, 108, 16502–16509.

Soto, F., Watkins, KL., Johnson, RE., Schottler, F., & Kerschensteiner, D. (2013). NGL-2 regulates pathway-specific neurite growth and lamination, synapse formation, and signal transmission in the retina. J

Neurosci, 33, 11949–11959.

Sousa, I., Clark, TG., Holt, R., Pagnamenta, AT., Mulder, EJ., Minderaa, RB., Bailey, AJ., Battaglia, A., Klauck, SM., Poustka, F., Monaco, AP.; & International Molecular Genetic Study of Autism Consortium (IMGSAC). (2010). *Polymorphisms in leucine-rich repeat genes are associated with autism spectrum disorder susceptibility in populations of European ancestry. Mol Autism, 1(1), 7.*

Stan, A., Pielarski, KN., Brigadski, T., Wittenmayer, N., Fedorchenko, O., Gohla, A., Lessmann, V., Dresbach, T., & Gottmann, K. (2010). *Essential cooperation of N-cadherin and neuroligin-1 in the transsynaptic control of vesicle accumulation. Proc Natl Acad Sci U S A, 107, 11116–11121.*

Stogmann, E., Reinthaler, E., Eltawil, S., El Etribi, MA., Hemeda, M., El Nahhas, N., Gaber, AM., Fouad, A., Edris, S., Benet-Pages, A., Eck, SH., Pataraia, E., Mei, D., Brice, A., Lesage, S., Guerrini, R., Zimprich, F., Strom, TM., & Zimprich, A. (2013). *Autosomal recessive cortical myoclonic tremor and epilepsy: association with a mutation in the potassium channel associated gene CNTN2. Brain, 136 (Pt 4), 1155–1160.*

Strauss, KA., Puffenberger, EG., Huentelman, MJ., Gottlieb, S., Dobrin, SE., Parod, JM., Stephan, DA., & Morton, DH. (2006). *Recessive symptomatic focal epilepsy and mutant contactin-associated protein-like 2. N Engl J Med, 354 (13), 1370–1377.*

Strekalova, H., Buhmann, C., Kleene, R., Eggers, C., Saffell, J., Hemperly, J., Weiller, C., Müller-Thomsen, T., & Schachner, M. (2006). *Elevated levels of neural recognition molecule L1 in the cerebrospinal fluid of patients with Alzheimer disease and other dementia syndromes. Neurobiol Aging, 27 (1), 1–9.*

Suda, S., Iwata, K., Shimmura, C., Kameno, Y., Anitha, A., Thanseem, I., Nakamura, K., Matsuzaki, H., Tsuchiya, KJ., Sugihara, G., Iwata, Y., Suzuki, K., Koizumi, K., Higashida, H., Takei, N., & Mori, N. (2011). *Decreased expression of axon-guidance receptors in the anterior cingulate cortex in autism. Mol Autism, 2(1), 14.*

Südhof, TC. (2008). *Neuroligins and neurexins link synaptic function to cognitive disease. Nature, 455, 903–911.*

Sun, C., Cheng, MC., Qin, R., Liao, DL., Chen, TT., Koong, FJ., Chen, G., & Chen, CH. (2011). *Identification and functional characterization of rare mutations of the neuroligin-2 gene (NLGN2) associated with schizophrenia. Hum Mol Genet, 20(15), 3042–3051.*

Supriyanto, I., Watanabe, Y., Mouri, K., Shiroiwa, K., Ratta-Apha, W., Yoshida, M., Tamiya, G., Sasada, T., Eguchi, N., Okazaki, K., Shirakawa, O., Someya, T., & Hishimoto, A. (2013). *A missense mutation in the ITGA8 gene, a cell adhesion molecule gene, is associated with schizophrenia in Japanese female patients. Prog Neuropsychopharmacol Biol Psychiatry, 40, 347–352.*

Sytnyk, V., Leshchyns'ka, I., Nikonenko, AG., & Schachner, M. (2006). *NCAM promotes assembly and activity-dependent remodeling of the postsynaptic signaling complex. J Cell Biol, 174, 1071–1085.*

Tabuchi, K., Blundell, J., Etherton, MR., Hammer, RE., Liu, X., Powell, CM., & Südhof, TC. (2007). *A neuroligin-3 mutation implicated in autism increases inhibitory synaptic transmission in mice. Science, 318, 71–76.*

Takahashi, H., Arstikaitis, P., Prasad, T., Bartlett, TE., Wang, YT., Murphy, TH., & Craig, AM. (2011). *Postsynaptic TrkC and presynaptic PTPσ function as a bidirectional excitatory synaptic organizing complex. Neuron, 69, 287–303.*

Takahashi, H., Katayama, K., Sohya, K., Miyamoto, H., Prasad, T., Matsumoto, Y., Ota, M., Yasuda, H., Tsumoto, T., Aruga, J., & Craig, AM. (2012). *Selective control of inhibitory synapse development by Slitrk3-PTPδ trans-synaptic interaction. Nat Neurosci, 15, 389–398.*

Takai, Y., Irie, K., Shimizu, K., Sakisaka, T., & Ikeda, W. (2003). Nectins and nectin-like molecules: roles in cell adhesion, migration, and polarization. Cancer Sci, 94, 655–667.

Takeichi, M. (1988). The cadherins: cell-cell adhesion molecules controlling animal morphogenesis. Development, 102, 639–655.

Takeichi, M. (2007). The cadherin superfamily in neuronal connections and interactions. Nat Rev Neurosci, 8, 11–20.

Taylor, AM., Wu, J., Tai, HC., & Schuman, EM. (2013). Axonal translation of β-catenin regulates synaptic vesicle dynamics. J Neurosci, 33, 5584–5589.

Thomas, LA., Akins, MR., & Biederer, T. (2008). Expression and adhesion profiles of SynCAM molecules indicate distinct neuronal functions. J Comp Neurol, 510, 47–67.

Tian, L., Nyman, H., Kilgannon, P., Yoshihara, Y., Mori, K., Andersson, LC., Kaukinen, S., Rauvala, H., Gallatin, WM., & Gahmberg, CG. (2000). Intercellular adhesion molecule-5 induces dendritic outgrowth by homophilic adhesion. J Cell Biol, 150 (1), 243–252.

Tian, L., Stefanidakis, M., Ning, L., Van Lint, P., Nyman-Huttunen, H., Libert, C., Itohara, S., Mishina, M., Rauvala, H., & Gahmberg, CG. (2007). Activation of NMDA receptors promotes dendritic spine development through MMP-mediated ICAM-5 cleavage. J Cell Biol, 178 (4), 687–700.

Ting, JT., & Feng, G. (2011). Neruobiology of obsessive compulsive disorder : insights into neural circuitry dysfunction through mousegenetics. Curr Opin Neurobiol, 21 (6), 842–848.

Torres, AR., Sweeten, TL., Cutler, A., Bedke, BJ., Fillmore, M., Stubbs, EG., & Odell, D. (2006). The association and linkage of the HLA-A2 class I allele with autism. Hum Immunol, 67 (4–5), 346–351.

Uchida, N., Honjo, Y., Johnson, KR., Wheelock, MJ., & Takeichi, M. (1996). The catenin/cadherin adhesion system is localized in synaptic junctions bordering transmitter release zones. J Cell Biol, 135, 767–779.

Uemura, M., Nakao, S., Suzuki, ST., Takeichi, M., & Hirano, S. (2007). OL-Protocadherin is essential for growth of striatal axons and thalamocortical projections. Nat Neurosci, 10, 1151–1159.

Uetani, N., Kato, K., Ogura, H., Mizuno, K., Kawano, K., Mikoshiba, K., Yakura, H., Asano, M., & Iwakura, Y. (2000). Impaired learning with enhanced hippocampal long-term potentiation in PTPdelta-deficient mice. EMBO J, 19, 2775–2785.

Uhász, GJ., Barkóczi, B., Vass, G., Datki, Z., Hunya, A., Fülöp, L., Budai, D., Penke, B., & Szegedi, V. (2010). Fibrillar Abeta (1–42) enhances NMDA receptor sensitivity via the integrin signaling pathway. J Alzheimers Dis, 19 (3), 1055–1067.

Vaags, AK., Lionel, AC., Sato, D., Goodenberger, M., Stein, QP., Curran, S., Ogilvie, C., Ahn, JW., Drmic, I., Senman, L., Chrysler, C., Thompson, A., Russell, C., Prasad, A.,Walker, S., Pinto, D., Marshall, CR., Stavropoulos, DJ., et al. (2012). Rare deletions at the neurexin 3 locus in autism spectrum disorder. Am J Hum Genet, 90 (1), 133–141.

van Daalen, E., Kemner, C., Verbeek, NE., van der Zwaag, B., Dijkhuizen, T., Rump, P., Houben, R., van 't Slot, R., de Jonge, MV., Staal, WG., Beemer, FA., Vorstman, JA., Burbach, JP., van Amstel, HK., Hochstenbach, R., Brilstra, EH., & Poot, M. (2011). Social Responsiveness Scale-aided analysis of the clinical impact of copy number variations in autism. Neurogenetics, 12, 315–323.

van Gool, D., Carmeliet, G., Triau, E., Cassiman, JJ., & Dom, R. (1994). Appearance of localized immunoreactivity for the alpha 4 integrin subunit and for fibronectin in brains from Alzheimer's, Lewy body dementia patients and aged controls. Neurosci Lett, 170 (1), 71–73.

van Harssel, JJ., Weckhuysen, S., van Kempen, MJ., Hardies, K., Verbeek, NE., de Kovel, CG., Gunning,

WB., van Daalen, E., de Jonge, MV., Jansen, AC.. Vermeulen, RJ., Arts, WF., Verhelst, H., Fogarasi, A., de Rijk-van Andel, JF., Kelemen, A., Lindhout, D., et al. (2013). Clinical and genetic aspects of PCDH19-related epilepsy syndromes and the possible role of PCDH19 mutations in males with autism spectrum disorders. Neurogenetics, 14 (1), 23–34.

Varoqueaux, F., Aramuni, G., Rawson, RL., Mohrmann, R., Missler, M., Gottmann, K., Zhang, W., Südhof, TC., & Brose, N. (2006). Neuroligins determine synapse maturation and function. Neuron, 51, 741–754.

Varoqueaux, F., Jamain, S., & Brose, N. (2004). Neuroligin 2 is exclusively localized to inhibitory synapses. Eur J Cell Biol, 83, 449–456.

Vawter, MP. (2000). Dysregulation of the neural cell adhesion molecule and neuropsychiatric disorders. Eur J Pharmacol, 405, 385–395.

Vawter, MP., Cannon-Spoor, HE., Hemperly, JJ., Hyde, TM., VanderPutten, DM., Kleinman, JE., & Freed, WJ. (1998a). Abnormal expression of cell recognition molecules in schizophrenia. Exp Neurol, 149, 424–432.

Vawter, MP., Hemperly, JJ., Hyde, TM., Bachus, SE., VanderPutten, DM., Howard, AL., Cannon-Spoor, HE., McCoy, MT., Webster, MJ., Kleinman, JE., & Freed, WJ. (1998b). VASE-containing N-CAM isoforms are increased in the hippocampus in bipolar disorder but not schizophrenia. Exp Neurol, 154, 1–11.

Vawter, MP., Howard, AL., Hyde, TM., Kleinman, JE., & Freed, WJ. (1999). Alterations of hippocampal secreted N-CAM in bipolar disorder and synaptophysin in schizophrenia. Mol Psychiatry, 4, 467–475.

Vincent, AK., Noor, A., Janson, A., Minassian, EA., Ayub, M., Vincent, JB., & Morel, CF. (2012). Identification of genomic deletions spanning the PCDH19 gene in two unrelated girls with intellectual disability and seizures. Clin Genet, 82 (6), 540–545.

Voikar, V., Kulesskaya, N., Laakso, T., Lauren, J., Strittmatter, SM., & Airaksinen, MS. (2013). LRRTM1-deficient mice show a rare phenotype of avoiding small enclosures--a tentative mouse model for claustrophobia-like behaviour. Behav Brain Res. 238, 69–78.

Vrijenhoek, T., Buizer-Voskamp, JE., van der Stelt, I., & Strengman, E., (2008). Genetic Risk and Outcome in Psychosis (GROUP) Consortium., Sabatti C., Geurts van Kessel A., Brunner HG., Ophoff RA., Veltman JA. Recurrent CNVs disrupt three candidate genes in schizophrenia patients. Am J Hum Genet, 83, 504–510.

Walsh, MT., Ryan, M., Hillmann, A., Condren, R., Kenny, D., Dinan, T., & Thakore, JH. (2002). Elevated expression of integrin alpha(IIb) beta(IIIa) in drug-naïve, first-episode schizophrenic patients. Biol Psychiatry, 52 (9), 874–879.

Wang, CY., Chang, K., Petralia, RS., Wang, YX., Seabold, GK., & Wenthold, RJ. (2006). A novel family of adhesion-like molecules that interacts with the NMDA receptor. J Neurosci, 26, 2174–2183.

Wang, K., Zhang, H., Ma, D., Bucan, M., Glessner, JT., Abrahams, BS., Salyakina, D., Imielinski, M., Bradfield, JP., Sleiman, PM., Kim, CE., Hou, C., Frackelton, E., Chiavacci, et al. (2009). Common genetic variants on 5p14.1 associate with autism spectrum disorders. Nature, 459, 528–533.

Wang, KS., Liu, X., Arana, TB., Thompson, N., Weisman, H., Devargas, C., Mao, C., Su, BB., Camarillo, C., Escamilla, MA., & Xu, C. (2013). Genetic association analysis of ITGB3 polymorphisms with age at onset of schizophrenia. J Mol Neurosci, 51 (2), 446–453.

Wang, PY., Seabold, GK., & Wenthold, RJ. (2008a). Synaptic adhesion-like molecules (SALMs) promote neurite outgrowth. Mol Cell Neurosci, 39, 83–94.

Wang, Q., Klyubin, I., Wright, S., Griswold-Prenner, I., Rowan, MJ., & Anwyl, R. (2008b). Alpha v integrins mediate beta-amyloid induced inhibition of long-term potentiation. Neurobiol Aging, 29 (10), 1485–193.

Wang, W., Wang, L., Luo, J., Xi, Z., Wang, X., Chen, G., & Chu, L. (2012). Role of a neural cell adhesion molecule found in cerebrospinal fluid as a potential biomarker for epilepsy. Neurochem Res, 37 (4), 819–825.

Wang, Z., Wang, B., Yang, L., Guo, Q., Aithmitti, N., Songyang, Z., & Zheng, H. (2009). Presynaptic and postsynaptic interaction of the amyloid precursor protein promotes peripheral and central synaptogenesis. J Neurosci, 29 (35), 10788–10801.

Willemsen, MH., Fernandez, BA., Bacino, CA., Gerkes, E., de Brouwer, AP., Pfundt, R., Sikkema-Raddatz, B., Scherer, SW., Marshall, CR., Potocki, L., van Bokhoven, H., & Kleefstra, T. (2010). Identification of ANKRD11 and ZNF778 as candidate genes for autism and variable cognitive impairment in the novel 16q24.3 microdeletion syndrome. Eur J Hum Genet, 18, 429–435.

Williams, ME., de Wit, J., & Ghosh, A. (2010). Molecular mechanisms of synaptic specificity in developing neural circuits. Neuron, 68, 9–18.

Wilson, GM., Flibotte, S., Chopra, V., Melnyk, BL., Honer, WG., & Holt, RA. (2006). DNA copy-number analysis in bipolar disorder and schizophrenia reveals aberrations in genes involved in glutamate signaling. Hum Mol Genet, 15 (5), 743–749.

Wong, M., & Guo, D. (2013). Dendritic spine pathology in epilepsy: cause or consequence? Neuroscience, 251, 141–150.

Woo, J., Kwon, SK., Choi, S., Kim, S., Lee, JR., Dunah, AW., Sheng, M., & Kim, E. (2009). Trans-synaptic adhesion between NGL-3 and LAR regulates the formation of excitatory synapses. Nat Neurosci, 12, 428–437.

Wu, Y., Wang, XF., Mo, XA., Li, JM., Yuan, J., Zheng, JO., Feng, Y., & Tang, M. (2011). Expression of laminin beta1 and integrin alpha2 in the anterior temporal neocortex tissue of patients with intractable epilepsy. Int J Neurosci, 121 (6), 323–328.

Wyszynski, M., Kim, E., Dunah, AW., Passafaro, M., Valtschanoff, JG., Serra-Pagès, C., Streuli, M., Weinberg, RJ., & Sheng, M. (2002). Interaction between GRIP and Liprin-α/SYD2 Is Required for AMPA Receptor Targeting. Neuron, 34, 39–52.

Xia, Y., Luo, C., Dai, S., & Yao, D. (2013). Increased EphA/ephrinA expression in hippocampus of pilocarpine treated mouse. Epilepsy Res, 105 (1–2), 20–29.

Xu, B., Li, S., Brown, A., Gerlai, R., Fahnestock, M., & Racine, RJ. (2003). EphA/ephrin-A interactions regulate epileptogenesis and activity-dependent axonal sprouting in adult rats. Mol Cell Neurosci, 24 (4), 984–999.

Xu, B., Woodroffe, A., Rodriguez-Murillo, L., Roos, JL., van Rensburg, EJ., Abecasis, GR., Gogos, JA., & Karayiorgou, M. (2009). Elucidating the genetic architecture of familial schizophrenia using rare copy number variant and linkage scans. Proc Natl Acad Sci U S A, 106 (39), 16746–16751.

Xu, NJ., & Henkemeyer, M. (2012). Ephrin reverse signaling in axon guidance and synaptogenesis. Semin Cell Dev Biol, 23, 58–64.

Yamada, A., Irie, K., Deguchi-Tawarada, M., Ohtsuka, T., & Takai, Y. (2003). Nectin-dependent localization of synaptic scaffolding molecule (S-SCAM) at the puncta adherentia junctions formed between the mossy fiber terminals and the dendrites of pyramidal cells in the CA3 area of the mouse hippocampus. Genes Cells, 8, 985–994.

Yamada, M., Hashimoto, T., Hayashi, N., Higuchi, M., Murakami, A., Nakashima, T., Maekawa, S., & Miyata, S. (2007). Synaptic adhesion molecule OBCAM., synaptogenesis and dynamic internalization. Brain Res, 1165, 5–14.

Yamazaki, T., Koo, EH., & Selkoe, DJ. (1997). Cell surface amyloid beta-protein precursor colocalizes with beta 1 integrins at substrate contact sites in neural cells. J Neurosci, 17 (3), 1004–1010.

Yan, J., Noltner, K., Feng, J., Li, W., Schroer, R., Skinner, C., Zeng, W., Schwartz, CE., & Sommer, SS. (2008). Neurexin 1alpha structural variants associated with autism. Neurosci Lett, 438, 368–370.

Yim, YS., Kwon, Y., Nam, J., Yoon, HI., Lee, K., Kim, DG., Kim, E., Kim, CH., & Ko, J. (2013). Slitrks control excitatory and inhibitory synapse formation with LAR receptor protein tyrosine phosphatases. Proc Natl Acad Sci U S A, 110, 4057–4062.

Zellinger, C., Hadamitzky, M., Bock, E., Berezin, V., & Potschka, H. (2011). Impact of the NCAM derived mimetic peptide plannexin on the acute cellular consequences of a status epilepticus. Neurosci Lett, 501 (3), 173–178.

Zhang, C., Milunsky, JM., Newton, S., Ko, J., Zhao, G., Maher, TA., Tager-Flusberg, H., Bolliger, MF., Carter, AS., Boucard, AA., Powell, CM., & Südhof, TC. (2009). A neuroligin-4 missense mutation associated with autism impairs neuroligin-4 folding and endoplasmic reticulum export. J Neurosci, 29, 10843–10854.

Zhang, R., Zhong, NN., Liu, XG., Yan, H., Qiu, C., Han, Y., Wang, W., Hou, WK., Liu, Y., Gao, CG., Guo, TW., Lu, SM., Deng, HW., & Ma, J. (2010). Is the EFNB2 locus associated with schizophrenia? Single nucleotide polymorphisms and haplotypes analysis. Psychiatry Res, 180 (1), 5–9.

Zhou, L., Barão, S., Laga, M., Bockstael, K., Borgers, M., Gijsen, H., Annaert, W., Moechars, D., Mercken, M., Gevaert, K., & De Strooper, B. (2012). The neural cell adhesion molecules L1 and CHL1 are cleaved by BACE1 protease in vivo. J Biol Chem, 287 (31), 25927–25940.

Chapter 3

Different Types of Tumor Vessels and Hypothesis of "Cavitary" Type of Angiogenesis on the Example of Gastric Cancer

Marina Senchukova[1], Andrew Ryabov[2], Alexander Stadnikov[3]

1 Introduction

Angiogenesis is one of the key factors of tumor progression (Folkman, 1998). Activation of angiogenesis is associated with a number of factors among which the special role belongs to vascular endothelial growth factor (VEGF), being expressed by tumoral and stromal cells and influencing the development of new blood vessels and survival of immature ones (Ferrara, 2002). In evaluating of angiogenesis in malignant growth it should be considered that the tumor vessels have some morphological features distinguishing them from usual vessels:

- The tumor vessels are often located chaotically. Typical for them are tortuosity, the formation of vascular rings and pathological partitions, abnormal arteriovenous shunts, vascular lacunae. The size of the vessels varies from a severe dilatation to a sharp narrowing with a possible alternation of expanded and constricted areas (Less *et al.*, 1991; Baluk *et al.*, 2005; Birau *et al.*, 2012; Fukumura *et al.*, 2010);

[1] Department of Oncology, Orenburg State Medical University, Russia.

[2] Department of Thoracoabdominal Oncosurgery, P.A. Hertsen Moscow Oncology Research Institute, Branch of National Medical Research Radiological Center, Russia.

[3] Department of Histology, Cytology and Embryology, Orenburg State Medical University, Russia.

- Some authors have noted the absence of pericytes in tumor vessels – the cells that are functionally related to the vascular endothelium and extremely important for the stabilization and maturation of vascular structures (Baluk *et al.*, 2003; Baluk *et al.*, 2005; Morikawa *et al.*, 2002);

- In tumors the vessels (mainly of capillary type) with impaired endothelial lining having a discontinuous basal membrane are frequently observed (Birau *et al.*, 2012; Ribatti *et al.*, 2007);

- The tumor vessels are characterized by the increased permeability playing an important role in the activation of tumor angiogenesis (Dvorak *et al.*, 1995; Nagy *et al.*, 2012);

- In the lumen of blood and lymph vessels of tumor there are often observed tumor emboli, the presence of which is an unfavorable prognostic factor (An *et al.*, 2007; Shen *et al.*, 2009; Yokota *et al.*, 2004).

It is worth noting that the assessment of angiogenesis activity in the tumor is one of the priority tasks in oncology. It is most often determined by the microvessel density (MVD) and the intensity of VEGF expression in tumor (Lazar *et al.*, 2008; Poon *et al.*, 2003; Zhao, 2006). The majority of researchers has pointed to the close relationship of these indicators with the depth of tumor invasion, the presence of metastases in regional lymph nodes (RLN) and the prognosis of the disease (Ding *et al.*, 2006; Ma *et al.*, 2007; Lazar *et al.*, 2008; Poon *et al.*, 2003; Wang *et al.*, 2007). At the same time, tumor vessels are known to be heterogeneous in its origin and morphology and various types of vessels may differ not only in clinical significance, but also in their sensitivity to the antiangiogenic therapy (Birau *et al.*, 2012; Nagy & Dvorak, 2012). Since there is no currently clear classification of tumor vessels by morphology and their role in tumor progression is obscure we decided to investigate this problem on the example of gastric cancer (GC).

2   The Different Types of Tumor Vessels in Gastric Cancer

We investigated samples of tumor and gastric mucosa (GM) in 73 patients with GC who had undergone radical surgery (R0) in the Orenburg Regional Clinical Oncology Center. The average age of the patients was 61.2±9.3 years (from 34 to 78 years, the median – was 61 years). The clinical features of patients included in this study are presented in Table 1.

All specimens were fixed in formalin and embedded in paraffin. Serial sections (4 μm) were stained with Mayer's hematoxylin and eosin, by van Gieson and immunohistochemically using antibodies to CD34, CD4, CD8, CD20 и CD68. The number of dilated capillaries and the cavitary structures (CS) type-1 were assessed by visual analog way using a low magnification (×100) as none, single (no more than two in the field of view) and multiple (more than two in the field of view). The same manner the presence of CS type-2 was defined. The density of the la-belled lymphocytes (CD4, CD8, CD20) and macrophages (CD68) was calculated on the relative area unit equal to 0.42 × 0.28 mm². MVD was assessed immunohistochemically using antibodies to CD34 (Vermeulen *et al.*, 2002).

Clinicopathologic variables		Number of cases (n)	Percent (%)
Gender	Male	43	58.9
	Female	30	41.1
Location of tumor	Upper third	14	19.2
	Middle third	18	24.7
	Lower third	39	53.4
	Total cancer	2	2.7
Lauren classification	Intestinal type	41	56.2
	Diffuse type	32	43.8
Differentiation	Well (G1)	27	36.9
	Moderate (G2)	14	19.3
	Poorly (G3 – G4)	9	12.3
	Signet ring cell carcinoma	23	31.5
Nodal status	pN0	43	59
	pN1	9	12.3
	pN2	21	28.8
Depth of invasion	pT1	16	21.9
	pT2	18	24.7
	pT3	36	49.3
	pT4	3	4.1
Stage (TNM)	T1-2N0M0	34	46.6
	T3N0M0	9	12.3
	T3-4N1M0	9	12.3
	T3-4N1M0	21	28.8

Table 1: Clinicopathologic characteristics of gastric carcinoma cases.

The obtained data were compared with clinical features of GC: stage, size, localization, histological type of tumor, 3-year overall survival (OS) and relapse-free survival (RFS).

The study of special features of angiogenesis by GC allowed us to establish the heterogeneity of vessels of tumor stroma and adjacent GM. We have singled out the following types of the vessels dissimilar in morphology and clinical significance:

2.1 Normal Vessels: Arteries, Veins, Arterioles, Venules and Capillaries

The normal arteries, veins, arterioles and venules were localized in gastric submucosa (GS) and had the average wall thickness 22.24±9.29, 13.26±3.65, 6.33±1.01 and 3.18±0.96 microns respectively. The normal capillaries were localized in both GM and GS and had 5 – 20 microns in diameter. The correlation of normal vessel density with clinical characteristics and long-term results of GC treatment was not revealed.

2.2   Dilated Capillaries of the Lamina Propria of Gastric Mucosa

The described vessels differed from usual capillaries by larger sizes (their diameter was more than 50 microns) and irregular form (Figure 1a). Both usual endothelial cells and the cells with large, light nuclei having a fine-netted chromatin structure took part in their formation. On a cross-section the nuclei of such cells were of the oval or round form (Figure 1b).

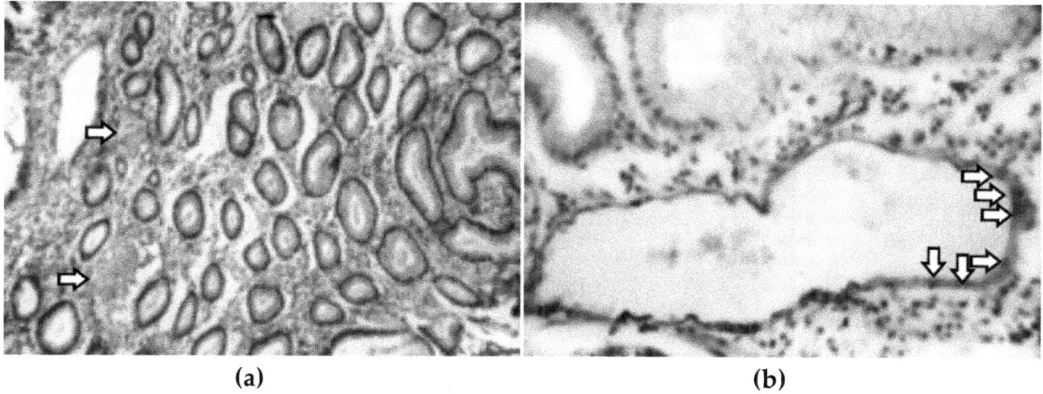

(a)   (b)

Figure 1: The dilated capillaries in the lamina propria of the gastric mucosa. **(a):** the dilated capillaries (arrows): H&E stain, bars = 100 μm; **(b):** the cells with large, light nuclei having a fine-netted chromatin structure (arrows) are seen in the endothelial lining of the dilated capillary: staining with CD34, bars = 20 μm.

The Spearman rank correlation analysis (ϱ) and gamma correlation coefficient test (gamma) showed that the presence of dilated capillaries in the lamina propria of the GM correlated with sizes tumor ($\varrho = 0.325$, $t = 2.79$, $p = 0.007$), TNM stage (gamma = 0.371, $z = 3.17$, $p = 0.001$), nodal stage (gamma = 0.387, $z = 2.88$, $p = 0.004$), 3-year OS (gamma = -0.467, $z = -2.18$, $p = 0.03$) and RFS (gamma = -0.435, $z = -2.64$, $p = 0.008$).

The increase of the number of the described vessels associated with the tumor size increasing (Table 2) and with the number of metastases in RLN (Table 3) was noted.

In the presence of multiple dilated capillaries in lamina propria of GM the decrease of 3-year OS and RFS of GC patients was recorded (Figure 2a and b).

Tumor size	The number of dilated capillaries			Statistics (LSD Test)
	No	Single	Multiple	
M±m$_x$ (см)	3.85 + 0.47	4.85 + 0.55	6.43 + 0.80	$p^{1-3} = 0.005$, $p^{2-3} = 0.08$

Table 2: The tumor sizes depending on the number of dilated capillaries in lamina propria of gastric mucosa.

Nodal stage	The number of dilated capillaries						Statistics
	No		Single		Multiple		
	n	%	n	%	n	%	
N0	21	47.7	17	38.6	6	13.6	$\chi^2 = 12.7$ $p = 0.02$
N1	2	25.0	6	75.0	0	0	
N2	6	28.6	6	28.6	9	42.8	

Table 3: The number of the dilated capillaries in lamina propria of gastric mucosa depending on the nodal stage.

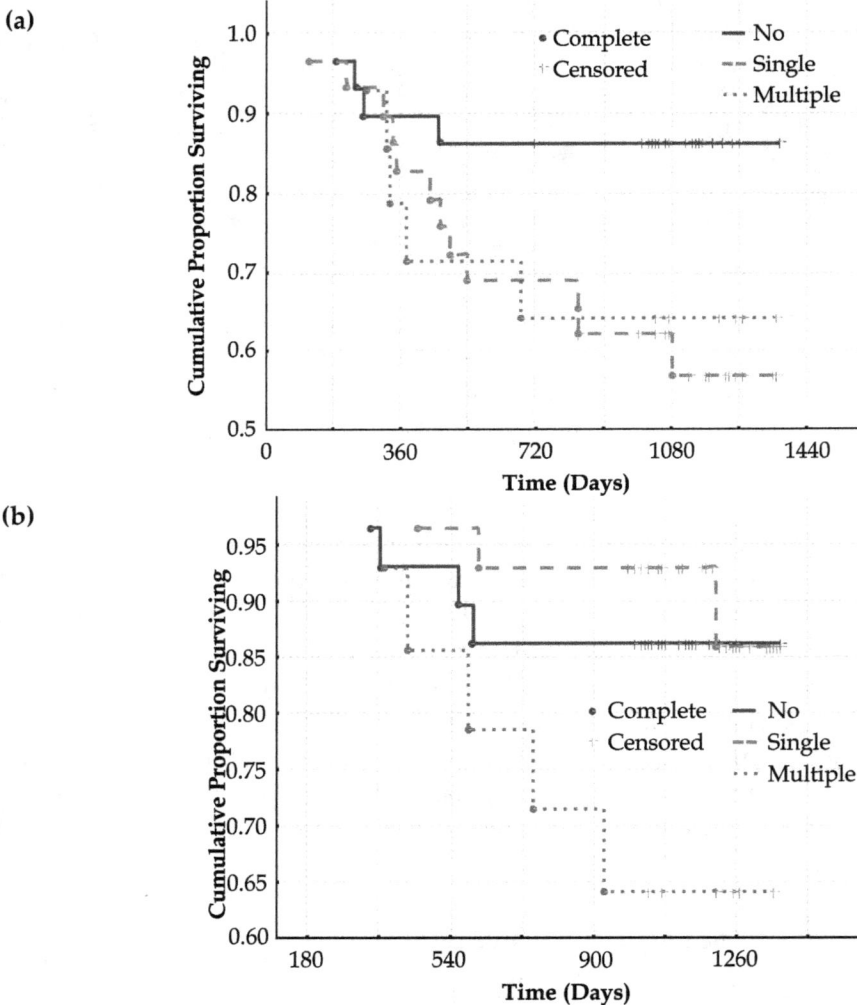

Figure 2: Survival of patients depending on the number of dilated capillaries in the lamina propria of gastric mucosa. **(a):** the curves of 3-year relapse-free surviving, **(b):** the curves of 3-year overall surviving.

There were no significant differences in the number of dilated capillaries in GM depending on the depth of invasion and histology of tumor.

2.3   The Venous Vessels of the Gastric Submucosa without Muscle Tissue in the Middle Layer

The extremely dilated vessels of this type were characterized by a lack of muscular tissue in the middle layer (Figure 3a). The wall thickness of such vessels ranged from 6.6 to 34.5 microns and the average was 17.43±4.05 microns. Tunica interna was formed by endothelial cells with flattened hyperchromatic nuclei. Vascular adventitia consisted of several layers of cells with elongated, curved nuclei and had a specific connective matrix with a predominance of fibrous structures in it (Figure 3b).

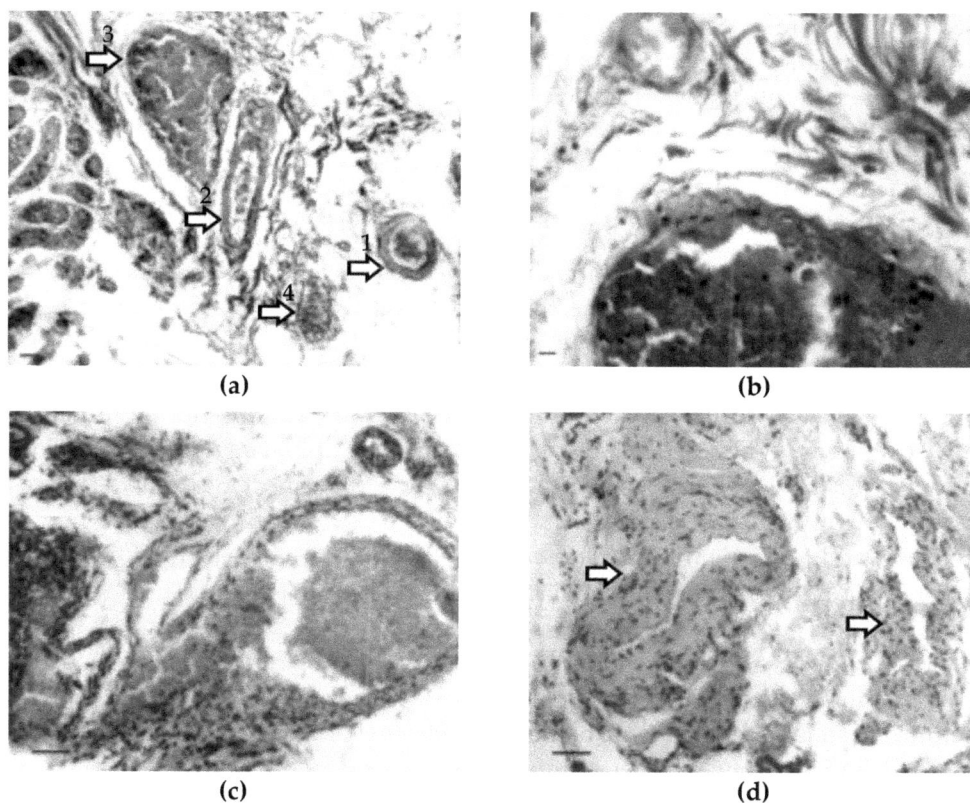

(a)   (b)

(c)   (d)

Figure 3: The vessels of gastric submucosa. (a): the normal arteriola (1) and venula (2), the dilated venous vessel without muscle tissue in the middle layer (3) and the dilated capillary (4): van Gieson's stain, bars = 100 μm; (b): the absence of muscle tissue in the middle layer of the venous vessel: van Gieson's stain, bars = 20 μm. (c): the dilated venous vessels of muscle type: H&E stain, bars = 100 μm; (d): the vessels of the arterial type with hypertrophied muscle layer (arrows): H&E stain, bars = 100 μm.

2.4   The Dilated Venous Vessels of Muscle-Type of the Gastric Submucosa

The vessels of this sort often had an irregular shape and formed the wide vascular lacunae with the stasis of formed elements in their lumen (Figure 3c). The wall thickness of such vessels varied within the wide limits from 18.8 to 54.5 microns and the average size was 32.8±7.1 micrometers.

2.5   The Vessels of the Arterial Type of the Gastric Submucosa with Hypertrophied Muscle Layer

The average wall thickness of these vessels was 56.2±2.6 micrometers. The arterial vessels that prevailed over all others in the number and occupied square were found in 9 samples (14.3%). The described vessels were more often full-blooded, less common - with collapsed walls (Figure 3d).

The correlation of the presence of dilated venous vessels and the vessels of arterial type with the clinical characteristics of GC and long-term results of treatment was not established.

2.6   The Dilated Vessels of Capillary Type of the Gastric Submucosa

In gastric GS adjacent to the tumor the dilated vessels of capillary type with diameter of 100 micron and more were often determined. A distinctive feature of the described vessels was the fact that both the endothelium of normal structure and the cells with large, pale nuclei having a fine-netted chromatin structure took part in their formation (Figure 4a and b). The cells with similar structure were observed not only in the lining of the described vessels but also next to them and around the capillaries located in the lamina propria of GM, and even in their lumen (Figure 4c). The important particularity of the described cells was their ability to form bands and closed structures (Figure 4d and e). Endothelial proliferations were also observed in the lumen of vessels (Figure 4f). The expression of CD34 was completely absent in the most of dilated capillaries (Figure 4g), sometimes it was barely visible or expressed fragmentary (Figure 4h).

The connective tissue surrounding the dilated capillaries was presented by the strands of thin, loose fibrils. The most vessels were free from the content, but there were sometimes vessels with plasma or blood cells. Stromal edema and diapedesis of blood cells were being observed in all the samples under study.

The correlation analysis demonstrated that the dilated capillaries of GS correlated with histologic type (gamma = 0.451, Z = 3.44, p = 0.0006), grade (gamma = 0.341, Z = 3.17, p = 0.002), N category (gamma = 0.536, Z = 4.75, p = 0.000002), 3-year OS (gamma = -0.344, Z = -2.23, p = 0.03) and RFS (gamma = -0.382, Z = -2.75, p = 0.006). The described type of vessels was significantly less common found in the intestinal type of GC, grade G1 and in the absence (N0) of lymph metastases (Table 4).

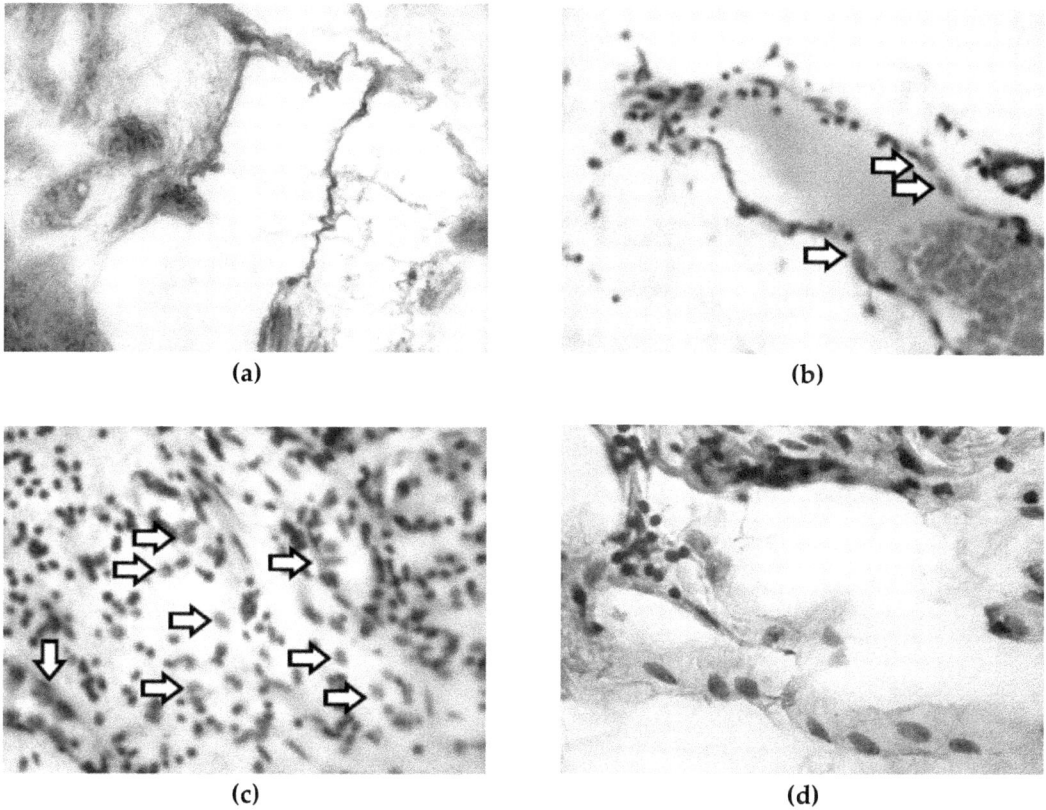

(a)

(b)

(c)

(d)

Figure 4 (a–d): The features of the dilated capillaries of gastric submucosa. **(a):** the dilated vessel of the capillary type in gastric submucosa: H&E stain, bars = 100 µm; **(b):** the endothelial cells with the large, pale nuclei having a fine-netted chromatin structure in the lining of the dilated capillary (arrows): H&E stain, bars = 20 µm; **(c):** the similar cells in the lumen of capillaries (thick arrows) and next to them (thin arrows) in the lamina propria of gastric mucosa: H&E stain, bars = 20 µm; The similar cells form the bands; **(d):** and the closed structures in gastric.

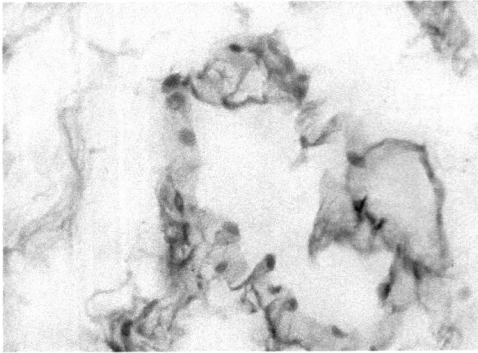

(e)

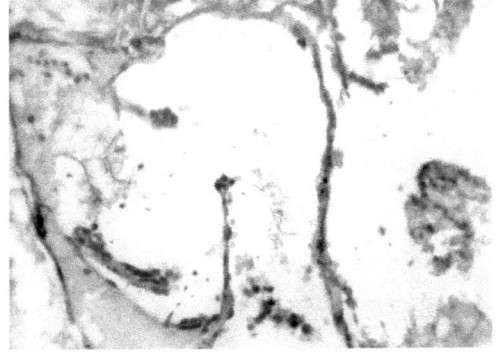

(f)

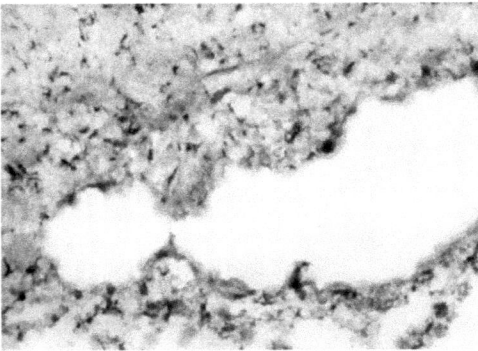

(g)

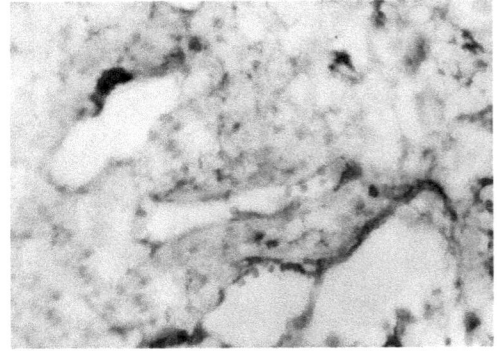

(h)

Figure 4 (e–h): The features of the dilated capillaries of gastric submucosa. **(e):** H&E stain, bars = 20 μm; **(f):** the endothelial proliferation in the lumen of dilated capillaries: staining with CD34, bars = 40 μm; The lack of the expression of CD34; **(g):** and the fragmented expression of CD34; **(h):** in the endothelial lining of dilated capillaries: staining with CD34, bars = 40 μm.

		The number of the dilated capillaries						Statistics
		no		single		multiple		
		n	%	n	%	n	%	
Histology	Intestinal type	20	66.7	6	20.0	4	13.3	$\chi^2 = 5.39$
	Diffuse-types	10	37.0	8	29.6	9	33.3	$p = 0.07$
Grade	G1	19	79.2	1	4.1	4	16.7	$\chi^2 = 13.18$
	G2	7	46.7	6	40.0	2	13.6	
	G3-4	7	36.8	5	26.3	7	36.8	$p = 0.04$
	Signet ring cell carcinoma	10	41.7	7	29.2	7	29.2	
Nodal Stage	N0	33	70.0	6	12.0	9	18.0	$\chi^2 = 13.49$
	N1	3	27.3	5	45.5	3	27.3	
	N2	5	23.8	8	38.1	8	38.1	$p = 0.01$

Table 4: The number of dilated capillaries in gastric submucosa depending on the patient characteristics: histology, grade, nodal stage.

The depth of tumor invasion (category T), the degree of atrophy, intestinal metaplasia and dysplasia of GM did not significantly influence the number of vessels of this type. However, the number of dilated capillaries of GS correlated with the MVD (ϱ = -0.519, t = -2.57, p = 0.02) and CD68 macrophages in GM (ϱ = -0.654, t = -2.87, p = 0.02). The decrease of the MVD (CD34 +) and the density of macrophages (CD68 +) in GM at the increase of the dilated capillaries number in GS was recorded.

In terms of prognosis more significant appeared to be the fact of the presence of dilated capillaries in GS than the fact of their quantity. The described vessels were detected in 24 of 32 (75%) patients with metastases in RLN and only in 15 out of 49 (30.6%) - without metastases (p = 0.0002). In the presence of dilated capillaries in GS the decrease of 3-year OS (p = 0.003) and RFS (p = 0.025) was noted (Figure 5a and b).

At the same time we did not detect the significant differences in the survival rates between the groups of patients with single and multiple dilated capillaries. The 3-year OS was 90.2%1, 61.1%2 and 80%3 (p^{1-2} = 0.008, p^{2-3} > 0.2 Log-Rank Test) and the RFS was 82.5%1, 58.8%2 and 60.0%3 (p^{1-2} = 0.049, p^{1-3} = 0.042 Log-Rank Test) in the absence[1], in the presence of single[2] and in the presence of multiple[3] vessels of this type respectively.

2.7   The Vessels of "Cavitary" Type

We had described before a new way of angiogenesis on the example of GC that consisted in the formation of CS in the tumor stroma and adjacent GM, being then lined by the be associated with the abruption of tumor cells from their underlying foundation (type-1), with the dilatation of tumor glands, flattening and thinning of the epithelial cells (type-2) and with the formation of CS directly into the GM or the tumor stroma without in-

(a)

(b)

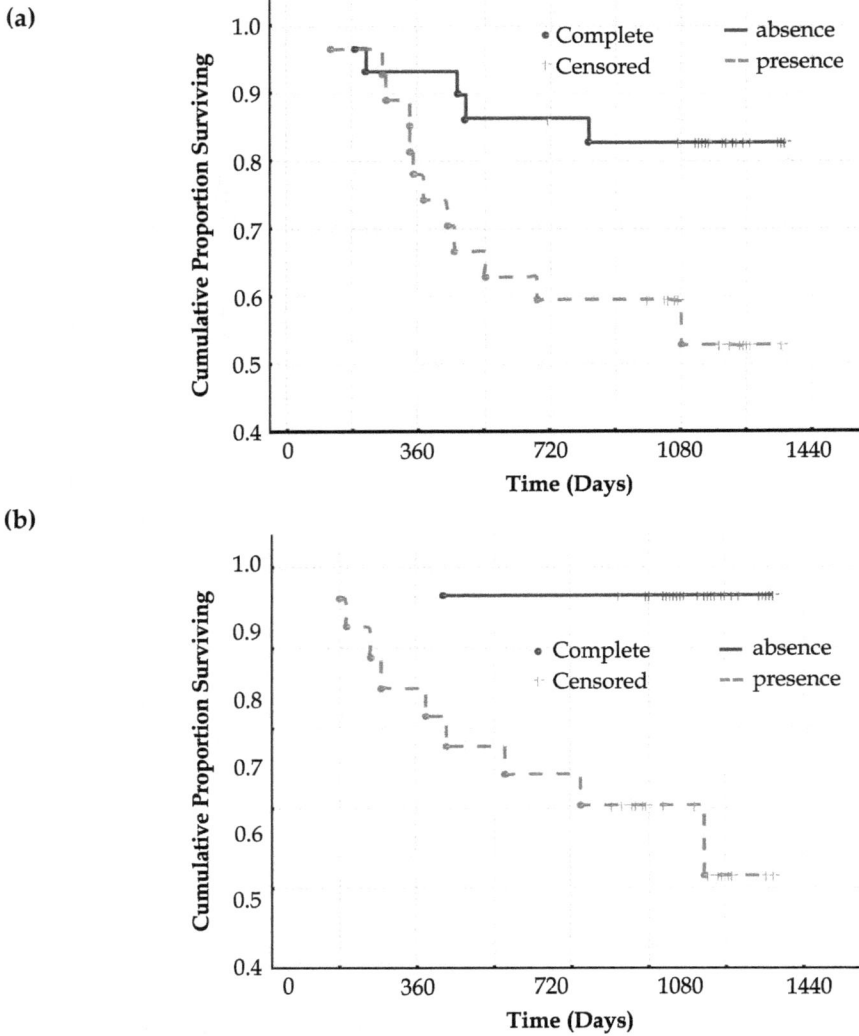

Figure 5: Survival of the patients depending on the presence of dilated capillaries in gastric submucosa. **(a):** the curves of 3-year relapse-free surviving; **(b):** the curves of 3-year overall surviving.

volvment of the tumor cells (type-3). However, in this work it was decided not to consider the features of cavitary" angiogenesis type-2 as only the CS type-1 and CS type-3 were associated with the clinical characteristics and prognosis of GC. Besides the existence of "cavitary" vessel type-2 is considered by us to demand an additional confirmation, for example by using double IHC staining. So in this chapter we described only two main types of CS formation corresponding to the first (CS type-1) and third (CS type-2) types of CS in our original work (Senchukova & Kiselevsky, 2014).

The first type of "cavitary" angiogenesis was associated with the abruption of layers of epithelial cells from their underlying foundation and their desquamation into the lumen of the "obliterated" gastric or tumor glands (Figure 6a). We have noted two main signs specific to this type of angiogenesis:

1.   The presence of CS with a partial endothelial lining. The cells of such lining are un-evenly stained by marker and have an uneven surface with a number of pro-tuberances (Figure 6b);

2.   The CS without endothelial lining and CS with a partial endothelial lining as well as the dilated vessels located next to them are simultaneously detected in the samples of tumor tissue by low ($\times$ 100) signification (Figure 6c). We believe that these vessels are directly related to "cavitary" angiogenesis type-1. In the lumen of such vessels the tumoral or epithelial emboli are often detected and erythrocyte margination is observed (Figure 6d).

We have also pointed out some differences in the morphology of CS type-1 in in-testinal and diffuse types of GC (Senchukova et al., 2015). In the intestinal type of GC the formation of CS type-1 was associated with tumor or normal glands where the flaking of epithelial cells from the basement membrane and their desquamation into the lumen of the "obliterated" gastric or tumor glands were being observed (see Figure 6a to c). The wall of such CS is most likely the basement membrane bordering the tumor stroma. In the diffuse type of GC the CS were presented by the structures limited from outside by the tumor cells (Figure 6e). In their lumen the fragments of tumor tissue having the same structure as the surrounding one were being detected. The cytoplasm of cells lining such CS did not often express CD34 and was difficult to be distinguished on the light-optical level. The cells with large, light, oval-shaped nuclei are sometimes observed in the struc-ture of such endothelial lining (Figure 6f).

The second type of "cavitary" angiogenesis was associated with the formation of CS directly into the GM or the tumor stroma. This supposition was due to the fact that in the some cases we had observed a characteristic cellular structure of the connective tissue of the lamina propria of GM (Figure 7a), often combining with the expressed phenomena of diapedesis of erythrocytes. Most often than not the described CS were observed in the GM at the level of gastric pits or directly in the stroma bordering upon tumor tissue. Sometimes the cavities with endothelial lining were revealed. The cytoplasm of the cells of such lining weakly expressed CD34 and was characterized by the presence of a number of protuberances and intracavitary growths (Figure 7b).

The Spearman rank correlation analysis (ϱ) and gamma correlation coefficient test (gamma) showed that the number of CS type-1 correlated with histological type (gamma = 0,344, z = 2.51, p = 0.01), degree of tumor differentiation (gamma = 0.318, z = 2.79, p = 0.005), TNM stage (gamma = 0,524, z =4.27, p < 0.0001), T stage (gamma = 0.666, z = 4.75, p < 0.0001), N stage (gamma = 0.520, z = 4.19, p < 0.0001), 3-year OS (gamma = -0.778, z = -4.64, p < 0.0001) and RFS (gamma = -0.766, z = -5.81, p < 0.0001). The correlation between the number of CS type-1 and CS type-2 was also noted (gamma = 0.577, z = 4.47, p < 0.0001).

The presence of multiple CS type-1 was the most significant factor associated with the prognosis of GC. The multiple CS type-1 were more frequently observed in diffuse type of GC (in 24,4% and 43,7% cases, respectively in intestinal and diffuse types of GC,

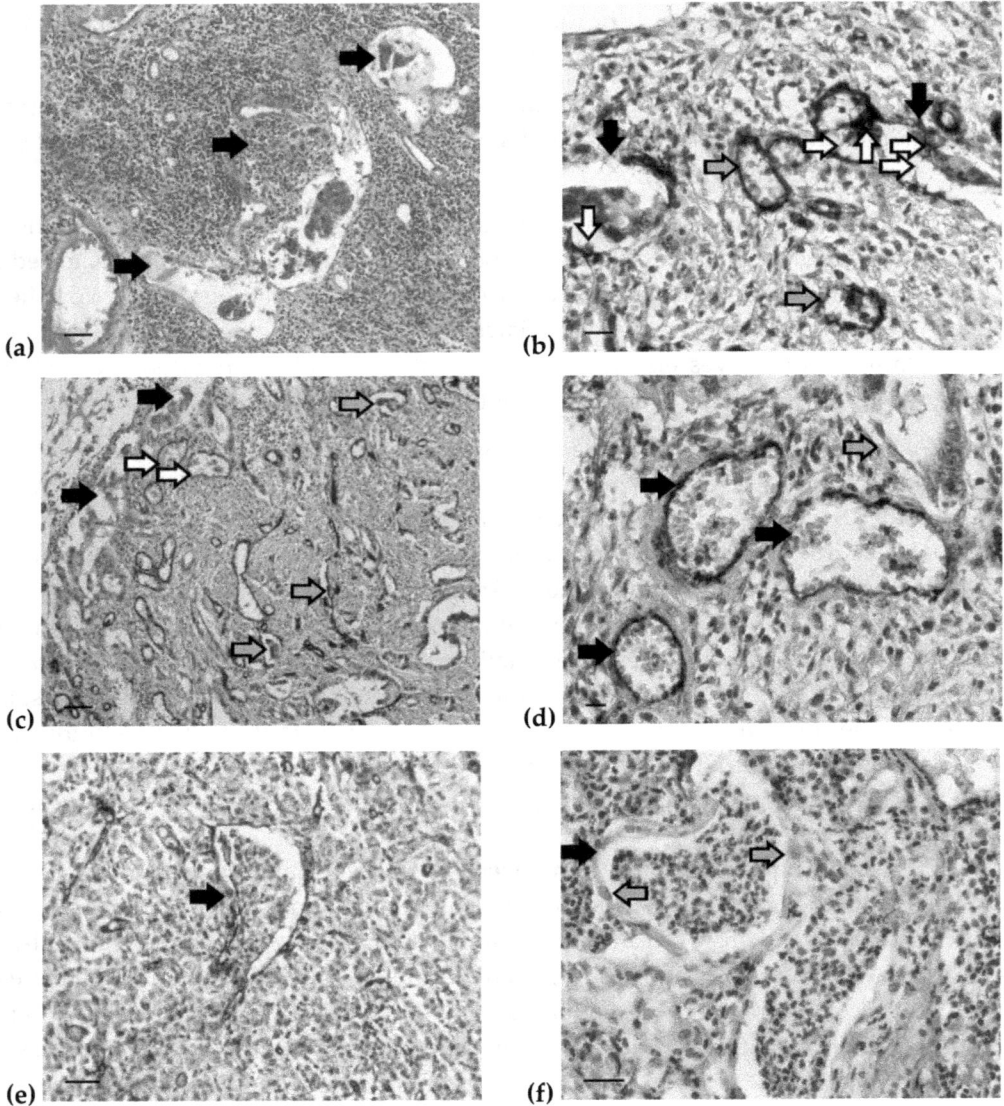

Figure 6: The morphological features of "cavitary" angiogenesis type-1. **(a):** the CS type-1 in tumor stroma: H&E stain, bars = 100 μm; **(b):** the CS type-1with a partial endothelial lining (black arrows) and dilated vessels located next to them (grey arrows). The cytoplasm of endothelial cells has an uneven surface with a number of protuberances (white arrows): staining with CD34, bars = 40 μm; **(c):** the CS type-1 without (black arrows) and partial (grey arrows) endothelial lining and the dilated vessels (grey arrows) with tumor emboli in their lumen: staining with CD34, bars = 100 μm; **(d):** the dilated vessels with tumor emboli in their lumen (black arrows) and tumor glands (grey arrow): staining with CD34, bars = 20 μm; **(e):** CS type-1 (arrow): staining with CD34, bars = 100 μm; **(f):** CS type-1 in diffuse type of GC (black arrow). The lining cells have the large, light, oval-shaped nuclei (grey arrow): staining with CD34, bars = 100 μm.

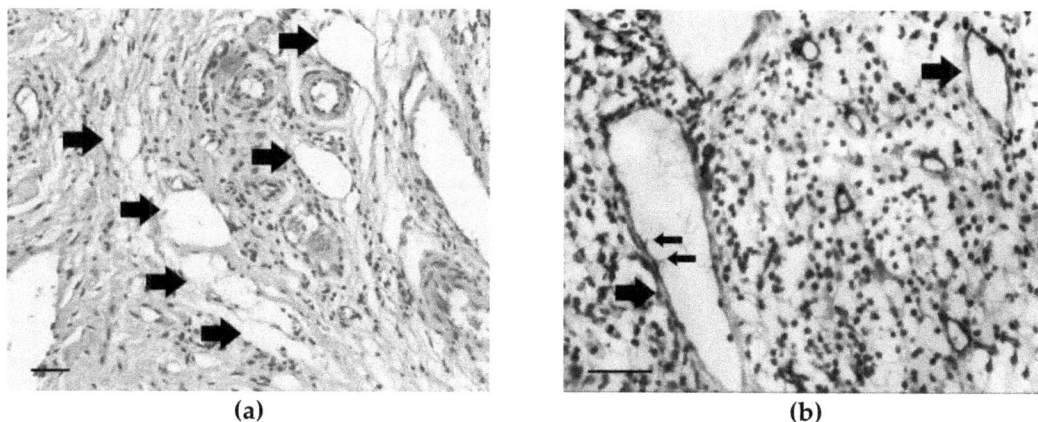

(a)   (b)

Figure 7: The morphological features of "cavitary" angiogenesis type-2. **(a):** the CS type-2 in the stroma bordering upon tumor tissue (arrows): H&E stain, bars = 100 μm; **(b):** the CS type-2 with endothelial lining (large arrows). The cytoplasm of the endothelial cells weakly expresses CD34 and has several protuberances growths (small arrows): staining with the anti-CD34, bars = 100 μm.

$\chi^2 = 3.42$, $p = 0,18$), in G3-G4 grade (in 14.8%, 42.9%, 62.5% and 37.5% cases, respectively in G1, G2, G3-4 and signet ring cell carcinoma, $\chi^2 = 9.64$, $p = 0.14$), in T3-4 stage (in 18.7%, 11.1%, 50% and 100% cases, respectively in T1, T2, T3 and T4 stage, $\chi^2 = 15.37$, $p = 0.001$) and in N2 stage (in 18.6%, 44.4% and 66.7% cases respectively in N0, N1 and N2 nodal stage, $\chi^2 = 15.74$, $p = 0.003$).

The increase of the number of CS type-1 was accompanied by the increasing of the density of CD68 in GM and tumor stroma. In the presence and absence of multiple CS type-1 the density of CD68 macrophages in GM was respectively 72.6±44.8 and 41.6±15.4 cells on area unit ($p = 0.06$) and in tumor stroma –68.3±41.7 and 27.2±20.2 cells on area unit ($p = 0.15$).

3-year OS and RFS were practically identical if the CS type-1 in tumor stroma were single or absent, and significantly worse when the CS type-1 were multiple (Figure 8a and b).

With or without the multiple CS type-1, the 3-year OS was 52.7% and 93.9% respectively ($p = 0.0013$, OR = 15.0, 95% CI = 2.96 – 76.31), and the RFS was 32.4% and 87.7% respectively ($p = 0.0001$, OR = 14.93, 95%CI = 4.34 – 51.38).

The CS type-2 correlated in its turn only with the histological type of tumor (gamma = 0.403, z = 2.68, $p = 0.008$). By the diffuse and intestinal type of GC they were revealed in 55.9% and 44.1% cases respectively ($\chi^2 = 3.24$, $p = 0.07$).

The multivariate Cox proportional hazard regression analysis indicated that TNM stage ($p = 0.003$), nodal stage ($p = 0.013$), the number of CV type-1 ($p = 0.005$) were significantly independent prognostic factors in patients with GC.

(a)

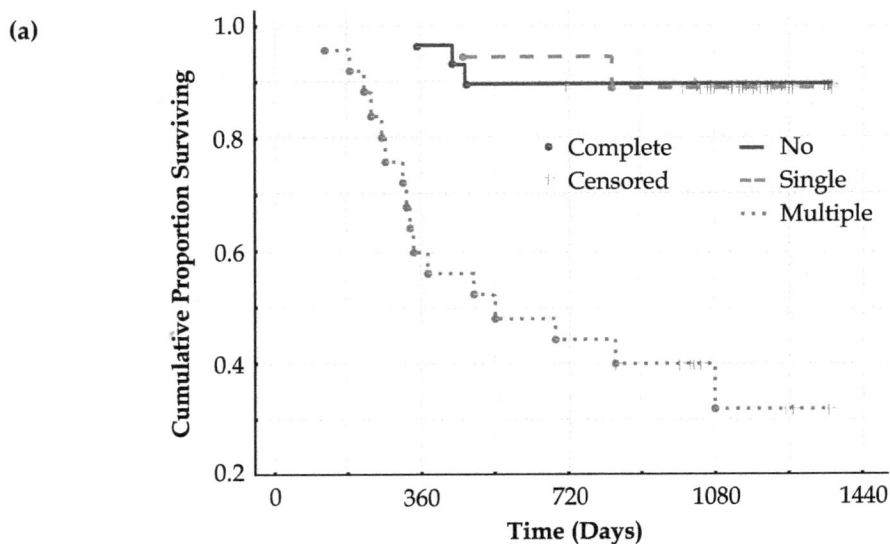

Continued on next page...

(b)   *...Continued from previous page*

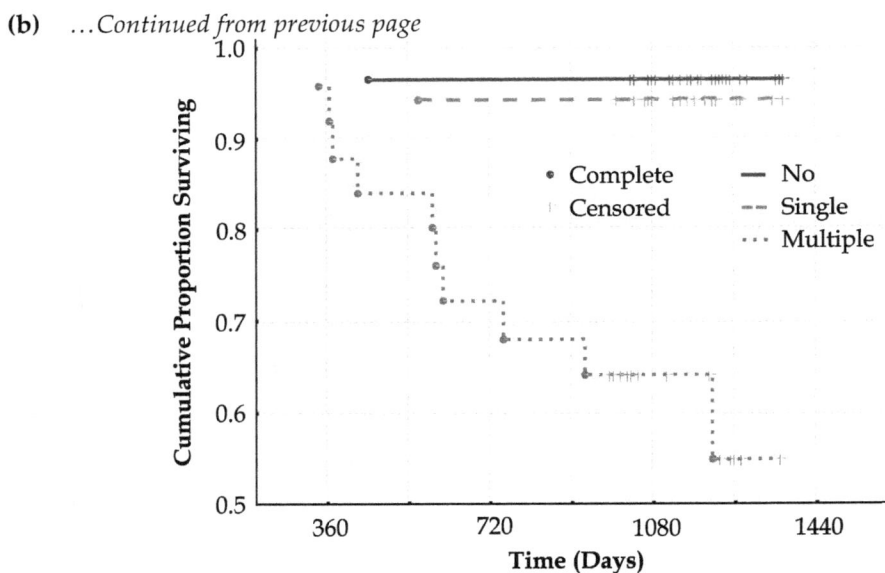

Figure 8: Survival of the patients depending on the presence of CS type-1 in tumor stroma. **(a):** the curves of 3-year relapse-free surviving; **(b):** the curves of 3-year overall surviving.

3   The Modern Concept of the Mechanisms of Tumor Vessel Formation, the Features of their Morphology and Role in Tumor Progression

Angiogenesis is a key factor in tumor progression, directly related to the invasion and metastasis of malignant tumors. The study of its mechanisms attracts attention of many scientists. However, it should be noted that the technical and methodological approaches to the solution of this problem significantly diverge in different researchers. Some researchers give preference to a quantitative evaluation of the angiogenesis activity in tumors, noting that a high MVD in the tumor and a high level of VEGF expression are more frequently observed in advanced malignancy in the presence of metastases and are correlated with poor prognosis (Ding *et al.*, 2006; Erenoglu *et al.*, 2000; Lazar *et al.*, 2008; Ma *et al.*, 2007; Millikan *et al.*, 2003; Poon *et al.*, 2003; Wang *et al.*, 2007).

Other researchers put more emphasis on the study of qualitative changes in the structure of vascular wall and microvasculature, pointing out that the tumor vascular network is heterogeneous in its structure and different types of vessels may respond differently to the use of angiogenesis blockers (Baluk *et al.*, 2005; Birau *et al.*, 2012; Gee *et al.*, 2003; Fukumura *et al.*, 2010; Morikawa *et al.*, 2002; Nagy & Dvorak, 2012; Nagy *et al.*, 2012).

In studies of peculiarities of angiogenesis in patients with GC we used both a quantitative assessment of the activity of tumor angiogenesis (Goddard *et al.*, 2002) and the study of the morphological features of the different types of tumor vessels. Such approach allowed us to single out some types of tumor vessels differed in morphology and their clinical importance, and to formulate a hypothesis of "cavitary" type of angiogenesis by GC (Senchukova & Kiselevsky, 2014).

In the quantitative evaluating of the angiogenesis activity, unlike a number of researchers (Lazar *et al.*, 2008; Poon *et al.*, 2003; Wang *et al.*, 2007), we did not reveal the relationships between MVD in tumor and factors of GC progression. From this point of view our results are closer to the results of the researchers who also found no correlation between MVD in tumor and prognosis by different malignancy (Torres *et al.*, 1999; Zeng *et al.*, 2010; Hillen *et al.*, 2006). Moreover, there is an opinion that the definition of MVD in the tumor is inappropriate to use widely in clinical practice because of apparent defects of this method (Brown *et al.*, 2008).

These limitations are related to the lack of clear standards in the technical aspect of the method based on the subjective assessment of optimal locations to determine "hot spots" as well as the lack of clear criteria for appraisal of the obtained results. A large number of histological types of GC having different ratio of parenchyma and stroma in the tumor makes it difficult to give not only a quantitative estimation of the MVD but the interpretation of the obtained data as well.

The study of the morphological features of tumor stroma vessels and the adjacent GM by GC allowed us to identify several types of abnormal vessels having different prognostic value. More often than others the clearly dilated venous vessels with and without muscle tissue in the middle layer were being defined in GS. We didn't reveal correlations between the vessels of this type and the factors of GC progression. It can be assumed that the described vessels are developing from normal vessels as a result of violations of the structure of their basement membrane. In some researches it was shown that the expression of VEGF-A by tumor and stroma cells caused a degradation of the basement membrane of vessels (Nagy *et al.*, 2012). This leads to the remodel of the existing arterioles and venules, to their sharp expansion and increase of vascular permeability playing an important role in tumor angiogenesis.

In contrast to the dilated venous vessels the dilated capillaries of the lamina propria of GM and GS were of great prognostic importance. A distinguishing feature of the described vessels was that both the endothelium of the normal structure and the cells with large, pale nuclei with fine-netted chromatin structure took part in their formation. The presence of dilated capillaries in GM was connected with more advanced stages of GC and with the worsening of the long-term results of GC treatment. As for the dilated capillaries of GS they were observed mainly in patients with lymphatic metastases. Their number was associated with histology, tumor grade, OS and RFS of patients with GC.

The obtained results allow us to suggest that angioblasts should be able to participate in the formation of dilated capillaries. Their involvement in tumor angiogenesis has been described by many researchers (Ahlskog *et al.*, 2003; Asahara *et al.*, 1997; Hillen & Griffioen, 2007; Sussman *et al.*, 2003). The following facts testify to the possible participation of angioblasts in the formation of the described vessels:

- the phenotypical features of the nuclei of cells lining the described vessels: large, pale with fine-netted chromatin structure;

- the lack of expression of CD34 in the newly formed vessels. This can be explained by the fact that the cells lining the dilated capillaries belong to negative CD34 progenitor cells, known as the precursors of CD34 positive cells (Kimura *et al.*, 2004.);

- the presence of the described cells not only in the endothelial lining of vessels, but also around the capillaries located in the lamina propria of GM and in their lumen;

- the ability to form the intravascular growing. This ability of tumor vascular endothelium has been also noted by other investigators who point to the fact that intravascular growing could participate in the formation of new vessels by dividing the capillary lumen (Nagy *et al.*, 2012).

We believe that the revealed changes in GS adjacent to tumor testifying about the active processes of angiogenesis are not casual. It is known that exactly at the border of the tumor and "normal" tissues there are being observed the most active processes associated with the formation of future tumor stroma that determine its further growth and metastasis of malignant neoplasm (Nagy *et al.*, 2012). We consider that a loose connective tissue of the GS is a favorable environment for the formation of a fibrin skeleton of future vessels and their growth as well.

Some scientists have presented evidence that a tumor vasculature is heterogeneous in its structure and different types of vessels may respond differently to the usage of angiogenesis blockers [Holash *et al.*, 1999; Chang *et al.*, 2000; Wang *et al.*, W., 2010; Burri *et al.*, 2004]. The differences in the structure of vessels may be associated with different mechanisms of their formation. These mechanisms include:

- **Sprouting angiogenesis** is a growth of new capillary vessels out of preexisting ones. The process of sprouting angiogenesis involves several sequential steps: the activation of endothelial cells by specific growth factors; the degradation of the extracellular matrix and basal membrane; the invasion of endothelial cells into the surrounding matrix and their migration to the problem areas: the focuses of inflammation, hypoxia, tumor growth (Morikawa *et al.*, 2002; Gee *et al.*, 2003; Baluk *et al.*, 2003; Hillen & Griffioen, 2007).

- **Vessel co-option** is a growth of tumor cells among existing vessels without evoking an angiogenic response (Dome *et al.*, 2002; Holash *et al.*, 1999).

- **Vasculogenic mimicry** is a process of vessel-like structure formation being partially or completely lined with tumor cells (Chang *et al.*, 2000; Folkman, 2001; Li *et al.*, 2010; Maniotis *et al.*, 1999; Wang *et al.*, 2010).

- **Intussusceptive angiogenesis** is a new concept of vessel formation when preexisting vessels split in two new vessels by the formation of transvascular tissue pillar into the lumen of the vessel (Burri *et al.*, 2004).

- **Vasculogenesis** is a formation of new blood vessels with the participation of «endothelial progenitor cells» (EPCs) circulating in blood. It is known that under the influence of tumor mediators, EPCs emerge from the bone marrow into the peripheral blood and can be included in the wall of the existing tumor vessels or participate in the formation of new blood vessels (Asahara *et al.*, 1997; Hillen & Griffioen, 2007; Sussman *et al.*, 2003).

Recently we described a new way of angiogenesis characterized by the formation of CS in the tumor stroma and adjacent GM then being lined by endothelial cells and merged into the blood vessels of the organ (Senchukova & Kiselevsky, 2014). We proposed that there are two main mechanisms of the formation of such CS. The first one is associated with the abruption of tumor cells from their underlying foundation, the second – with the formation of CS directly into the GM or the tumor stroma without involvement of the tumor cells. Analysis of the received data has showed that the first type of "cavitary" angiogenesis plays perhaps a key role in progression of GC. So, the presence of multiple CS type-1 was associated with the diffuse type of GC, grade G3-G4, T3-4 and N2 stages of GC and with the reduction of 3-year RFS and OS. In turn, the presence of CS type-2 was associated with the histological type of GC.

We have also pointed out some differences in the morphology of CS type-1 in intestinal and diffuse types of GC (Senchukova *et al.*, 2015).

We believe that the important role in the formation of the described "cavitary" structures can play inflammatory changes in the tumor stroma and the adjacent GM. It has been known that an active inflammatory process is connected with the increased secretion by immune cells of cytokines, chemokines, growth factors and proteases (Eiro & Vizoso, 2012; Wu & Zhou, 2009) that promote the activation of tumor angiogenesis on the one hand (De Narddo *et al.*, 2008; Pollard, 2009) and influence the adhesive properties of tumor cells on the other (Mantur & Wojszel, 2008; Reiss *et al.*, 2006). Besides some studies have shown that the immune cells may be directly associated with tumor progression and invasion (Man, 2010; Man *et al.*, 2010; Man *et al.*, 2013; Pawelek & Chakraborty, 2008) and that the type and density of immune cells in the tumor tissue may be one of the most reliable parameters for predicting a patient's clinical outcome in certain types of cancer (Schreiber *et al.*, 2011).

In our research, the presence of CS type-1 was associated only with the density of CD68 macrophages. It has been documented that the tumor-infiltrating macrophages (TIM) are favorable to the activation of tumor angiogenesis at the expense of the increasing production of mediators that promote angiogenesis, such as vascular endothelial growth factor (VEGF) and cyclo-oxygenase-2 – derived prostaglandin E2. The activation of TIM is modulated by local signals within the tumor microenvironment such as tumor necrosis factor-α and hypoxia (Ohta *et al.*, 2004; Sica *et al.*, 2006). They are often found in the vicinity of tumor glands basement membranes, in the places where its integrity is destroyed (Peng *et al.*, 2010). It is logical to assume that the main mechanism of the damaging effect may be associated with the synthesis of matrix metalloprotease (MMP) that are proteolytic enzymes used by cancer to degrade the extracellular matrix (Kamoshida *et al.*, 2012, Kamoshida *et al.*, 2013).

We believe that the previously described "Retraction Artifact" (it is a space between tumor cells and their surrounding stroma) has a direct relationship to the type-1 of "cavitary" angiogenesis. The prognostic significance of "Retraction Artifact" as a factor associated with tumor progression has been mentioned in a number of studies (Acs *et al.*, 2007; Acs *et al.*, 2012; Zaorsky *et al.*, 2012). However, in contrast to the cited sources, we succeeded to link this phenomenon to a previously undocumented type of angiogenesis and to show that tumoral emboli in blood vessels can be formed at the expense of the abruption of tumor cells from their adjacent stroma and of their desquamation directly into the lumen of the vessels of "cavitary" type. It could be assume that the disorder of the adhesive properties of tumor cells is of the key importance in the formation of CS type-1. The focal disruptions in the tumor capsule (Man**, 2010; Man***, 2010) associated with increased immune cell infiltration (Man, 2010; Man *et al.*, 2013) are most likely related to this processes.

It is possible that another important factor associated with the formation of CS type-1 and type-2 is a phenomenon of the increased vascular permeability that on the one hand may influence the process of stroma retraction and on the other - promote the formation of a fibrin matrix and a migration of endothelial cells (Nagy *et al.*, 2012). There is a good reason to believe that parallel processes of formation and lysis of stroma that more actively occurring at the boundary between tumor and adjacent tissue may contribute to the formation of CS type-2.

Concluding the discussion, we would like to point out some differences in the morphology of CS type-1 in intestinal and diffuse types of GC (Senchukova et al, 2015):

- In the intestinal type of GC the desquamated epithelium of tumor glands was observed in the lumen of CS, while in the diffuse type – there were fragments of tumor tissue.

- In the intestinal type of GC the wall of CS was likely the basement membrane bordering the tumor stroma, while in the diffuse one - the tumor cells. We believe that the revealed features are associated with the differences of the biological properties of the tumor cells themselves and their microenvironment. Worthy of note are some features of intestinal and diffuse types of GC which, in our opinion, are able to influence the mechanism of the formation of CS type-1:

- The increased synthesis of thrombospondin in diffuse adenocarcinomas. Thrombospondin-4 is a glycoprotein of the extracellular matrix involved in the regulation of the adhesive properties of tumor cells. Its highest intensity of expression was observed within the extracellular matrix surrounding the tumor cells in the fields of high tumor cell density and invasion (Forster, 2011).

- The significantly higher levels of MMP-1, MMP-7, VEGF and E-cadherin in diffuse type of GC (Zhou *et al.*, 2010; Kuang *et al.*, 2013).

- A higher incidence of positive expression of integrin beta3 mRNA in diffuse type of GC (Li *et al.*, 2008). It must be noted that integrins are cell adhesion molecules, which mediate cell-cell adhesion or cell-extracellular matrix adhesion and are essential for invasion and metastasis of carcinoma cells. These authors have demonstrated the relationship between integrin β3 mRNA and VEGF protein expression, MVD and 5-year survival rate of gastric carcinoma patients.

4   Conclusion

The results of this study testify that the vessels in the tumor stroma and adjacent GM differ both in structure and clinical significance.

From scientific and practical points of view, two types of vessels the presence of which correlates with clinical characteristics and long-term results of GC treatment are of the most interest: the dilated capillaries of GM and GS and the vessels of "cavitary" type. A distinguishing feature of the dilated capillaries is that both the endothelium of normal structure and the cells with large, pale nuclei with fine-netted chromatin structure take part in their formation. The phenotypical features of the nuclei of cells lining dilated capillaries testify that EPCs could participate in the formation of these vessels. The relationship of the described vessels with the presence of lymph metastases allows them to be considered as a factor in the progression of GC.

As for our hypothesis of the "cavitary" type of angiogenesis, the obtained data indicate that this type of vascular formation possibly plays a key role in the progression of GC. This follows from the fact that the presence of multiple CS type-1 is closely associated with the presence of metastases in RLN and the decrease of RFS and OS of patients with GC. It is conceivable that a violation of the adhesive properties of tumor cells, inflammatory changes in the tumor stroma and the adjacent GM and microvascular hyperpermeability is associated with the formation of CS type-1. We believe that further studies should be carried out to investigate the mechanism of the formation of the described vessels and their role in progression of GC.

Abbreviations

CS: "cavitary" structures; EPCs: endothelial progenitor cells; GC: gastric cancer; GM: gastric mucosa; GS: gastric submucosa; MMP: matrix metalloprotease; MV: microvessels; MVD: microvessel density; RLN: OS: overall survival; regional lymph nodes; RFS: relapse-free survival; VEGF: TIM: tumor-infiltrating macrophages; vascular endothelial growth factor

References

Acs, G., Dumoff, K.L., Solin, L.J., Pasha, T., Xu, X., & Zhang, P.J. (2007). *Extensive Retraction Artifact Correlates With Lymphatic Invasion and Nodal Metastasis and Predicts Poor Outcome in Early Stage Breast Carcinoma. Am J Surg Pathol, 31, 129–140.*

Acs, G., Paragh, G., Rakosy, Z., Laronga, C., & Zhang, P.J. (2012). *The extent of retraction clefts correlates with lymphatic vessel density and VEGF-C expression and predicts nodal metastasis and poor prognosis in early-stage breast carcinoma. Mod Pathol, 25(2), 163–177.*

Ahlskog, J., Paganelli, G., & Neri, D. (2006). *Vascular tumor targeting. Q J Nucl Med Mol Jmaging, 50, 296–309.*

An, J.Y., Baik, Y.H., Choi, M.G., Noh, J.H., Sohn, T.S., & Kim, S. (2007). *Predictive factors for lymph node metastasis in early gastric cancer with submucosal invasion: analysis of a single institutional experience. Ann Surg, 246(5), 749–53.*

Asahara, T., Masuda, H., Takahashi, T., Kalka, C., Pastore, C., Silver, M., Kearne, M., Magner, M., & Isner, J.M. (1999). *Bone marrow origin of endothelial cell progenitor cells responsible for postnatal vasculogenesis in physiological and pathological neovascularization. Circ Res, 85, 221–228.*

Baluk, P., Hashizume, H., & McDonald, D.M. (2005). *Cellular abnormalities of blood vessels as targets in cancer. Curr Opin Genet Dev, 15, 102–111.*

Baluk, P., Morikawa, S., Haskell, A., Mancuso, M., & McDonald, D.M. (2003). *Abnormalities of Basement Membrane on Blood Vessels and Endothelial Sprouts in Tumors. American Journal of Pathology, 163 (5), 1801–1815.*

Birau, A., Ceausu, R.A., Gaje, P., Raica, M., & Olariu, T. (2012). *Assessement of angiogenesis reveals blood vessel heterogeneity in lung carcinoma. Oncol Lett, 4(6), 1183–1186.*

Brown, A.P., Citrin, D.E., & Camphausen, K.A. (2008). *Clinical biomarkers of angiogenesis inchibichion. Cancer Metastasis Rev, 27 (3), 415–434.*

Burri, P.H., Hlushchuk, R., & Djonov, V. (2004). *Intussusceptive Angiogenesis: Its Emergence, Its Characteristics, and Its Significance. Developmental Dinamics, 231, 474–478.*

Chang, Y.S., di Tomaso, E., McDonald, D.M., Jones, R., Jain, R.K., & Munn, L.L. (2000). *Mosaic blood vessels in tumors: Frequency of cancer cells in contact with flowing blood. PNAS, 97(26), 14608–14613.*

De Narddo, D.G., Johansson, M., & Coussens, L.M. (2008). *Immune cells as mediators of solid tumor metastasis. Cancer Metastasis Rev, 27, 11–18.*

Ding, S., Li, C., Lin, S., Yang, Y., Liu, D., Han, Y., Zhang, Y., Li, L., Zhou, L., & Kumar, S. (2006). *Comparative evaluation of microvessel density determined by CD34 or CD105 in benign and malignant* gastric lesions. Hum Pathol, 37(7), 861–6.

Dome, B., Paku, S., Somlai, B., & Tímár, J. (2002). Vascularization of cutaneous melanoma involves vessel co-option and has clinical significance. J Pathol, 197(3), 355–62.

Dvorak, H.F., Brown, L.F., Detmar, M., & Dvorak, A.M. (1995). Vascular permeability factor/vascular endothelial growth factor, microvascular hyperpermeability, and angiogenesis. Am J Pathol, 146, 1029–1039.

Eiro, N. & Vizoso F.J. (2012). Inflammation and cancer. World J Gastrointest Surg, 4(3), 62–72.

Erenoglu, C., Akin, M.L., Uluutku, H., Tezcan, L., Yildirim, S., & Batkin, A. (2000). Angiogenesis predicts poor prognosis in gastric carcinoma. Dig Surg, 17(6), 581–586.

Ferrara, N. (2002). Timeline: VEGF and the quest for tumour angiogenesis factors. Nat Rev Cancer. 2, 795–803.

Folkman, J. (1998). Is tissue mass regulated by vascular endothelial cells? Prostate as the first evidence. Endocrinology, 139(2), 441–442.

Folkman. J. (2001). Can mosaic tumor vessels facilitate molecular diagnosis of cancer? Proc Natl Acad Sci U S A, 98(2), 398–400.

Forster, S., Gretschel, S., Jons, T., Yashiro, M., & Kemmner, W. (2011). THBS4, a novel stromal molecule of diffuse-type gastric adenocarcinomas, identified by transcriptome-wide expression profiling. Mod Pathol, 24(10): 1390–403.

Fukumura, D., Duda, D.G., Munn, L.L., & Jain, R.K. (2010). Tumor Microvasculature and Microenvironment: Novel Insights Through Intravital Imaging in Pre-Clinical Models. Microcirculation, 17(3), 206–225.

Gee, M.S., Procopio, W.N., Makonnen, S., Feldman, M.D., Yeilding, N.M., & Lee, W.M. (2003). Tumor Vessel Development and Maturation Impose Limits on the Effectiveness of AntiVascular Therapy. Am J Pathol, 162, 183–193.

Goddard, J.C., Sutton, C.D., Furness ,P.N., Kockelbergh, R.C., & O'Byrne, K.J. (2002). A computer image analysis system for microvessels density measurement in solid tumours. Angiogenesis, 5(1–2), 15–20.

Hillen F. & Griffioen A. (2007). Tumour vascularization: sprouting angiogenesis and beyond. Cancer and Metastasis Reviews, 26 (3–4), 489–502.

Hillen, F., van de Winkel, A., Creytens, D., Vermeulen, A.H., & Griffioen, A.W. (2006). Proliferating endothelial cells, but not microvessel density, are a prognostic parameter in human cutaneous melanoma. Melanoma Res, 16(5), 453–7.

Holash, J., Maisonpierre, P.C., Compton, D., Boland, P., Alexander, C.R., Zagzag, D., Yancopoulos, G.D., & Wiegand, S.J. (1999). Vessel cooption, regression, and growth in tumors mediated by angiopoietins and VEGF. Science, 5422, 1994–1998.

Kamoshida, G., Matsuda, A., Miura, R., Takashima, Y., Katsura, A., & Tsuji, T. (2013). Potentiation of tumor cell invasion by co-culture with monocytes accompanying enhanced production of matrix metalloproteinase and fibronectin. Clin Exp Metastasis, 30(3), 289–97.

Kamoshida, G., Matsuda, A., Sekine, W., Mizuno, H., Oku, T., Itoh, S., Irimura, T., & Tsuji, T. (2012). Monocyte differentiation induced by co-culture with tumor cells involves RGD-dependent cell adhesion to extracellular matrix. Cancer Let, 315(2), 145–52.

Kimura, T., Wang, J., Matsui, K., Imai, S., Yokoyama, S., Nishikawa, M., Ikehara, S., & Sonoda, Y. (2004). Proliferative and migratory potentials of human cord blood-derived CD34- severe combined *immunodeficiency repopulating cells that retain secondary reconstituting capacity. Int J Hematol, 79(4), 328–33.*

Kuang, R.G., Wu, H.X., Hao, G.X., Wang, J.W. & Zhou, C.J. (2013). Expression and significance of IGF-2, PCNA, MMP-7, and α-actin in gastric carcinoma with Lauren classification. Turk J Gastroenterol, 24(2): 99–108.

Lazar, D., Taban, S., Raika, M., Sporea, I., Cornianu, M., Goldiş, A., & Vernic, C. (2008). Immunohistochemical evaluation of the tumor neoangiogenesis as a prognostic factor for gastric cancers. Romanian Journal of Morphology and Embryology, 49(2), 137–148.

Less, J.R., Skalak, T.C., Sevick, E.M., & Jain, R.K. (1991). Microvascular architecture in a mammary carcinoma: branching patterns and vessel dimensions. Cancer Res, 5, 265–273.

Li, M., Gu, Y., Zhang, Z., Zhang, S., Zhang, D., Saleem, A.F., Zhao, X., & Sun, B. (2010). Vasculogenic mimicry: a new prognostic sign of gastric adenocarcinoma. Pathol Oncol Res, 16(2), 259–66.

Li, S.G., Ye, Z.Y., Zhao, Z.S., Tao, H.Q., Wang, Y.Y., & Niu, C.Y. (2008). Correlation of integrin beta3 mRNA and vascular endothelial growth factor protein expression profiles with the clinicopathological features and prognosis of gastric carcinoma. World J Gastroenterol, 14(3): 421–7.

Ma, J., Zhang, L., Ru, G.Q., Zhao, Z.S., & Xu, W.J. (2007). Upregulation of hypoxia inducible factor 1α mRNA is associated with elevated vascular endothelial growth factor expression and excessive angiogenesis and predicts a poor prognosis in gastric carcinoma. World J Gastroenterol, 13(11), 1680–1686.

Man, Y.G., Harley, R., Mason, J., & Gardner, W.A. (2010). Contributions of leukocytes to tumor invasion and metastasis: the "piggy-back" hypothesis. Cancer Epidem, 34, 3–6.

Man*, Y.G. (2010). Aberrant leukocyte infiltration: a direct trigger for breast tumor invasion and metastasis. Int J Biol Sci, 6(2), 129–32.

Man**, Y.G. (2010). Tumor cell budding from focally disrupted tumor capsules: a common pathway for all breast cancer subtype derived invasion? J Cancer, 1, 32–37.

Man***, Y.G. (2010). A seemingly most effective target for early detection and intervention of prostate tumor invasion. J Cancer, 1, 63–69.

Man, Y.G., Stojadinovic, A., Mason, J., Avital, I., Bilchik, A., Bruecher, B., Protic, M., Nissan, A., Izadjoo, M., Zhang, X., & Jewett, A. (2013). Tumor-Infiltrating Immune Cells Promoting Tumor Invasion and Metastasis: Existing Theories. J Cancer, 4(1), 84–95.

Maniotis, A.J., Folberg, R., Hess, A., Seftor, E.A., Gardner, L.M., Pe'er, J., Trent, J.M., Meltzer, P.S., & Hendrix, M.J. (1999). Vascular Channel Formation by Human Melanoma Cells in Vivo and in Vitro: Vasculogenic Mimicry. American Journal of Pathology, 155(3), 739–752.

Mantur, M. & Wojszel, J.(2008). Cell adhesion molecules and their participation in the process of inflammation and cancerogenesis. Pol Merkur Lekarski, 24(140), 177–80.

Millikan, K.W., Mall, J.W., Myers, J.A., Hollinger, E.F., Doolas, A., & Saclarides, T.J. (2000). Do angiogenesis and growth factor expression predict prognosis of esophageal cancer? Am Surg, 66, 401–405.

Morikawa, S., Baluk, P., Kaidoh, T., Haskell, A., Jain, R.K., & McDonald, D.M. (2002). Abnormalities in Pericytes on Blood Vessels and Endothelial Sprouts in Tumors. American Journal of Pathology, 160(3), 985–1000.

Nagy, J.A. & Dvorak, H.F. (2012). Heterogeneity of the tumor vasculature: the need for new tumor blood vessel type-specific targets. *Clin Exp Metastasis, 29(7), 657–62.*

Nagy, J.A., Dvorak, A.M., & Dvorak, H.F. (2012). *Vascular hyperpermeability, angiogenesis, and stroma generation. Cold Spring Harb Perspect Med, 2(2), a006544.*

Ohta, M., Kitadai, Y., & Tanaka, S. (2003). *Monocyte chemoattractant protein-1 expression correlates with macrophage infiltration and tumor vascularity in human gastric carcinomas. Int J Oncol, 22 (4), 773–8.*

Pawelek, J.M. & Chakraborty, A.K. (2008). *The cancer cell-leukocyte fusion theory of metastasis. Adv Cancer Res, 101, 397–444.*

Peng, C.W., Liu, X.L., Liu, X., & Li, Y. (2010). *Co-evolution of cancer microenvironment reveals distinctive patterns of gastric cancer invasion: laboratory evidence and clinical significancePollard J.W. (2009). Trophic macrophages in development and disease. Nat Rev Immunol, 9(4), 259–70.*

Poon, R.T., Fan, S.T., & Wong, J. (2003). *Clinical significance of angiogenesis in gastrointestinal cancers: a target for novel prognostic and therapeutic approaches. Ann Surg, 238, 9–28.*

Reiss, K., Ludwig, A., & Saftig P. (2006). *Breaking up the tie: disintegrin-like metalloproteinases as regulators of cell migration in inflammation and invasion. Pharmacol Ther, 111(3), 985–1006.*

Ribatti, D., Nico, B., Crivellato, E., & Vacca, A. (2007). *The structure of the vascular network of tumors. Cancer Lett,248(1), 18–23.*

Schreiber, R.D., Old, L.J., & Smyth M.J. (2011). *Cancer immunoediting: integrating immunity's roles in cancer suppression and promotion. Science, 331 (6024): 1565–70.*

Senchukova, M. & Kiselevsky, M.V. (2014). *The "Cavitary" type of angiogenesis by gastric cancer. Morphological characteristics and prognostic value, J Cancer, 5 (5), 311–319.*

Senchukova, M., Ryabov, A., Karmakova, T., Tomchuk, O., & Stadnikov, A. (2015) *The morphological features of "cavitary" type angiogenesis in diffuse and intestinal types of gastric cancer and its relationship with tumor-infiltrating immune cells. BJMMR, 7 (4), 272–284.*

Shen, L., Huang, Y., Sun, M., Xu, H., Wei, W., & Wu, W. (2009). *Clinicopathological features associated with lymph node metastasis in early gastric cancer: analysis of a single-institution experience in China. Can J Gastroenterol, 23(5), 353–6.*

Sica, A., Schioppa, T., Mantovani, A., Allavena, F. (2006). *Tumour-associated macrophages are a distinct M2 polarised population promoting tumour progression: potential targets of anti-cancer therapy. Eur J Cancer, 42, 717–27.*

Sussman, L. K., Upalakalin, J. N., Roberts, M. J., Kocher, O., & Benjamin, L.E. (2003). *Blood markers for vasculogenesis increase with tumor progression in patients with breast carcinoma. Cancer Biology Therapy, 2, 255–256.*

Torres, C., Wang, H., Turner, J., Shahsafaei, A., & Odze, R.D. (1999). *Prognostic significance and effect of chemoradiotherapy on microvessel density (angiogenesis) in esophageal Barrett's esophagus-associated adenocarcinoma and squamous cell carcinoma. Hum Pathol, 30, 753–758.*

Vermeulen, P.B., Gasparini, G., Fox, S.B., Colpaert, C., Marson, L.P., Gion, M., Beliën, J.A., de Waal, R.M., Van Marck, E., Magnani, E., Weidner, N., Harris, A.L., & Dirix, L.Y. (2002). *Second international consensus on the methodology and criteria of evaluation of angiogenesis quantification in solid human tumours. Eur J Cancer, 38, 1564–1579.*

Wang, W., Lin, P., Han, C., Cai, W., Zhao, X., & Sun, B. (2010). *Vasculogenic mimicry contributes to lymph node metastasis of laryngeal squamous cell carcinoma. J Exp Clin Cancer Res, 29, 60.*

Wang, Y.D., Wu, P., Mao, J.D., Huang, H., & Zhang, F. (2007). *Relationship between vascular invasion and microvessel density and micrometastasis. World J Gastroenterol, 46 (13), 6269–6273.*

Wu Y. & Zhou B.P. (2009). *Inflammation: a driving force speeds cancer metastasis. Cell Cycle, 8(20), 3267–3273.*

Yokota, T., Ishiyama, S., Saito, T., Teshima, S., Narushima, Y., Murata, K., Iwamoto, K., Yashima, R., Yamauchi, H., & Kikuchi, S. (2004). *Lymph node metastasis as a significant prognostic factor in gastric cancer: a multiple logistic regression analysis. Scand J Gastroenterol, 39(4), 380–4.*

Zaorsky, N.G., Patil, N., Freedman, G.M., & Tuluc, M. (2012). *Differentiating lymphovascular invasion from retraction artifact on histological specimen of breast carcinoma and their implications on prognosis. J Breast Cancer, 15(4), 478–80.*

Zeng, W., Gouw, A.S., van den Heuvel, M.C., Molema, G., Poppema, S., van der Jagt, E.J., & de Jong, K.P. (2010). *Hepatocellular carcinomas in cirrhotic and noncirrhotic human livers share angiogenic characteristics. Ann Surg Oncol, 17(6), 1564–71.*

Zhao, H.E., Qin, R., Chen, X.X., Sheng, X., Sheng, X., Wu, J.F., Wang, D.B., & Chen, G.H. (2006). *Microvessel density is a prognostic marker of human gastric cancer. World J Gastroenterol, 47 (12), 7598–7603.*

Zhou, Y., Li, G., Wu, J., Zhang, Z., Wu, Z., Fan, P., Hao, T., Zhang, X., Li, M., Zhang, F., Li, Q., Lu, B., & Qiao, L. (2010). *Clinicopathological significance of E-cadherin, VEGF, and MMPs in gastric cancer. Tumour Biol, 31(6): 549–58.*

Chapter 4

Tumor Regression – A Capital Feature in Rectal Cancer Therapy Decision Tree

Marisa D. Santos[1] and Carlos Lopes[1]

1 Introduction

Treatment of locally advanced rectal cancer (LARC) is one of the biggest challenges in digestive oncology. Results depend on appropriate plan based on neoadjuvant therapy and/or curative surgery. Customized therapy must consider also biological data and tumor chemoradiotherapy response, although their real utility is not yet well known and they are poorly predictable. Until new advances in knowledge come, neoadjuvant chemoradiation followed by TME surgery and systemic chemotherapy still remains standard care for LARC. To identify prognostic factors in LARC treated with neoadjuvant chemoradiation has become a major goal of several studies and may contribute to clarify some issues that remain open, such as: which patients actually benefit from neoadjuvant CRT, how to identify CRT "bad responders", how to identify patients at high risk of recurrence.

Tumor regression grades are important scales to assess tumor chemoradiotherapy response. They allow the identification of patients groups with "good" and "poor" response according different prognosis of each one. So, Tumor Regression Grades can influence locally advanced rectal cancer therapy decision tree.

2 Colorectal Cancer and Locally Advanced Rectal Cancer (LARC)

---

[1] Department of Surgery, Centro Hospitalar do Porto, I.C.B.A.S., University of Porto, Portugal.

Colorectal cancer is a major cause of mortality throughout the World. It accounts for over 9% of all cancer incidences, being the third most common cancer in developed countries and the fourth most common cause of death.

About one third of colorectal cancer is located in the rectum. This location, especially if in the middle or lower rectum, has therapeutic and survival implications.

Surgery remains the primary therapeutic tool in the treatment of rectal cancer, and with the practice of mesorectum complete excision (TME) in cancers of the middle and lower rectum, it was possible to reduce the locoregional recurrence (Heald et al., 1982; Kiss et al., 2011; Maurer et al., 2011; MacFarlane et al., 1993). However, concerning locally advanced rectal cancer (LARC) this approach has proved insufficient in maintaining levels of locoregional recurrence between 4 and 6% (Kapiteijn et al., 2001; Sauer et al., 2004) and neoadjuvant therapeutic should be considered before surgery.

3   Neoadjuvant Therapy in LARC

Neoadjuvant chemoradiation (CRT) followed by total mesorectum excision (TME) surgery and systemic chemotherapy remains the standard of care for locally advanced rectal cancer, but not all cases benefit from this treatment modality.

Sauer et al. (2012) reported a persisting significant improvement of pre, versus postoperative CRT on local control, although without improving overall survival. Improved survival is achieved only in situations of good or complete pathological response to chemoradiation (Lee et al., 2013b; Martin et al., 2012a). Neoadjuvant CRT allows reduction of regional recurrences (improves pelvic disease control), and survival increases when there is complete pathological response (ypCR) (Martin et al., 2012b). The rate of response is better in neoadjuvant CRT compared with long course RT, and possibly absent in short course RT with immediate surgery. In fact, maximal response of the radiation occurs only several weeks after its end (de Campos-Lobato et al., 2011a). For that reason surgery has been delayed until 8–12 weeks following neoadjuvant CRT (Pettersson et al., 2010; 2012; Siegel et al., 2009).

The use of neoadjuvant CRT leading to tumor shrinkage increases the likelihood of performing a sphincter preserving surgery and increases circumferential and distal margins in surgical specimen with reduction of lymphatic and vascular invasion (Bernstein et al., 2009; Das et al., 2007; Gosens et al., 2008; Kim et al., 2002; Lindebjerg et al., 2009; Rullier et al., 2005). Chemoradiation induces a tumor downstaging effect, which potentially improves the feasibility of a complete resection with benefits in local disease control. However the type and remission rate to neoadjuvant CRT remains considerably variable. While some patients may not respond, others may even have progression of disease. Other group of patients experience downstaging and 15–25% has surgical specimens without any viable tumor cells, a condition referred to as pathologic complete response (ypCR) (Bateman et al., 2009; Rodel et al., 2005).

4   Tumor Regression Grading Systems

Tumor response to neoadjuvant CRT can induce cytoreduction and downstaging of the lesion and can also cause histological changes that can be assessed by tumor regression systems, which in turn offer another method for evaluating tumor regression.

Tumor regression grades evaluate tumor response to neoadjuvant treatment, mainly in CRT. There are several tumor regression systems trying to quantify the response to CRT and ultimately to have a prognostic value (Bateman et al., 2009; Dworak et al., 1997; Jacobi et al., 1997).

In order to quantify neoadjuvant CRT response, several grades can be used, being particularly important in situations where the pathological response is not complete (Dworak et al., 1997; Glynne-Jones et al., 2006; Junker, 2004; Mandard et al., 1994; Rodel et al., 2005; Wheeler et al., 2002; Williams et al., 2009;). Most have 3 to 5 levels, allowing group creation according to the responses (Table 1) (Bateman et al., 2009; Dworak et al., 1997; Mandard et al., 1994).

There is no consensual regression grading system for surgical specimens with resected tumor specimens after neoadjuvant chemoradiotherapy. A common, largely accepted, standardized and validated TRG system does not exist, so the published systems vary in the definition of categories, interfering with studies results.This lack of consensus impeaches clinical management and leaves clinicians without a uniform scoring regression system that could guide their decisions.

In our experience definition of "near complete response" makes the difference in terms of accuracy of prognosis. "Good responders" are the patients with complete or near complete response, all the others are "bad responders". TRG Mandard proved to be a good system for that definition as we try to demonstrate.

5   The Association of Tumor Response and Prognosis

The value of tumor regression grading systems, as an independent prognostic factor for disease-free survival has been demonstrated in several studies (Dhadda et al., 2011; Lee et al., 2013b; Suarez et al., 2008; Vecchio et al., 2005).

Association of tumor response and prognosis has been previously reported. Previous reports have focused on specific T or N downstaging and included in their analysis ypCR (Chan et al., 2005; de Campos-Lobato et al., 2010; Park et al., 2012). Other authors have emphasized the value of tumor regression grade, which could more accurately reflect tumor response at a cellular level (Dworak et al., 1997; Mandard et al., 1987; Wheeler et al., 2004).

In our series we evaluated the accuracy of Mandard and Dworak systems in rectal cancer neoadjuvant chemoradiotherapy (CRT) as a prognostic factor, mainly for patients who achieved a near complete response (Santos et al., 2014). Between 2003 and 2011, we treated 139 patients with locally advanced rectal cancer (LARC) who received neoadjuvant CRT followed by total mesorectum excision (TME).

Mandard et al.	Becker et al.	Rectal Cancer Regression Grading (RCRG) system	RCPath dataset for colorectal cancer (Royal College of Pathologits)	Dworak et al.	Rödel et al.
1. No viable cancer cells, complete response	1.A No residual tumor/tumor bed and chemotherapy effect	1. Sterilisation or only microscopic foci of adenocarcinoma remaining, with marked fibrosis	A. No residual tumor cells and/or mucus lakes only	0. No regression	0. No regression
2. Single cells or small groups of cancer cells	1.B <10% Residual tumor/tumor bed and chemotherapy effect	2. Marked fibrosis but macroscopic disease present	B. Minimal residual tumor, that is, only occasional microscopic foci are identified with difficulty	1. Dominant tumor mass with obvious fibrosis and/or vasculopathy	1. Regression of <25% of tumor mass
3. Residual cancer outgrown by fibrosis	2. 10–50% Residual tumor/tumor bed and chemotherapy effect	3.Little or no fibrosis, with abundant macroscopic disease	c. No marked regression	2. Dominant tumor mass with obvious fibrosis and/or vasculopathy	2. Regression of 25–50% tumor mass
4. Significant fibrosis outgrown by cancer	3. >50% Residual tumor/tumor bed ± chemotherapy effect			3. Very few (difficult to find microscopically) tumor cells in fibrotic tissue with or without mucus substance	3. Regression of >50% tumor mass
5. No fibrosis with extensive residual cancer				4. Complete regression	4. Complete regression

Table 1: Examples for tumor regression grading systems. (dark tone – complete or near complete response; light tone – incomplete or absent response).

Aspects of this series, namely characteristics of the patients, surgical results, pathological findings, as well as the detailed protocols of CRT are described elsewhere (Santos et al., 2013, 2014).

They were reassessed for disease recurrence and survival; the specimens' slides were reviewed and classified according to two tumor regression grading (TRG) systems: Mandard and Dworak. Based on these TRG scores, two patient groups were created: patients with good response versus patients with poor response (Mandard TRG1+2 versus Mandard TRG3+4+5 and Dworak TRG4+3 versus Dworak TRG2+2+10) (Figure 1 and 2).

Overall survival (OS), disease-free survival (DFS), and disease recurrence were then evaluated. The mean age was 64.2 years and median follow up was 56 months. No significant survival difference was found when comparing patients with Dworak TRG 4+3 versus Dworak TRG2+1+0(p = 0.10). MandardTRG1+2 presented significantly better OS and DFS than Mandard TRG3+4+5 (OS p = 0.013; DFS p = 0.007).

Mandard system provides higher accuracy over Dworak system in predicting rectal cancer prognosis when neoadjuvant CRT is applied for tumor regression. Mandard TRG proved effective in identifying subgroups with different responses. In our studies Mandard system was applied, which essentially counts the number of residual tumor cells in TGR2. (Figure 1). TRG1 identifies a complete response (ypCR).

In our series the application of the Mandard system allowed identification of two subgroups of patients with different impact in terms of survival (Figure 3 and 4).

5.1 Complete Pathological Response and "Near Complete"

Tumor regression can range from zero evidence of treatment efficacy, to a complete response (ypCR) with no viable tumor cells identified. It is well established that patients with pCR after chemoradiation have better long-term outcomes than those without pCR (Capirci et al., 2008; Maas et al., 2010; Martin et al., 2010a). Complete pathological response leads to excellent locoregional management as it provides an increase in survival for stage I values, i.e. 90% at 5 years (Bosset et al., 2005, 2006; Capirci et al., 2006, 2008; Stipa et al., 2006). Based on these data there are centers that in case of a ypCR advocate a policy of "wait and see" reserving surgical resection only for cases of "tumor escape". The published results of these centers refer survival rates equal to or greater than those achieved in ypCR patients with resection (de Campos-Lobato et al., 2011b; Habr-Gama et al., 2009, 2010, 2011).

Complete response, however, accounts for less than one third of the patients, and the majority of patients present either partial or no response at all. The prognostic value of partial or near complete response is an important topic and research is underway (Lee et al., 2013b; Valentini, 2011).

While there is substantial data regarding the relationship between ypCR and improved oncologic outcomes, the prognostic significance of "near complete" re-

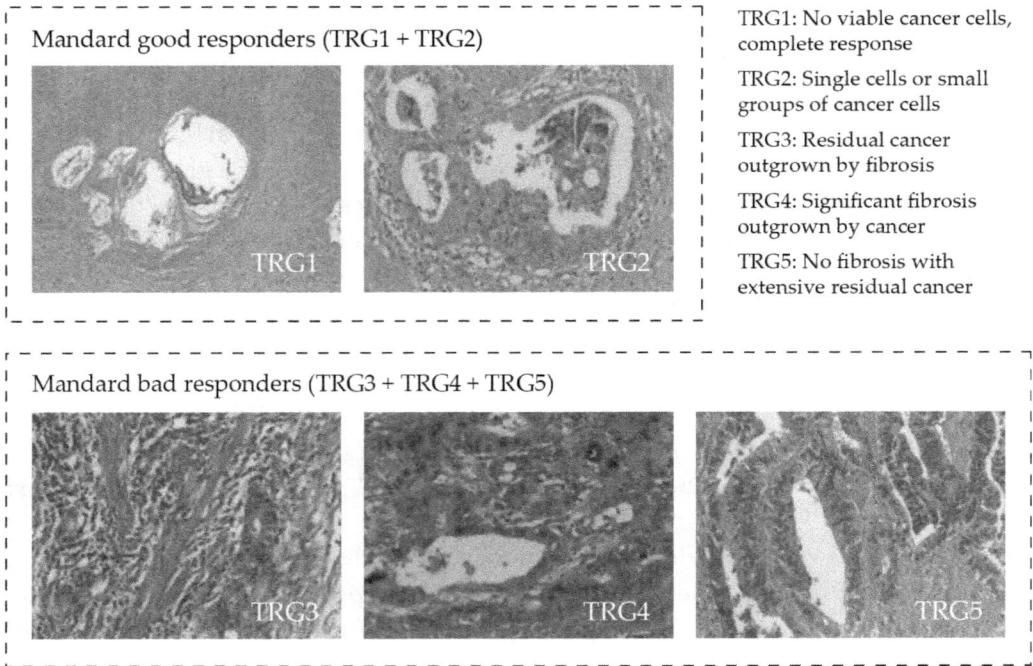

TRG1: No viable cancer cells, complete response

TRG2: Single cells or small groups of cancer cells

TRG3: Residual cancer outgrown by fibrosis

TRG4: Significant fibrosis outgrown by cancer

TRG5: No fibrosis with extensive residual cancer

Figure 1: Mandard TRG system.

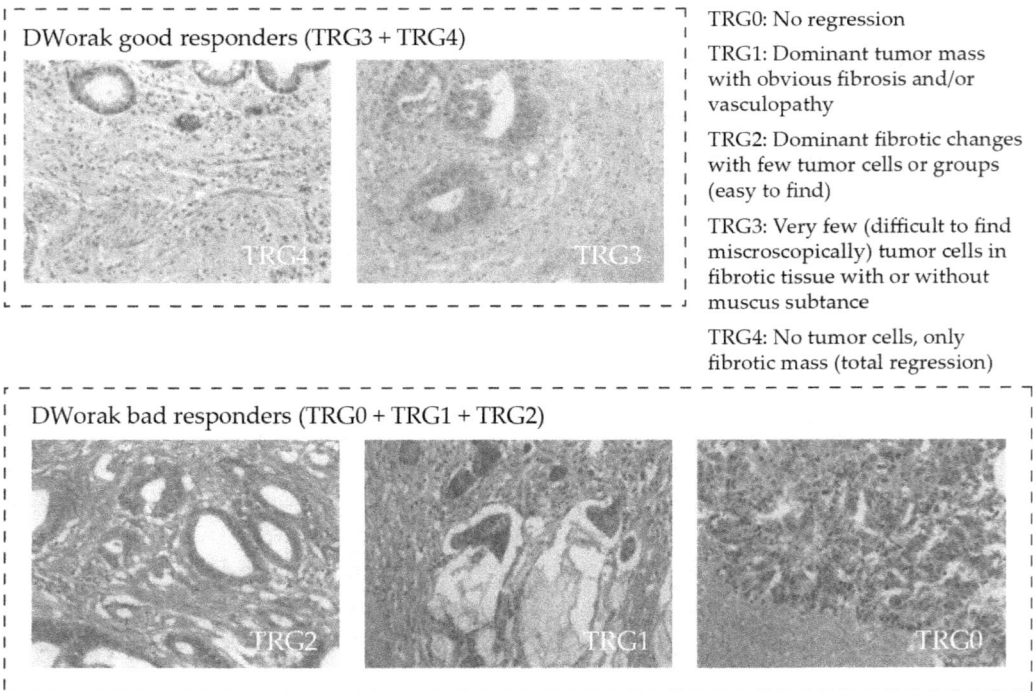

TRG0: No regression

TRG1: Dominant tumor mass with obvious fibrosis and/or vasculopathy

TRG2: Dominant fibrotic changes with few tumor cells or groups (easy to find)

TRG3: Very few (difficult to find miscroscopically) tumor cells in fibrotic tissue with or without muscus subtance

TRG4: No tumor cells, only fibrotic mass (total regression)

Figure 2: Dworak TRG system.

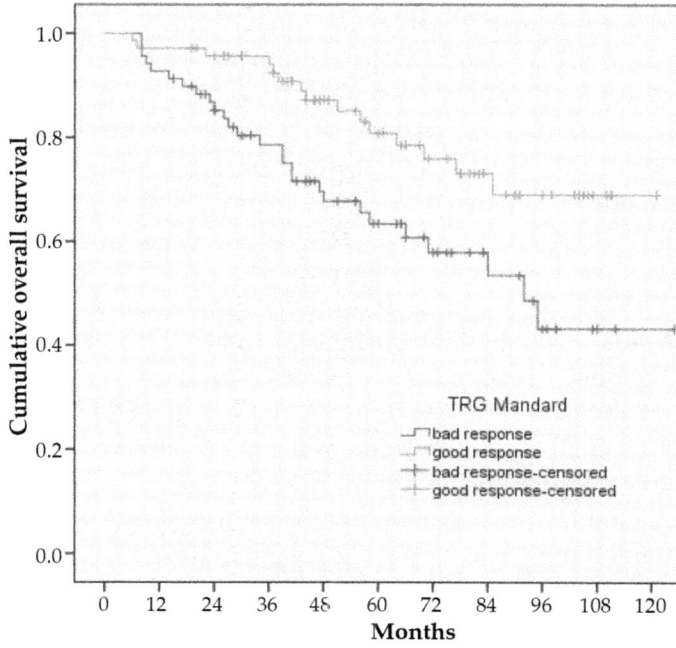

Figure 3: Five–year Overall survival (OS).

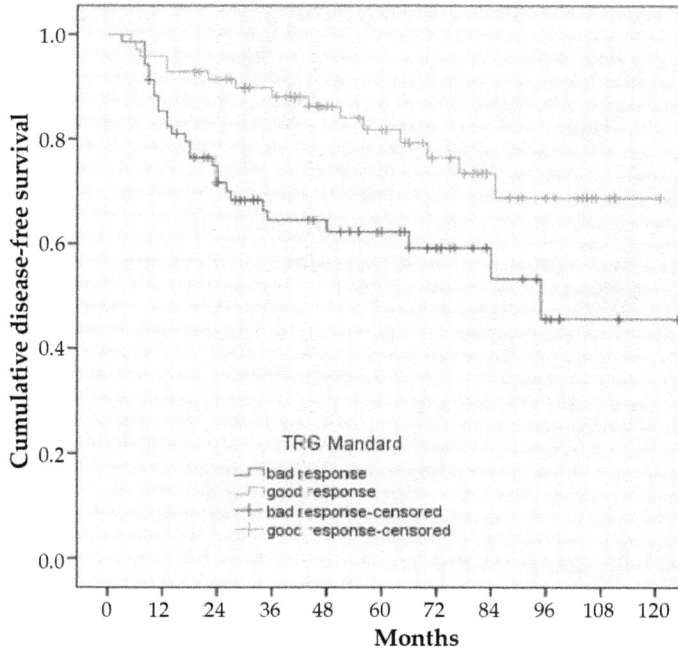

Figure 4: Five-year disease free survival (DFS).

sponse to CRT has not been extensively evaluated (Lee et al., 2013b). In the most studies only the presence of a pathological complete response is correlated to better long outcome and survival improvement (Martin et al., 2012a).

In our data the outcome for patients with a near complete response (Mandard TRG2 or Dworak TRG3) is almost similar to the outcome for patients with complete response (Mandard TRG1 or Dworak TRG4). This result suggests that it may be possible to combine tumors into a group of good responders (Mandard TRG1+2/Dworak TRG4+3) and a group of poor responders (Mandard TRG3+4+5/Dworak TRG2+1+0), since those who show significant histopathological regression and complete pathologic regression have a similarly better prognosis than the remaining poorly responding patients.

This kind of division was also used by other authors (Arredondo et al., 2013; Dhadda et al., 2011; Rodel et al., 2005; Suarez et al., 2008). Beddy et al. (2008) used Mandard TRG and observed better DFS in the combined group of patients having either complete response or near complete response (TRG0 + TRG1) when compared with the remaining patients. Dhadda et al. (2011) applied Mandard system and the results obtained suggested improved DFS and OS after preoperative CRT in TRG2 versus TRG3 in Cox regression analysis. Others series with different TGR system and multivariate analyses failed to demonstrate the prognostic value of TRG for DFS (Bujko et al., 2010; Rodel et al., 2005).

In our opinion, Mandard TRG2 (near complete response) identifies a larger number of patients with better prognosis than Dworak TRG3. This finding may explain the better correlation between Mandard grading and disease prognosis, rather than with Dworak grading.

Good responders have higher 5-year overall survival and 5-year disease free survival than poor responders, albeit these results are statistically significant only when Mandard system is considered. In our analysis a good response, defined as Mandard 1 and 2 classifications, was present in 70 of the 139 patients receiving CRT (50.4%). These patients were associated with lower locoregional recurrence and improved survival when compared with Mandard bad responders.

Therefore, association of ypCR with near complete response (good responders) maintains similar prognostic to ypCR alone in patients with LARC (Table 2).

In previews studies, Mandard system proved to be a good determinant of outcome, when cases were grouped into TRG1+2 (good responders) and TRG3+4+5 (poor responders). This methodology proved superior than division in groups ypCR (TRG1) versus all other (TRG2–5) regarding DFS and OS (Santos et al., 2013).

5.2   Poor Pathological Response

Chemoradiation induces a tumor downstaging effect, which potentially improves the probability of complete resection and sphincter-preserving surgery, with benefit in local control. However, some patients still develop distant and/or local recurrence with survival compromise, particularly those with a poor pathological tumor response. According to data we identified a subset of patients where the neoadju-

CRT (n=139)		
Five years overall survival	Mandard good response (TRG1-2)	80.8% (se =5.3%)
	Mandard bad response (TRG3-5)	63.4% (se=6.4%) p=0.013[a]
	ypCR (Mandard TRG1)	80.4% (se=8.9)
	Mandard partial response (TRG2)	81.0% (se=6.7) p=0.77[a]
Five years DFS	Mandard good response (TRG1-2)	81.7% (se=5.1%)
	Mandard bad response (TRG3-5)	61.7% (se=6.3%) p=0.007[a]
	ypCR (Mandard TRG1)	80.1% (se=9.1%)
	Mandard partial response (TRG2)	82.8% (se=6.1%) p=0.71[a]

Table 2: TRG and clinical long term outcome. Univariable analysis. Follow-up: mean – 56 months (range : 6–125); (se – standard error ; [a] Log Rank test).

vant CRT has the maximum effect and better prognosis (subgroup with higher number of patients than ypCR) and a subgroup of poorer prognosis where other therapeutic regimens will be need to improved survival.

The ability to predict a response, either before treatment or during its early stages, could spare "poor responders" patients to stress and expense of undergoing treatment from which they will derive no benefit. Instead, these patients would be candidates for more intensive treatment strategies. Identifying "poor responders" only in post-treatment may also be an indicator for a different and more intensive adjuvant therapy. Nowadays, individualizing the treatment approach in locally advanced rectal cancer is a demanding goal to achieve.

6   Mandard Good/Poor Responders and other Potential Prognostic Factors

In LARC, traditional pretreatment clinical prognostic factors identified in others studies such as age, gender, clinical stage, tumor mobility, circumference of the rectal wall involved in the tumor, tumor distance from anal verge, are poorly associated with survival, except preoperative CEA levels and surgery procedure (Kim et al., 2012; Lee et al., 2013a; Reshef et al., 2012; Wallin et al., 2013; Yeo et al., 2012).

When neoadjuvant CRT is used, the prognosis factors are usually related with downstaging and tumor response.

Tumor downstaging, pathological TNM stage, CMR of surgical specimen and TGR value reflected on neoadjuvant CRT tumor response and are considered in several studies the main prognostic factors of survival (Capirci et al., 2008; Martin et al., 2012a, 2012c; Luna-Perez et al., 2003; Quah et al., 2008; Rullier et al., 2010; Yeo et al., 2010, 2012).

In most studies, pathologic T category and nodal status after neoadjuvant CRT still remain the most important independent prognostic factors for DFS (Kim et al., 2010b; Klos et al, 2011; Madbouly et al., 2013; Rodel et al., 2005). The reason for these different results in literature can be related to several differences: number of patients of the studies, follow-up interval, inclusion criteria of patients, regimens of neoadjuvant CRT, time- interval between CRT and surgery, R1 definition, TRG system used and different adjuvant therapy protocols.

In our series we analyzed those variables in the TRG groups created. The presence of a good response in either one of the two systems did not have an impact in terms of sphincter preservation surgery. When response was good in both TRG , an estimated 78.5% reduction of positive lymph nodes was achieved when clinical values were compared (uN + = 28) against pathological ones (ypN + = 6). These aspects contributed to lowering locoregional and distant recurrence in good responders. It is possible that the impact of a good response in obtaining radial margins greater than 1 mm and the reduction of the number of positive lymph nodes and the pathological T stage have contributed in an effective way to increase the survival of this subgroup (Santos et al., 2013).

In our latest data (study with the same drawing but with more patients 167 and not yet published) the clinical parameters and biopsies characteristics don`t have prognostic value (Table 3 and 4) only pathological parameters (Table 5).

We identified independent significance for overall disease (Mandard TRG response) and also for disease-free survival in Mandard TRG response and ypN stage. Patients with bad response (Mandard TRG3-5) had HR of death 3.79 higher than patients with good response for overall survival (p=0.013); patients with Mandard bad response (TRG3-5) and ypN+ had HR of death 3.90 higher than patients with Mandard good response and ypN0 (p=0. 017 and p=0.021, respectively).

Mandard TRG response, which shows the CRT effect, seems to be a prognostic factor that, along with TNM stage, predicts the survival and recurrence rates.

7   Predictive Factors to Mandard Response

The influence of clinical parameters in tumor response has been widely studied. In some studies, tumor size, tumor circumferential extent, poor differentiation, mucinous tumor, distance from anal verge, clinical T stage, nodal clinical stage, tumor downstaging, pretreatment carcinoembryonic antigen (CEA) level and or interval of time between surgery and radiotherapy completion were associated with CRT tumor response (Das et al., 2007; Farnault et al., 2011; Huh et al., 2013; Moureau-Zabotto et al., 2011; Oberholzer et al., 2012; Qiu et al., 2011; Tulchinsky et al., 2008; Yan et al., 2011; Yang et al., 2013).

Magnetic resonance imaging (MRI) and positron emission tomography-computed tomography (PET-CT) also may be useful to predict the response at early stages (Dietz et al., 2008; Everaert et al., 2011; Ippolito et al., 2012; Jung et al., 2012; Meng et al., 2014; Shanmugan et al., 2012). Emerging evidence has shown the prognostic importance of reassessing rectal cancers using high-resolution T2- weighted MRI after completion of CRT (Dresen et al., 2009; Franklin et al., 2012; Patel et al.,

Variable		N (%)
Age	Mean	64.62
	Range	(29–83)
Gender	Male	105 (62.9)
	Female	62 (37.1)
Tumor lengh	< 4 cm	41 (24.6)
	≥ 4 cm and < 6 cm	85 (50,8)
	≥ 6 cm	41 (24.6)
Tumor circumference	≤ 1/3	27 (16.2)
	> 1/3 and ≤ 1/2	59 (35.3)
	> 1/2 and ≤ 2/3	39 (23.4)
	> 2/3 and ≤ 3/3	42 (25.1)
Distance from anal verge	> 6cm	79 (47.3)
	≤ 6cm	88 (52.7)
CEA pre-CRT	< 5	116 (69.5)
	≥ 5	44 (26.3)
	missing	7 (4.2)
cT stage	2–3	152 (91.0)
	4	15 (9.0)
Clinical stage	II	75 (44.9)
	III	92 (55.1)
CEA post-CRT	< 5	141 (84.4)
	≥ 5	14 (8.4)
	missing	12 (7.2)
Surgery procedure	AAR/SSO	108 (64.7)
	AAP /others	59 (35.3)
Surgery	open	129 (77.2)
	laparoscopic	38 (22.8)
Perioperative complications	morbidity	42 (25.1)
	abdominal or pelvic abscess	16 (9.5)
	anastomose leak	3 (1,7)
	reoperation	6 (3.5)
	readmission	3 (1.7)

Table 3: Clinical parameters.

Variable		N (%)
grade	1	46 (27.5)
	2	98 (58.7)
	3	8 (4.8)
	missing	15 (9.0)
mucinous presence	no	145 (86.8)
	yes	7 (4.2)
	missing/not applied	15 (9.0)
mitosis number	≤ 9,5	34 (20.4)
	≥ 9,6	117 (70.0)
	missing /not applied	16 (9.6)
inflammatory infiltrate	scarce	33 (19.8)
	moderated	66 (39.5)
	marked	52 31.1)
	missing/not applied	16 (9.6)
desmoplastic reaction	scarce	44 (26.3)
	moderated	80 (47.9)
	marked	27 (16.2)
	missing/not applied	16 (9.6)
necrosis degree	scarce	79 (47.3)
	moderated	40 (23.9)
	marked	32 (19.2)
	missing/ not applied	16 (9.6)

Table 4: Biopsies characteristics.

Variables		n	5-year Overall survival (standard error)	P value (Log rank test)	5-Year Disease free survival (standard error)	P value (Log rank test)
Mandard response	TRG1-2 good response	86	0.850 (0.044)		0.836(0.046)	
	TRG3-5 bad response	81	0.559 (0.067)	<0.001	0.566(0.065)	<0.001
CRM distance	>2 mm	159	0.737(0.041)		0.723(0.041)	
	≤2 & >1mm	8	0.281(0.222)	0.066	0.500(0.177)	0.089
ypT stage	0–2	62	0.828(0.055)		0.826(0.056)	
	3–4	105	0.551(0.077)	0.031	0.641(0.054)	0.055
ypN stge	0	110	0.806(0.044)		0.786(0.046)	
	1–2	57	0.551(0.077)	0.002	0.569(0.073)	<0.001
T downstaging	Yes	67	0.793(0.059)		0.790(0.050)	
	No	100	0.670(0.055)	0.110	0.656(0.054)	0.053
Pathological TNM downstaging	Yes	96	0.802(0.050)		0.795(0.050)	
	No	71	0.619(0.064)	0.091	0.597(0.064)	0.019
Differentiation grade in resected specimen	0 + 1	52	0.852(0.061)		0.852(0.070)	
	2 + 3	115	0.665(0.050)	0.033	0.649(0.050)	0.015

Table 5: Shows survival variables with p value <0.15 (Log Rank test)

2012;). Reassessment of MRI scans after preoperative therapy has implications for surgical planning, the timing of surgery, sphincter preservation, deferral of surgery for good responders, and development of further preoperative treatments for radiologically identified poor responders. However MRI findings depends when is realized and the ability of MRI to differentiate tumor from fibrosis post-treatment. On post-CRT T2- weighted MRI, we found that areas of fibrosis have very low signal intensity, whereas areas of residual tumor have intermediate signal-intensity, which can be difficult to interpret. We haven't yet in our data sufficient number of MRI pre and post chemoradiation capable of predict tumor response and we do not use PET-CT as routine .

However, no clinical parameters with prediction value of CRT response have been consistently identified. The results are often unlike (Choi et al., 2012; Kim et al., 2010a; Kim et al., 2013; Qiu et al., 2011; Yang et al., 2013).

In our last series (study with 167 patients not yet published), distance from anal verge is the only clinical parameter in univariate analysis with predictive value for Mandard response: distal tumors (≤ 6 cm from anal verge) show a better response according to Mandard (Table 6).

Variables		n	Bad responders % (Mandard TRG3–5)	Odds ratio	p
Distance from anal verge	≤6 cm	86	58.0	1.00	
	>6 cm	81	39.5	2.11 (1.14–3.92)	0.017
Mitosis number in resected spec-imen	≤ 9,5	73	32.9	1.00	
	≥ 9,6	68	77.9	7.21 (3.40–15.32)	<0.001
Necrosis grade in resected speci-men	scarce	27	77.8	10.36 (3.76–28.57)	<0.001
	moderate	38	92.1	34.53 (9.76–122.41)	<0.001
	marked	99	25.3	1.00	<0.001
CRM distance	≥2 mm	159	45.9	1.00	
	<2 & >1mm	8	100	2.18 (1.84–2.58)	0.003
ypT stage	0–1	38	7.9	1.00	
	2–4	129	60.5	17.84 (5.21–61.09	<0.001
ypN stge	0	110	32.7	1.00	
	1–2	57	78.9	7.71 (3.64–16.34)	<0.001
Pathological stage	0–I	58	15.5	1.00	<0.001
	II	58	55.2	6.70 (2.78–16.14)	<0.001
	III	51	78.4	19.80 (7.47–52.48)	<0.001
T downstaging	Yes	67	23.9	1.00	
	No	100	65.0	5.92	<0.001
Pathological TNM downstag-ing	Yes	96	34.4	1.00	
	No	70	67.1	3.90	<0.001
Reduction of number mitosis	Yes	83	41.0	1.00	
	No	52	73.1	3.91 (1.84–8.30)	<0.001
Differentiation grade in resected specimen	0 + 1	52	15.4	1.00	
	2 + 3	115	63.5	9.56	<0.001

Table 6: Preditive value of clinical and pathological characteristics to Mandard response

This result is concordant with the described by Das et al. (2007) The opposite is described by Restivo et al. (2013) The delay of surgery after radiotherapy completion in 8 to 12 weeks seems to increase tumor necrosis grade and pathological complete response (ypCR) rate up to 30 to 40% (de Campos-Lobato et al., 2011a; Habr-Gama et al., 2008; Garcia-Aguilar et al., 2011; Willett & Czito, 2008). We have 18.5% of ypCR but we can't study this variable because our patients were operated around 8 weeks after radiotherapy conclusion.

Pretreatment CEA level is probably the most cited clinical parameter as having tumor response predictive value (Das et al., 2007; Kim et al., 2012; Moureau-Zabotto et al., 2011; Tural et al., 2013Wallin et al., 2013; Yan et al., 2011). In our study CEA level, other clinical parameters and the biopsy characteristics analyzed, did not predict tumor response to CRT (study with 167 patients not yet published).

The biopsy characteristics, namely differentiation grade, mitoses number, necrosis, inflammatory and desmoplastic reaction amount, had no utility to recognize or predict tumor behavior (study with 167 patients not yet publish) .

Tumor hypoxia and proliferative cell activity reduces the effectiveness of both radiation in therapy and chemotherapy and are a well-known risk factor for tumor radio resistance. We thought that biopsy necrosis grade and mitotic counts (number of mitoses per ten high-powered fields) could interfere with CRT tumor response but it was not possible to find a statistically significant correlation in our last data.

All predictive factors found are, one way or another, related with tumor donwstaging and/or neoadjuvant chemoradiation tumor response in pathological variables found post-treatment (Table 5). This is an expected result.

In our last study the post-treatment differentiation, feasibility and proliferative activity of tumor cells show greater impact as predictors of Mandard response (more than pathological TNM stage or tumor downstaging). The presence of accentuated necrosis, mitosis number>9.5 for 10 high-powered fields and moderate or poorly differentiated grade in resected specimen had a predictive value for Mandard response of 85%. Those variables had a significant predictive value of Mandard response in multivariate analysis (study with 167 patients not yet published – Table 7).

Thus, the only process for assessing neoadjuvant CRT response is obtained from post treatment variables. The absence of reliable clinical predictors of response to CRT, emphasizes the need to find molecular factors able to predict response and thus individualize the treatment approach in locally advanced rectal cancers. On this series the Mandard grade response proved useful to modify the adjuvant treatment plan in patients who were "bad responders" into a more aggressive treatment.

8   Conclusions

Neoadjuvant chemoradiation (CRT) followed by total mesorectum excision (TME) surgery, and systemic chemotherapy still remains the standard of care for locally

Variable		Odds ratio	Confidence interval 95%	P
Differentiation grade in resected specimen	0 + 1	1.00	–	
	2 + 3	10.45	3.38–32.30	<0.001
Necrosis grade in resected specimen	marked	1.00	–	
	scarce/ moderate	8.82	3.04–25.54	<0.001
Mitosis number in resected specimen	≤ 9,5	1.00	–	
	≥ 9,6	4.07	1.52–10.90	0.005

Table 7: Multivariate stepwise model – dependent variable Mandard response: "0" good response and "1" bad response

advanced rectal cancer, but not all cases benefit from this treatment modality. This multimodal treatment improves disease pelvic control but better survival is achieved only if pathological response is present.

TRG scales provides a system to assess tumor chemoradiotherapy response. This response can range from absent – no fibrosis with extensive residual cancer (zero evidence of treatment efficacy) – to a complete response (ypCR) with no viable tumor cells identified. The pathological response to neoadjuvant CRT has been reported in several studies to be closely related to oncologic outcomes.

Mandard tumor regression grade (TRG) proved to be a good system to measure neoadjuvant CRT response. To identify the group of patients with better prognosis, Mandard TRG seems more effective than Dworak TGR. Mandard was the one that better correlated with the presence of therapeutic response and prognosis.

In our research, the Mandard system proved to be a good determinant of outcome, when cases were grouped into TRG1–2 (good responders) and TRG3–5 (poor responders). This methodology proved superior than division in groups ypCR (TRG1) versus all others (TRG2–5) regarding DFS and OS. The presence of a good response in terms of Mandard tumor regression grade was associated with a lower incidence of locoregional recurrence and improved survival. Mandard system provides an important tool for survival analysis.

None of the clinical or the biopsy characteristics assessed, had a predictive value of Mandard response, except the distance from anal verge. Only pathological parameters related with tumor response to chemoradiotherapy have predictive value for Mandard response. There's a lack of clinical and pathological preoperative variables able to predict Mandard response, only postoperative pathological parameters related with nCRT tumor response have a predictive value. Based on these results it's impossible at this moment, to identify the group of patients who truly benefits of neoadjuvant CRT, but we can identify the group of patients (the Mandard bad responders) that will benefit with a more aggressive adjuvant treatment.

References

Arredondo J, Baixauli J, Beorlegui C et al. (2013). Prognosis factors for recurrence in patients with locally advanced rectal cancer preoperatively treated with chemoradiotherapy and adjuvant chemotherapy. Dis Colon Rectum 2013; 56: 416–421.

Bateman AC, Jaynes E, Bateman AR. (2009). Rectal cancer staging post neoadjuvant therapy – how should the changes be assessed? Histopathology 2009; 54: 713–721.

Beddy D, Hyland JM, Winter DC et al. (2008). A simplified tumor regression grade correlates with survival in locally advanced rectal carcinoma treated with neoadjuvant chemoradiotherapy. Ann Surg Oncol 2008; 15: 3471–3477.

Bernstein TE, Endreseth BH, Romundstad P, Wibe A. (2009). Circumferential resection margin as a prognostic factor in rectal cancer. Br J Surg 2009; 96: 1348–1357.

Bosset JF, Calais G, Mineur L et al. (2005). Enhanced tumorocidal effect of chemotherapy with preoperative radiotherapy for rectal cancer: preliminary results – EORTC 22921. J Clin Oncol 2005; 23: 5620–5627.

Bosset JF, Collette L, Calais G et al. (2006). Chemotherapy with preoperative radiotherapy in rectal cancer. N Engl J Med 2006; 355: 1114–1123.

Bujko K, Kolodziejczyk M, Nasierowska-Guttmejer A et al. (2010). Tumour regression grading in patients with residual rectal cancer after preoperative chemoradiation. Radiother Oncol 2010; 95: 298–302.

Capirci C, Rubello D, Chierichetti F et al. (2006). Long-term prognostic value of 18F-FDG PET in patients with locally advanced rectal cancer previously treated with neoadjuvant radiochemotherapy. AJR Am J Roentgenol 2006; 187: W202–208.

Capirci C, Valentini V, Cionini L et al. (2008). Prognostic value of pathologic complete response after neoadjuvant therapy in locally advanced rectal cancer: long-term analysis of 566 ypCR patients. Int J Radiat Oncol Biol Phys 2008; 72: 99–107.

Chan AK, Wong A, Jenken D et al. (2005). Posttreatment TNM staging is a prognostic indicator of survival and recurrence in tethered or fixed rectal carcinoma after preoperative chemotherapy and radiotherapy. Int J Radiat Oncol Biol Phys 2005; 61: 665–677.

Choi CH, Kim WD, Lee SJ, Park WY. (2012). Clinical predictive factors of pathologic tumor response after preoperative chemoradiotherapy in rectal cancer. Radiat Oncol J 2012; 30: 99-107.

Das P, Skibber JM, Rodriguez-Bigas MA et al. (2007). Predictors of tumor response and downstaging in patients who receive preoperative chemoradiation for rectal cancer. Cancer 2007; 109: 1750–1755.

de Campos-Lobato LF, Geisler DP, da Luz Moreira A et al. (2011a). Neoadjuvant therapy for rectal cancer: the impact of longer interval between chemoradiation and surgery. J Gastrointest Surg 2011; 15: 444–450.

de Campos-Lobato LF, Stocchi L, da Luz Moreira A et al. (2010). Downstaging without complete pathologic response after neoadjuvant treatment improves cancer outcomes for cIII but not cII rectal cancers. Ann Surg Oncol 2010; 17: 1758–1766.

de Campos-Lobato LF, Stocchi L, da Luz Moreira A et al. (2011b). Pathologic complete response after neoadjuvant treatment for rectal cancer decreases distant recurrence and could eradicate local recurrence. Ann Surg Oncol 2011; 18: 1590–1598.

Dhadda AS, Dickinson P, Zaitoun AM et al. (2011). Prognostic importance of Mandard tumour regression grade following pre=operative chemo/radiotherapy for locally advanced rectal cancer. Eur J Cancer 2011; 47: 1138–1145.

Dietz DW, Dehdashti F, Grigsby PW et al. (2008). Tumor hypoxia detected by positron emission tomography with 60Cu-ATSM as a predictor of response and survival in patients undergoing Neoadjuvant chemoradiotherapy for rectal carcinoma: a pilot study. Dis Colon Rectum 2008; 51: 1641-1648.

Dresen RC, Beets GL, Rutten HJ et al. (2009). Locally advanced rectal cancer: MR imaging for restaging after neoadjuvant radiation therapy with concomitant chemotherapy. Part I. Are we able to predict tumor confined to the rectal wall? Radiology 2009; 252: 71-80.

Dworak O, Keilholz L, Hoffmann A. (1997). *Pathological features of rectal cancer after preoperative radiochemotherapy. Int J Colorectal Dis 1997; 12: 19–23.*

Everaert H, Hoorens A, Vanhove C et al. (2011). *Prediction of response to neoadjuvant radiotherapy in patients with locally advanced rectal cancer by means of sequential 18FDG-PET. Int J Radiat Oncol Biol Phys 2011; 80: 91-96.*

Farnault B, Moureau-Zabotto L, de Chaisemartin C et al. (2011). *Predictive factors of tumour response after neoadjuvant chemoradiation for locally advanced rectal cancer and correlation of these factors with survival]. Cancer Radiother 2011; 15: 279-286.*

Franklin JM, Anderson EM, Gleeson FV. (2012). *MRI features of the complete histopathological response of locally advanced rectal cancer to neoadjuvant chemoradiotherapy. Clin Radiol 2012.*

Garcia-Aguilar J, Smith DD, Avila K et al. (2011). *Optimal timing of surgery after chemoradiation for advanced rectal cancer: preliminary results of a multicenter, nonrandomized phase II prospective trial. Ann Surg 2011; 254: 97-102.*

Glynne-Jones R, Anyamene N. (2006). *Just how useful an endpoint is complete pathological response after neoadjuvant chemoradiation in rectal cancer? Int J Radiat Oncol Biol Phys 2006; 66: 319–320.*

Gosens MJ, Klaassen RA, Tan-Go I et al. (2007). *Circumferential margin involvement is the crucial prognostic factor after multimodality treatment in patients with locally advanced rectal carcinoma. Clin Cancer Res 2007; 13: 6617–6623.*

Habr-Gama A, Oliva Perez R. (2009). *The strategy "wait and watch" in patients with a cancer of bottom stocking rectum with a complete clinical answer after neoadjuvant radiochemotherapy. J Chir (Paris) 2009; 146: 237–239.*

Habr-Gama A, Perez RO, Proscurshim I et al. (2008). *Interval between surgery and neoadjuvant chemoradiation therapy for distal rectal cancer: does delayed surgery have an impact on outcome? Int J Radiat Oncol Biol Phys 2008; 71: 1181-1188.*

Habr-Gama A, Perez RO, Sao Juliao GP et al. (2011). *Nonoperative approaches to rectal cancer: a critical evaluation. Semin Radiat Oncol 2011; 21: 234–239.*

Habr-Gama A, Perez RO, Wynn G et al. (2010). *Complete clinical response after neoadjuvant chemoradiation therapy for distal rectal cancer: characterization of clinical and endoscopic findings for standardization. Dis Colon Rectum 2010; 53: 1692–1698.*

Heald RJ, Husband EM, Ryall RD. (1982). *The mesorectum in rectal cancer surgery – the clue to pelvic recurrence? Br J Surg 1982; 69: 613–616.*

Huh JW, Kim HR, Kim YJ. (2013). *Clinical prediction of pathological complete response after preoperative chemoradiotherapy for rectal cancer. Dis Colon Rectum 2013; 56: 698-703.*

Ippolito D, Monguzzi L, Guerra L et al. (2012). *Response to neoadjuvant therapy in locally advanced rectal cancer: assessment with diffusion-weighted MR imaging and 18FDG PET/CT. Abdom Imaging 2012.*

Jacobi K, Walther A, Kuhn R et al. (1997). *Advantages and limitations of intraoperative mechanical autotransfusion in al prostatectomies. Anaesthesist 1997; 46: 101–107.*

Jung SH, Heo SH, Kim JW et al. (2012). *Predicting response to neoadjuvant chemoradiation therapy in locally advanced rectal cancer: diffusion-weighted 3 Tesla MR imaging. J Magn Reson Imaging 2012; 35: 110-116.*

Junker K. (2004). *Therapy-induced morphological changes in lung cancer. Pathologe 2004; 25: 475–480.*

Kapiteijn E, Marijnen CA, Nagtegaal ID et al. (2001). *Preoperative radiotherapy combined with total mesorectal excision for resectable rectal cancer. N Engl J Med 2001; 345: 638–646.*

Kim DJ, Kim JH, Lim JS et al. (2010a). *Restaging of Rectal Cancer with MR Imaging after Concurrent Chemotherapy and Radiation Therapy. Radiographics 2010; 30: 503-516.*

Kim JS, Cho MJ, Song KS, Yoon WH. (2002). *Preoperative chemoradiation using oral capecitabine in locally advanced rectal cancer. Int J Radiat Oncol Biol Phys 2002; 54: 403–408.*

Kim JW, Kim HC, Park JW et al. (2013). *Predictive value of (18)FDG PET-CT for tumour response in patients with locally advanced rectal cancer treated by preoperative chemoradiotherapy. Int J Colorectal Dis 2013; 28: 1217-1224.*

Kim TH, Chang HJ, Kim DY et al. (2010b). Pathologic nodal classification is the most discriminating prognostic factor for disease-free survival in rectal cancer patients treated with preoperative chemoradiotherapy and curative resection. Int J Radiat Oncol Biol Phys 2010; 77: 1153-1165.

Kim YJ, Park SC, Kim DY et al. (2012). No correlation between pretreatment serum CEA levels and tumor volume in locally advanced rectal cancer patients. Clin Chim Acta 2012; 413: 511-515.

Kiss L, Kiss R, Porr PJ et al. (2011). Pathological evidence in support of total mesorectal excision in the management of rectal cancer. Chirurgia (Bucur) 2011; 106: 347–352

Klos CL, Bordeianou LG, Sylla P et al. (2011). The prognostic value of lymph node ratio after neoadjuvant chemoradiation and rectal cancer surgery. Dis Colon Rectum 2011; 54: 171-175.

Lee JH, Kim SH, Jang HS et al. (2013a). Preoperative elevation of carcinoembryonic antigen predicts poor tumor response and frequent distant recurrence for patients with rectal cancer who receive preoperative chemoradiotherapy and total mesorectal excision: a multi-institutional analysis in an Asian population. Int J Colorectal Dis 2013; 28: 511-517.

Lee YC, Hsieh CC, Chuang JP. (2013b). Prognostic Significance of Partial Tumor Regression After Preoperative Chemoradiotherapy for Rectal Cancer: A Meta-analysis. Dis Colon Rectum 2013; 56: 1093–1101.

Lindebjerg J, Spindler KL, Ploen J, Jakobsen A. (2009). The prognostic value of lymph node metastases and tumour regression grade in rectal cancer patients treated with long-course preoperative chemoradiotherapy. Colorectal Dis 2009; 11: 264–269.

Luna-Perez P, Bustos-Cholico E, Alvarado I et al. (2005). Prognostic significance of circumferential margin involvement in rectal adenocarcinoma treated with preoperative chemoradiotherapy and low anterior resection. J Surg Oncol 2005; 90: 20-25.

Maas M, Nelemans PJ, Valentini V et al. (2010). Long-term outcome in patients with a pathological complete response after chemoradiation for rectal cancer: a pooled analysis of individual patient data. Lancet Oncol 2010; 11: 835–844.

MacFarlane JK, Ryall RD, Heald RJ. (1993). Mesorectal excision for rectal cancer. Lancet 1993; 341: 457–460.

Madbouly KM, Abbas KS, Hussein AM. (2013). Metastatic lymph node ratio in stage III rectal carcinoma is a valuable prognostic factor even with less than 12 lymph nodes retrieved: a prospective study. Am J Surg 2013.

Mandard AM, Dalibard F, Mandard JC et al. (1994). Pathologic assessment of tumor regression after preoperative chemoradiotherapy of esophageal carcinoma. Clinicopathologic correlations. Cancer 1994; 73: 2680–2686.

Mandard AM, Duigou F, Marnay J et al. (1987). Analysis of the results of the micronucleus test in patients presenting upper digestive tract cancers and in non-cancerous subjects. Int J Cancer 1987; 39: 442–444.

Martin ST, Heneghan HM, Winter DC. (2012a). Systematic review and meta-analysis of outcomes following pathological complete response to neoadjuvant chemoradiotherapy for rectal cancer. Br J Surg 2012.

Martin ST, Heneghan HM, Winter DC. (2012b). Systematic review of outcomes after intersphincteric resection for low rectal cancer. Br J Surg 2012.

Martin ST, Heneghan HM, Winter DC. (2012c). Systematic review and meta-analysis of outcomes following pathological complete response to neoadjuvant chemoradiotherapy for rectal cancer. Br J Surg 2012; 99: 918-928.

Maurer CA. Renzulli P, Kull C et al. (2011). The impact of the introduction of total mesorectal excision on local recurrence rate and survival in rectal cancer: long-term results. Ann Surg Oncol 2011; 18: 1899–1906.

Meng X, Huang Z, Wang R, Yu J. (2014). Prediction of response to preoperative chemoradiotherapy in patients with locally advanced rectal cancer. Biosci Trends 2014; 8: 11-23.

Moureau-Zabotto L, Farnault B, de Chaisemartin C et al. (2011). Predictive factors of tumor response after neoadjuvant chemoradiation for locally advanced rectal cancer. Int J Radiat Oncol Biol Phys 2011; 80: 483-491.

Oberholzer K, Menig M, Kreft A et al. (2012). Rectal cancer: mucinous carcinoma on magnetic resonance imaging indicates poor response to neoadjuvant chemoradiation. Int J Radiat Oncol Biol Phys 2012; 82: 842-848.

Park IJ, You YN, Agarwal A et al. (2012). Neoadjuvant treatment response as an early response indicator for patients with rectal cancer. J Clin Oncol 2012; 30: 1770–1776.

Patel UB, Blomqvist LK, Taylor F et al. (2012). MRI after treatment of locally advanced rectal cancer: how to report tumor response--the MERCURY experience. AJR Am J Roentgenol 2012; 199: W486-495.

Pettersson D, Cedermark B, Holm T et al. (2010). Interim analysis of the Stockholm III trial of preoperative radiotherapy regimens for rectal cancer. Br J Surg 2010; 97: 580–587.

Pettersson D, Holm T, Iversen H et al. (2012). Preoperative short-course radiotherapy with delayed surgery in primary rectal cancer. Br J Surg 2012; 99: 577–583.

Qiu HZ, Wu B, Xiao Y, Lin GL. (2011). Combination of differentiation and T stage can predict unresponsiveness to neoadjuvant therapy for rectal cancer. Colorectal Dis 2011; 13: 1353-1360.

Quah HM, Chou JF, Gonen M et al. (2008). Pathologic stage is most prognostic of disease-free survival in locally advanced rectal cancer patients after preoperative chemoradiation. Cancer 2008; 113: 57-64.

Reshef A, Lavery I, Kiran RP. (2012). Factors associated with oncologic outcomes after abdominoperineal resection compared with restorative resection for low rectal cancer: patient- and tumor-related or technical factors only? Dis Colon Rectum 2012; 55: 51-58.

Restivo A, Zorcolo L, Cocco IM et al. (2013). Elevated CEA levels and low distance of the tumor from the anal verge are predictors of incomplete response to chemoradiation in patients with rectal cancer. Ann Surg Oncol 2013; 20: 864-871.

Rodel C, Martus P, Papadoupolos T et al. (2005). Prognostic significance of tumor regression after preoperative chemoradiotherapy for rectal cancer. J Clin Oncol 2005; 23: 8688–8696.

Rullier A, Laurent C, Capdepont M et al. (2010). Impact of tumor response on survival after radiochemotherapy in locally advanced rectal carcinoma. Am J Surg Pathol 2010; 34: 562-568.

Rullier A, Laurent C, Vendrely V et al. (2005). Impact of colloid response on survival after preoperative radiotherapy in locally advanced rectal carcinoma. Am J Surg Pathol 2005; 29: 602–606.

Santos MD, Silva C, Rocha A et al. (2013). Tumor regression grades: can they influence rectal cancer therapy decision tree? Int J Surg Oncol 2013; 2013: 572149.

Santos MD, Silva C, Rocha A et al. (2014). Prognostic value of mandard and dworak tumor regression grading in rectal cancer: study of a single tertiary center. ISRN Surg 2014; 2014: 310542.

Sauer R, Becker H, Hohenberger W et al. (2004). Preoperative versus postoperative chemoradiotherapy for rectal cancer. N Engl J Med 2004; 351: 1731–1740.

Sauer R, Liersch T, Merkel S et al. (2012). Preoperative versus postoperative chemoradiotherapy for locally advanced rectal cancer: results of the German CAO/ARO/AIO-94 randomized phase III trial after a median follow-up of 11 years. J Clin Oncol 2012; 30: 1926–1933.

Shanmugan S, Arrangoiz R, Nitzkorski JR et al. (2012). Predicting Pathological Response to Neoadjuvant Chemoradiotherapy in Locally Advanced Rectal Cancer Using (18)FDG-PET/CT. Ann Surg Oncol 2012.

Siegel R, Burock S, Wernecke KD et al. (2009). Preoperative short-course radiotherapy versus combined radiochemotherapy in locally advanced rectal cancer: a multi-centre prospectively randomised study of the Berlin Cancer Society. BMC Cancer 2009; 9: 50.

Stipa F, Chessin DB, Shia J et al. (2006). A pathologic complete response of rectal cancer to preoperative combined-modality therapy results in improved oncological outcome compared with those who achieve no downstaging on the basis of preoperative endorectal ultrasonography. Ann Surg Oncol 2006; 13: 1047–1053.

Suarez J, Vera R, Balen E et al. (2008). Pathologic response assessed by Mandard grade is a better prognostic factor than down staging for disease-free survival after preoperative radiochemotherapy for advanced rectal cancer. Colorectal Dis 2008; 10: 563–568.

Tulchinsky H, Shmueli E, Figer A et al. (2008). An interval >7 weeks between neoadjuvant therapy and surgery improves pathologic complete response and disease-free survival in patients with locally advanced rectal cancer. Ann Surg Oncol 2008; 15: 2661-2667.

Tural D, Selcukbiricik F, Dztfcrk MA et al. (2013). The relation between pathologic complete response and clinical outcome in patients with rectal cancer. Hepatogastroenterology 2013; 60.

Valentini V. (2011). The right study design is needed to find out which patients benefit from preoperative chemoradiotherapy for intermediate staged rectal cancer. Onkologie 2011; 34: 6–8.

Vecchio FM, Valentini V, Minsky BD et al. (2005). The relationship of pathologic tumor regression grade (TRG) and outcomes after preoperative therapy in rectal cancer. Int J Radiat Oncol Biol Phys 2005; 62: 752–760.

Wallin U, Rothenberger D, Lowry A et al. (2013). CEA - a predictor for pathologic complete response after neoadjuvant therapy for rectal cancer. Dis Colon Rectum 2013; 56: 859-868.

Wheeler JM, Dodds E, Warren BF et al. (2004). Preoperative chemoradiotherapy and total mesorectal excision surgery for locally advanced rectal cancer: correlation with rectal cancer regression grade. Dis Colon Rectum 2004; 47: 2025–2031.

Wheeler JM, Warren BF, Mortensen NJ et al. (2002). Quantification of histologic regression of rectal cancer after irradiation: a proposal for a modified staging system. Dis Colon Rectum 2002; 45: 1051–1056.

Willett CG, Czito BG. (2008). Impact of time duration after neoadjuvant therapy to surgery on response and outcome in rectal cancer patients. Ann Surg Oncol 2008; 15: 2636-2638.

Williams GT QP, Shepherd NA. (2008). 2nd edn. London: Dataset for colorectal cancer, The Royal College of Pathologists. Available at http://www.rcpath.org/resources/pdf/G049--ColorectalDataset-Sep07.pdf. Last accessed 24 April 2008.

Yan H, Wang R, Zhu K et al. (2011). Predictors of sensitivity to preoperative chemoradiotherapy of rectal adenocarcinoma. Tumori 2011; 97: 717-723.

Yang KL, Yang SH, Liang WY et al. (2013). Carcinoembryonic antigen (CEA) level, CEA ratio, and treatment outcome of rectal cancer patients receiving pre-operative chemoradiation and surgery. Radiat Oncol 2013; 8: 43.

Yeo SG, Kim DY, Kim TH et al. (2010). Pathologic complete response of primary tumor following preoperative chemoradiotherapy for locally advanced rectal cancer: long-term outcomes and prognostic significance of pathologic nodal status (KROG 09-01). Ann Surg 2010; 252: 998-1004.

Yeo SG, Kim DY, Park JW et al. (2012a). Stage-to-stage comparison of preoperative and postoperative chemoradiotherapy for T3 mid or distal rectal cancer. Int J Radiat Oncol Biol Phys 2012; 82: 856-862.

Yeo SG, Kim DY, Park JW et al. (2012b). Tumor volume reduction rate after preoperative chemoradiotherapy as a prognostic factor in locally advanced rectal cancer. Int J Radiat Oncol Biol Phys 2012; 82: e193-199.

Chapter 5

Magnetic Resonance Imaging in Guidance and Assessement of Cardiovasular Interventions

Maythem Saeed[1] and Mark W. Wilson[1]

1 Introduction

X-ray fluoroscopy is routinely used in patients to guide vascular and cardiac interventions, because of the ability to perform real-time imaging and easy access to patients during interventions (Athanasoulis, 2001; Lakhan et al., 2009; Sousa et al., 2005). X-ray fluoroscopy, however, is limited for defining soft tissue and obtaining functional information. The poor contrast between pathologic and healthy surrounding tissue hinders X-ray fluoroscopy in defining targets (Peters, 2006), which subsequently leads to blind delivery of therapies to the targets (Saeed et al., 2006, 2008a).

On the other hand, MRI uses low energy and no ionizing radiation. It does not require the injection of iodinated contrast, which has been associated with complications, including nephrotoxicity and anaphylaxis. Several studies also showed that exposure to ionizing radiation from X-ray procedures is associated with an increased risk of cancer (Berrington et al., 2004; Frush, 2004; Prasad et al., 2004). A study showed that high dose or repeated administration of gadolinium-based MR contrast media might be a concern, especially in patients with impaired renal function (Sadowski et al., 2007). This problem can be reduced by ensuring a glomerular filtration rate of > 30 ml/min/1.73 m^2 and contrast agents with high molecular stability (Bongartz et al., 2008).

The recently developed real-time MR sequences offer high temporal/spatial resolution images, safety, accuracy, flexibility and functionality. It also offers rapid recon-

---

[1] Department of Radiology and Biomedical Imaging, School of Medicine, University of California San Francisco, San Francisco, California, USA.

struction and display of 3D images. These features are crucial for minimally invasive vascular and cardiac interventions. Recent improvements in signal processing, tissue characterization and angiographic integration have allowed for MR-guidance in complex interventional procedures (de Silva et al., 2006; Saybasili et al., 2010). Therefore, it has been used in focused ultrasound (Cline et al., 1994, 1995), MRI thermometry (Chung et al., 1999; Cline et al., 1994; Kuroda et al., 2000), functional imaging integrated into MR guided neurosurgical interventions (Yang et al., 2001), local drug delivery (Saeed et al., 2008a; Yang et al., 2006), endoscopy (Hsu et al., 1998), intravascular interventions (Atalar et al., 1998; Bakker et al., 1997, 1998; Ladd et al., 1998; Leung et al., 1995; Smits eta l., 1998; van der Weide et al., 1998; Wendt & Wacker, 2000) and intra-operative imaging (Hall et al., 2000; Martin et al., 2000; Samset & Hirschberg, 1999; Schwartz et al., 1999; Yang et al, 2001).

2 MRI Scanners

Open and closed bore MR scanners have been designed for cardiovascular interventions (Hushek et al., 2008). Open scanners were designed to ease patient access/observation and increase comfort for the interventionists. These scanners have low field strength (0.5T), thus offer suboptimal image quality and slow switching speeds that do not meet the need of cardiovascular interventions. Wacker et al. (2005a) found that higher field strength (1.0T) scanners halved the intervention time during stent deployment compared with 0.2T open-bore scanners. The hybrid XMR system consists of an angiographic laboratory adjacent to closed-bore 1.5T MR scanners, wherein an on-track patient table could be moved rapidly between the two imaging modalities (Hushek et al., 2003; Martin et al., 2003). More recently, another XMR hybrid system has been developed that has a side-by-side 1.5T magnet and C-arm X-ray system (Personal communication). The in-suite operation consoles and display monitors are of great help in instant image acquisition and monitoring (Figure 1).

The advantages of hybrid XMR systems are: 1) intermodal movement is minimized because a patient will remain on the same sliding table throughout the intervention and imaging session; 2) unlike single system, the XMR hybrid system permits evaluation of the impact of interventional procedures via MR monitoring; 3) it permits rapid deployment of catheters, and efficient execution of desired interventions without the obligation of using MR compatible devices; 4) it reduces radiation exposure and 5) offers the convenience of a single visit. However, currently XMR systems are available only in few medical centers.

3 Interventional Catheters and Devices

In general endovascular catheters, guide wires and cardiac devices are optimized for their mechanical properties and visibility under projection X-ray imaging. They contain substantial metallic components, such as ferromagnetic material, which is not MR com-

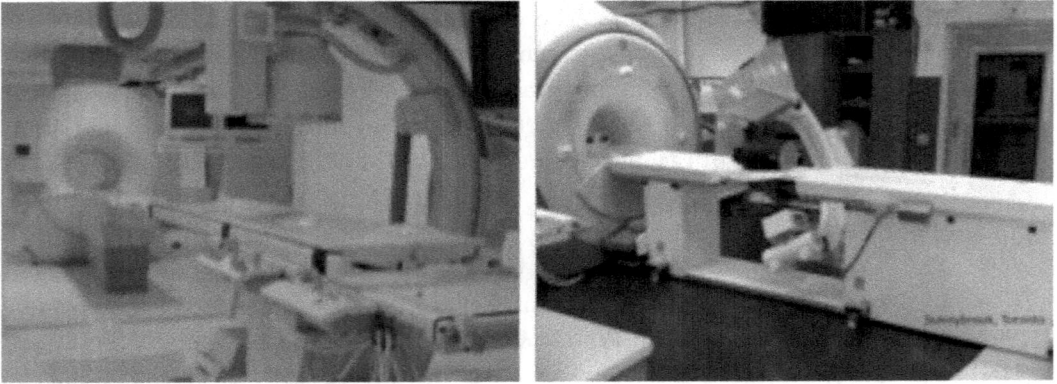

Figure 1: These two XMR suites couple a state-of-the-art MR scanner (background) with a fully functional catheter laboratory (foreground). Hybrid XMR suite equipped with a closed-bore 1.5T MR scanner and C-arm X-ray fluoroscopy. The suite consists of 2 rooms separated by a sliding door. The suite features a floating patient table that can slide a patient quickly and smoothly from one imaging system to the other. (left, Phillips Medical Systems). On the right side, the recently developed hybrid system, where both C-arm X-ray fluoroscopy and 1.5T MR systems are in the same room, thereby making interventional procedures shorter and more efficient (courtesy of Dr. Graham Wright, Sunnybrook, Toronto).

patible. Therefore, their visualization on MRI has been difficult due to susceptibility artifacts derived from the ferromagnetic material, geometry and design (Klemm et al., 2000; Kuehne et al., 2003). Special MR compatible endovascular catheters, guide wires and cardiac devices that are made of nickel-titanium alloy (nitinol), platinum, gold, copper, nonbraided or plastic catheters have been recently developed cause substantially less susceptibility artifacts (Buecker et al., 2004; Kuehne et al., 2002, 2003) and produce less radiofrequency heating in vivo (Nitz et al., 2001). Mekle et al. (2009) used a synthetic MR friendly polymer-based guide-wire for dilatation of an artificial stenosis in phantoms and in the carotid artery, aorta, and iliac arteries of swine. Other investigators manufactured a guide wire based on micropultruded fiber-reinforced material doped with iron particles to improve visibility (Krueger et al., 2008).

Investigators used three approaches for endovascular catheter tracking and navigation, namely passive tracking, active tracking and magnetic catheter steering (Figure 2). The contrast between the catheter and background blood can be improved by injecting MR contrast media, which prevents flow artifacts because steady state is reached earlier (Maes et al., 2005; Martin et al., 2003). Bakker et al. (1997) were the first to use passive tracking approach for steering basilica veins of healthy volunteers. Later, Manke et al and Razavi et al. adapted this passive approach in patients (Manke et al., 2000 Razavi et al., 2003). Contrast media were mounted on non-braided catheters and used as markers for tracking. The advantage of catheter labeling is that it requires no hardware

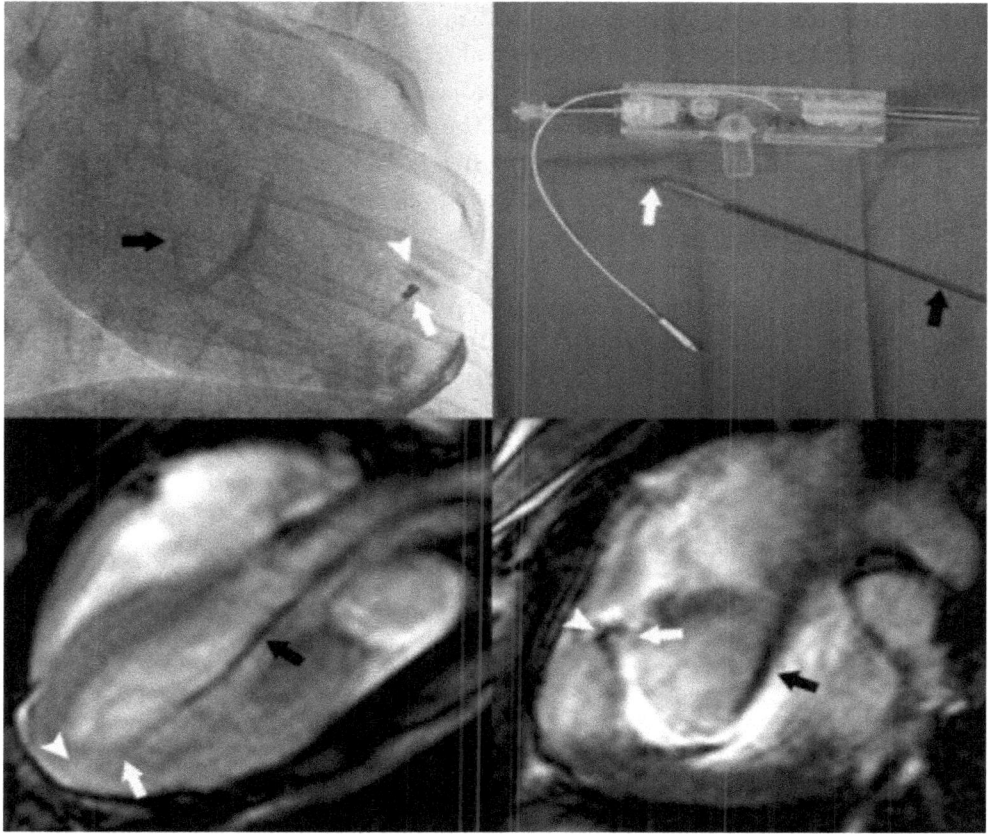

Figure 2: Selected X-ray photograph (top left), an active MRI catheter (top right) with the coil at the tip (white arrow) embedded in the shaft of the catheter (black arrow) and shoots of MR-guided imaging using passive catheter (bottom left) and active catheter (bottom right). These transendocardial procedures were used to deliver locally different genes or stem cells in infarcted myocardium to enhance angiogenesis and myogenesis.

or instrument modifications and the disadvantage is that the catheter disappears when out of the imaging plane.

Active tracking relies on specially designed micro-coils, electrified wire loop and self-resonant radiofrequency circuits. The coils pick up signal during slice excitation and generate a frequency-encoded recall echo, which can be detected in 3D at a spatial resolution of approximately 1 mm. The micro-coils provide robust tracking of the catheter shaft and tip that allows the user to identify its position and target (Figure 2) (Bock et al., 2004; Saeed et al., 2006; Wacker et al., 2005b). Quick et al. (2002) used antennas for active catheter tracking and imaging of the abdominal aorta, superior mesenteric artery, renal arteries, hepatic artery and celiac trunk.

The safety of active endovascular devices is still a major concern in MR-guided interventions. The conductive nature of the long metallic braids creates a safety hazard in the MR environment, as the braided shaft can interact with incident RF energy and the electric field transmitted from the RF coil (Park et al., 2007). The heat created by the active coils causes necrosis of the tissue adjacent to the catheter and blood clotting, which may lead to vascular embolization. The methods for mitigating the potential for heating include using unbraided catheters, insulating the conductive structure, limiting the RF power to which it is exposed, or altering its interaction with the RF energy source (Kocaturk et al., 2009). The FDA limits the allowable power deposition via MR imaging to 8 W/kg and temperature change to 2°C.

Magnetic catheter steering is a new approach for tracking endovascular catheters using remote control (Bernhardt et al., 2011; Settecase et al., 2011). This approach relies on a small magnetic moment created by application of an electrical current to copper coils on the catheter tip, which results in alignment of the catheter in the direction of the B0 field. Magnetic catheter steering approach allows for more efficiency in navigating small, tortuous blood vessels, which are currently difficult to catheterize due to build-up of friction at vascular bends. In addition to improved visualization of the endovascular catheter at low power levels, this technology permits deposition of thermal energy for ablation of tissues at higher power levels. This approach is currently under extensive work in our laboratory.

3.1   Contrast Media

MR-guided intervention can also benefit from using MR contrast media. MR contrast media represents alternative diagnostic option in patients at risk for adverse reactions to iodinated contrast media. In the early phase of using MR contrast media, the main problem was toxicity because investigators used pure paramagnetic heavy metal ions. Later paramagnetic ions were chelated with DTPA, DOTA or BOPTA to reduce their toxicity at the same time it reduces some of the paramagnetic properties of the free ions. In the late 1980 and early 1990 the first extracellular MR contrast media (Gadopentetate Dimeglumine, Magnevist) was approved for clinical routine. Intravascular contrast media are available for preclinical use only. Extravasation and elimination of intravascular contrast media are very slow compared with extracellular contrast media.

The most common classification of MR contrast media is based on their distribution in the tissue, namely the extracellular (low molecular weight; < 2 kDa), intravascular (high molecular weight; > 50 kDa), and/or intracellular compartment. Unlike extracellular and intracellular, intravascular contrast media remain in the intravascular compartment for a prolonged period due to their size and composition, therefore they provided extended delineation of vascular tree during MR-guided interventions. MR contrast media have been used on MR-guided procedures to improve visualization of devices (Hsu et al., 1998; Saeed et al., 2008a; Yang et al., 2001, 2006) in road mapping blood vessels (Buecker et al., 2004; Maes et al., 2005; Martin et al., 2005; Smits et al., 1998;) and defining pathologic targets (Hsu et al., 1998; Saeed et al., 2006, 2008a; Samset et al., 1999; Yang et al., 2006).

3.2 Real-Time MRI Sequences

MR-guided interventions became possible because of major advancements in the speed of data acquisition, data transfer, and interactive control and display. Other factors include highly uniform magnetic fields, rapidly changeable magnetic field gradients, multi-channel receivers and computing systems. Real-time MR sequences achieve high speeds by maximizing the switching rates of gradients and RF pulses. The speed of imaging is determined by how quickly spatial encoding can be performed and how fast k-space data can be acquired. Actively shielded, strong, fast-switching gradients and fast electronics have allowed data acquisition intervals to be reduced.

Most modern real-time MR implementations employ balanced steady state free precession techniques because of efficient use of magnetization, high SNR, and short repetition times (Bock et al., 2006; Busse et al., 2001; Duerk et al., 1998; Elgort & Duerk, 2005). The performance of these sequences is currently in the range needed to perform MR guided procedures at >5 frame per second (Bock et al., 2006). The steady state free precession acquisitions have been performed using radial (Peters et al., 2003), and spiral (Spielman et al., 1995) k-space trajectories; ie the readout MR signal is stored in K-space, which is equivalent to a Fourier plane. These acquisition techniques in conjunction with spiral or radial filling of the k-space are considered very reliable for high spatial and temporal resolutions. These imaging sequences also benefit from the use of multiple receiver coil elements (Pruessmann et al., 1999; Rasche et al., 1997). Parallel imaging accelerates acquisition by using the different spatial sensitivities of the coils to correct for under-sampling of image data (Niendorf & Sodickson, 2006). Other sequences that can improve imaging speed while simultaneously balancing image quality include non-Cartesian k-space sampling, temporal data sharing between images, and adjusting the tradeoff between region of interest coverage, temporal and spatial resolution (Elgort & Duerk, 2005). The use of 32 channel receiver arrays that will perform rapid 3D cardiac imaging and parallel transmission techniques to permit more efficient data collection, are also under active investigation (Kyriakos et al., 2006). It should be noted that real-time MR sequences are not free of limitations. For example, the closed configuration of MR scanners >1.5T limit access to the patient and RF pulses induce heating when conductive material is applied in devices; MR imaging is sensitive to magnetic field inhomogeneity, pulsatility/motion of spins and chemical shift.

Pre and post-intervention, the following MR sequences were used: (a) balanced fast field echo cine MR imaging for measuring LV volumes, ejection fraction, cardiac output, stroke volume, LV mass, wall thickness and radial strain (Carlsson et al., 2008; Carlsson et al., 2011; Dicks et al., 2009, 2010; Jacquier et al., 2007; Saeed et al., 2008b, (b) tagged gradient echo planar imaging for measuring circumferential strain and LV rotation (Carlsson et al., 2011; Dicks et al., 2009), (c) phase-contrast velocity-encoded gradient echo planar imaging for measuring longitudinal strain (Bergvall et al., 2006), (d) T2-weighted turbo spin echo sequence for measuring interstitial edema after ablation, (e) T2* multi-echo gradient echo sequence for measuring vascular and myocardial hemorrhage after intervention (Saeed et al., 2010), (f) T1-weighted gradient echo (radiofrequency spoiled) perfusion imaging sequence for measuring myocardial perfusion changes after delivery of therapy and (g) delayed contrast enhanced T1-weighted gradient echo sequence for assessing tissue viability.

4   Applications of MR-Guidance

4.1   Vascular Interventions

In the last decade MR imaging has been extended from a diagnostic to dynamic modality by tracking intravascular guide-wires and catheters in real-time. It should be noted that only a few investigators have performed vascular stenting in patients under MR guidance (Manke et al., 2001; Paetzel et al., 2005). In 1997 the first human MR-guided study was performed and showed excellent visualization of an endovascular catheter labeled with dysprosium ring markers (Bakker et al., 1997). In this study, investigators did not use guide wires during the movement of the catheter in the cephalic vein of healthy volunteers. Later, MR-guided percutaneous transluminal angioplasty was conducted without complications in 13 patients with iliac stenosis (Manke et al., 2001) and in 15 patients with femoral and popliteal artery stenosis (Paetzel et al., 2005). Furthermore, MR imaging provides detailed information on vascular layers and is able to differentiate between plaque components, such as fibrous, lipid rich and calcified tissue (Choudhury et al., 2004; Kramer et al., 2007).

Stenting and/or angioplasty have been performed using MR-guidance for dilatation of the aorta, pulmonary, coronary, renal iliac and femoral arteries (Boll et al., 2004; Buecker et al., 2000; Choudhury et al., 2004; Dion et al., 2000; Hamer et al., 2006; Kramer et al., 2007; Kuehne et al., 2003; Mahnken et al., 2004; Manke et al., 2001; Omary et al., 2000; Paetzel et al., 2005; Raman et al., 2005; Raval et al., 2005; Saeed et al., 2006; Spuentrup et al., 2002a). Kos et al. (2009) used a polyetheretherketone-based MR imaging-compatible guide-wire for aortic stenting and vena cava filter placement in swine. Several groups have successfully used MR-guidance for placement of vena cava filters (Bartels et al., 2001; Bucker et al., 2001). Pulmonary artery stents have also been accurately implanted across the pulmonary valve (Kuehne et al., 2001, 2002, 2003). Mahnken et al. (2004) used MR-guided procedures for placement of aortic stents grafts and Manke et al. (2001) successfully deployed stents under MR-guidance in iliac arterial stenosis in patients. Post-interventional MR imaging confirmed the location and functionality of the stents.

MR-guidance has also been used for assessment of the pulmonary arterial pressure in pediatric and adult patients with congenital heart disease (Kuehne et al., 2004b; Razavi et al., 2003). A variety of MR-guided interventions have been performed in patients with congenital heart diseases including; placing transjugular, intrahepatic portosystemic stents, radiofrequency ablation, aortic coarctation, atrio-septal defect and cardiac catheterization. In 2006, Krueger et al. (2006) performed the first MR-guided study using balloon angioplasty for treating aortic coarctation in 5 patients. This was an important step toward MR-guided treatment of congenital diseases.

Kuehne et al. (2004a) demonstrated successful implant of a self-expanding stent valve in the aorta via percutaneous access under MR-guidance. Transcatheter aortic valve implantation, either retrograde through a transfemoral approach or antegrade through a transapical approach, has become a clinical reality in the treatment of critical aortic stenosis in high-risk patients. MR-guidance plays an important role in transcatheter aortic valve implantation and replacement of insufficient aortic or pulmonic valves (Buecker et al., 2004; Kuehne et al., 2001, 2002). MR imaging enables accurate and reproducible quantifications of regurgitate fraction before and after valve placement. Under MR-guidance, McVeigh et al. (2006) used apical access to guide the placement of a prosthetic aortic valve in beating heart.

4.2   Cardiac Interventions

MR imaging is a technique that provides high-resolution 3D images of the heart. Percutaneous closure of atrio-septal defects under MR-guidance has been proven in animals (Rickers et al., 2003), but is hampered by image artifacts produced by the closure devices and the use of fast sequences for cardiac imaging (Shellock & Valencerina, 2005). Atrial septal defect (ASD) is another congenital defect common in children, leading to heart failure and pulmonary hypertension. Percutaneous transcatheter delivery of an ASD occluder has been performed on X-ray fluoroscopy (Omeish & Hijazi, 2001). MR imaging provides reliable diagnosis of ASD (Kersting-Sommerhoff et al., 1990) and MR-guidance was used for delivery (Figure 3) and sizing of ASD closure (Figure 4) (Buecker et al., 2002a, 2002b Schalla et al., 2005). The occluder was made of a nitinol mesh to reduce the distortion of artifacts in the images (Schalla et al., 2003).

Others used a commercial nitinol snare coaxial cathetersystem for delivering septal occluders (Schalla et al., 2005). The advancement of the delivery system through the IVC to the right atrium was monitored under MR-guidance (Figure 3). Other studies used active catheters to approach the left atrium and ventricle from the right atrium and ventricle and measure flow and pressure changes resulted from defects (Razavi et al., 2003; Schalla et al., 2003). Measurements of flow on velocity encoded MR imaging and blood pressure were used to calculate pulmonary resistance. The flow and resistance data obtained on Fick and MR cardiac catheterization methods were in agreement.

A clinical study in 10 patients and 5 volunteers showed that MR-guidance is suited to guide flow directed catheters for measurement of invasive pulmonary artery pressures (Kuehne et al., 2005). Pulmonary vascular flow was noninvasively measured using velocity-encoded cine MR imaging, while pulmonary pressure was measured invasively through a catheter guided into the pulmonary artery under MR-guidance. The results indicate that MR imaging is a promising tool for measurement of pulmonary vascular resistance in patients with different degrees and forms of pulmonary hypertension. MR-guidance has also been used in connecting cardiac chambers and blood vessels in a swine model, where Arepally et al. connected the right and left atrium by puncturing the interatrial septum using an active Brockenbrough-style needle (Arepally et al., 2006). In a clinical study in seven patients, Dick et al. conducted trans-septal puncture and balloon septostomy under MR-guidance (Dick et al., 2005).

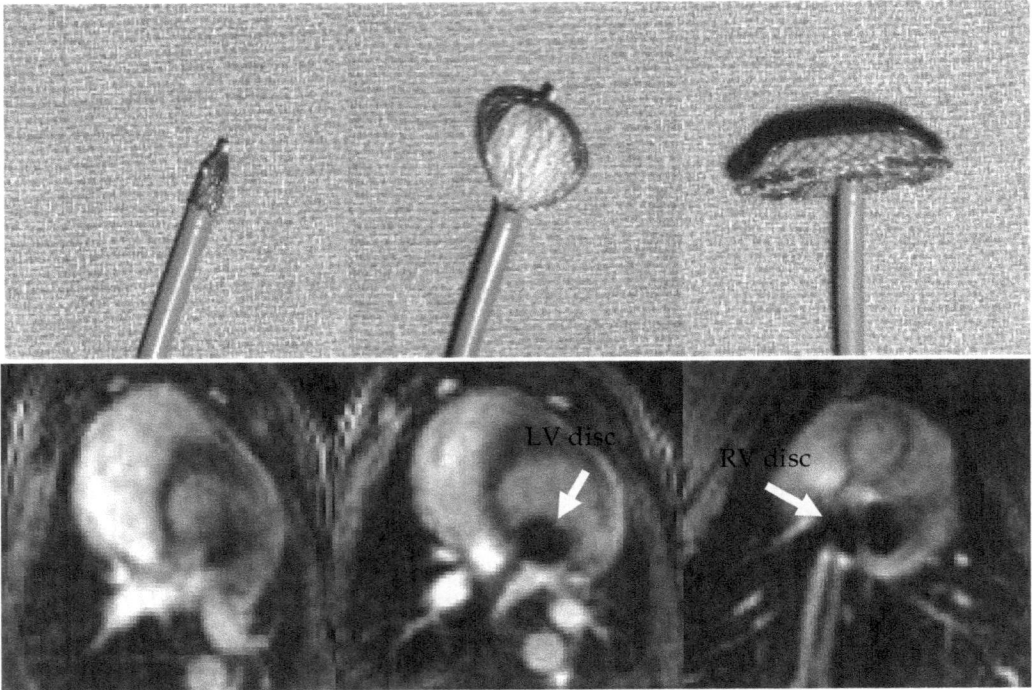

Figure 3: Percutaneous transcatheter delivery of an ASD occluder device at different phases of expansion in vitro (top) and MR images showing the advancement of the ASD closure into the site of the defect in in vivo (bottom, arrows).

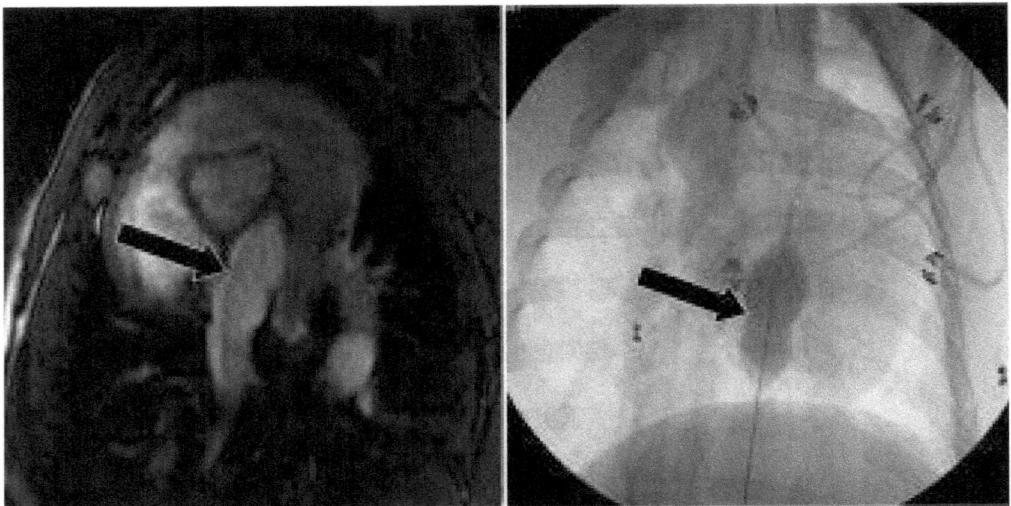

Figure 4: MR (left) and X-ray fluoroscopy images (right) were used to measure the diameter of anASD defect. The images show the close relation between the sizes of the defect on both modalities.

5   MR-Guidance for Delivering Local Therapies

Recently, angiogenic growth factor proteins, gene and stem cell therapies have been delivered, during coronary artery bypass grafting, as an alternative treatment to restore myocytes and blood vessels in end stage patients (Allen et al., 1999; Kleiman et al., 2003; Laham et al., 1999; Ruel et al., 2002; Simons et al., 2000; Stamm et al., 2007;). Others used catheter-based local delivery approaches (Figure 5).

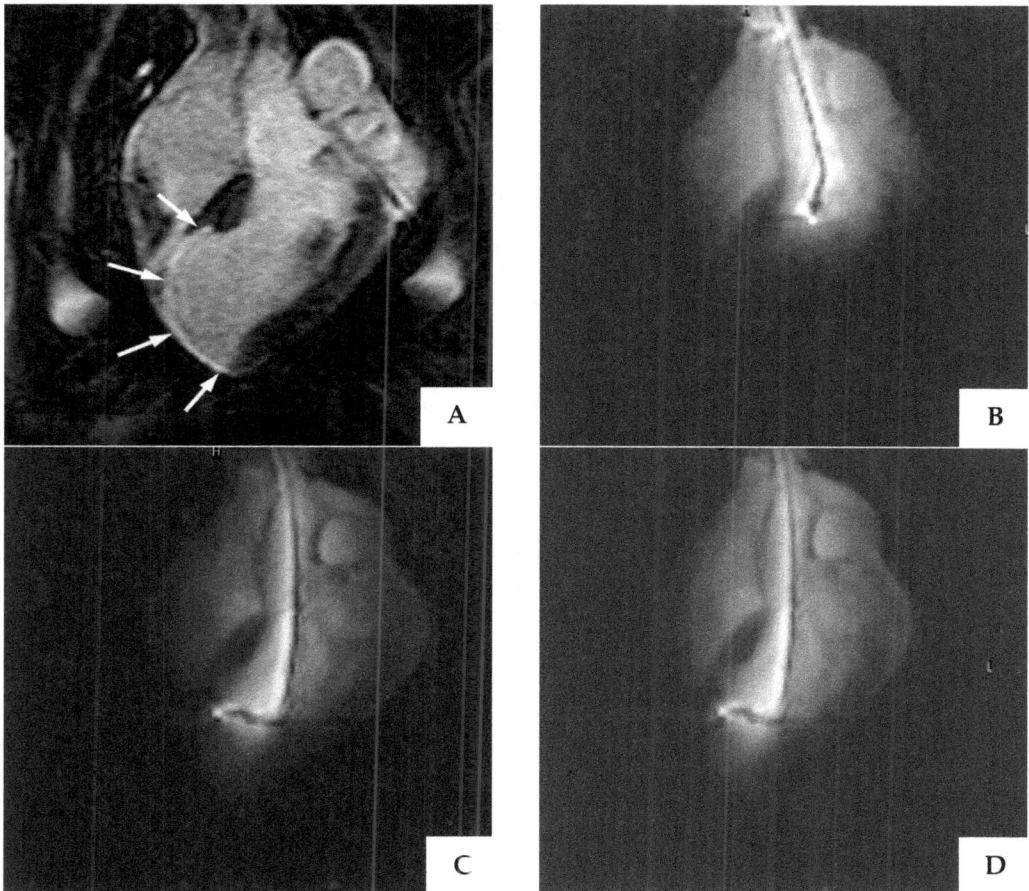

Figure 5: Contrast enhanced MR image shows the scar in the left ventricle (A, arrows). Real time snapshots of the advancement of the active catheter into the aorta (B), left ventricle (C) and injection of therapy into the target (D). This procedure was used to deliver angiogenic genes and labeled stem cells.

Preclinical and clinical studies have shown that the percutaneous local delivery approach (intramyocardial and intraarterial) is visible under MRI-guidance (Assmus et al., 2006; Freyman et al., 2006; Menasche et al., 2008; Narazaki et al., 2008; Saito et al.,

2003). Animal studies confirmed the success of catheter-based transendocardial delivery of genes in infarcted myocardium. The benefits of catheter-based local delivery of therapies are: 1) targeting only the diseased region, 2) delivering a high local dose, 3) eliminating a high systemic dose and side effects and 4) reducing the chance of angiogenesis in hidden tumor sites especially in elderly patients (Allen et al., 1999; Kleiman et al., 2003; Laham et al., 1999; Ruel et al., 2002; Simons et al., 2000; Simonetti et al., 2002; Stamm et al., 2007).

Preclinical studies have indicated that MR imaging provides quantitative data on myocardial viability, infarct transmurality, microvascular obstruction and hemorrhage. These capabilities have positioned MR imaging as an important approach to pursue for assessing the benefits of locally delivered genes (Saeed et al., 2008a; Yang et al., 2006). Another MR study showed the increase in collateral blood flow of infarcted myocardium after delivering vascular endothelial growth factor, which was confirmed on histology (Figure 6) (Pearlman et al., 2000).

Post et al. (2006) demonstrated an improvement in regional radial strain after intramyocardial injection of adenovirus coding for P39 gene. Furthermore, Liu et al. (2006) found improvement in LV ejection fraction and smaller number of segments with wall motion abnormality after intramyocardial injection of fibroblast growth factor.

Local stem cell transplantation is another therapy for treating ischemic heart disease. The therapeutic effect of stem cells seems to be related to the release of angiogenic factors rather than trans-differentiation of delivered stem cells. Two predominant routes for stem cell delivery to infarcted myocardium are intracoronary infusion and direct intramyocardial injection. Each of these delivery routes attempts to maximize the retention of delivered cells to infarcted myocardium. Early clinical studies indicated that cell transplantation, delivered under MR-guidance, is safe and feasible (Dick et al., 2003, 2005; Hill et al., 2003; Kraitchman et al., 2003). MR imaging has been used not only to track stem cells in the myocardium, but also to non-invasively evaluate ventricular function, perfusion and viability (Ebert et al., 2007). Cell tracking on MR imaging is based on labeling injected cells with FDA approved super paramagnetic iron oxide particles (Budde et al., 2009; Kraitchman et al., 2003). It has been shown that iron labeled cells maintain their viability, proliferation and differentiation (Hill et al., 2003). The cluster of iron labeled cells appear dark on T2* and T2 MR images (Arbab et al., 2005; Budde et al., 2009; Ebert et al., 2007; Kraitchman et al., 2003). Several factors affect the detection of iron labeled cells, which include magnetic field strength, labeling efficiency, type of cells and time of imaging after delivery. Investigators found that the duration of MR detection varies between cells; up to 5 weeks for stem cells (Himes et al. 2004) and up to 16 weeks for skeletal myoblasts (Cahill et al., 2004). Investigators also found hypointense tiny regions far from the site of injection, indicative of migration of stem cells within the infarction several weeks after delivery. MR imaging was used to evaluate changes in LV remodeling following the delivery of cellular therapy (Amado et al., 2005; Arai et al., 2006; Grauss et al., 2008; Hashemi et al., 2008; Moelker et al., 2006; Ziebart et al., 2008). Amado et al. (2006) were able to identify a time-dependent recovery of local contractility associated with the appearance of new tissue resulting from transplantation of allogeneic stem cells in a pig model of infarct.

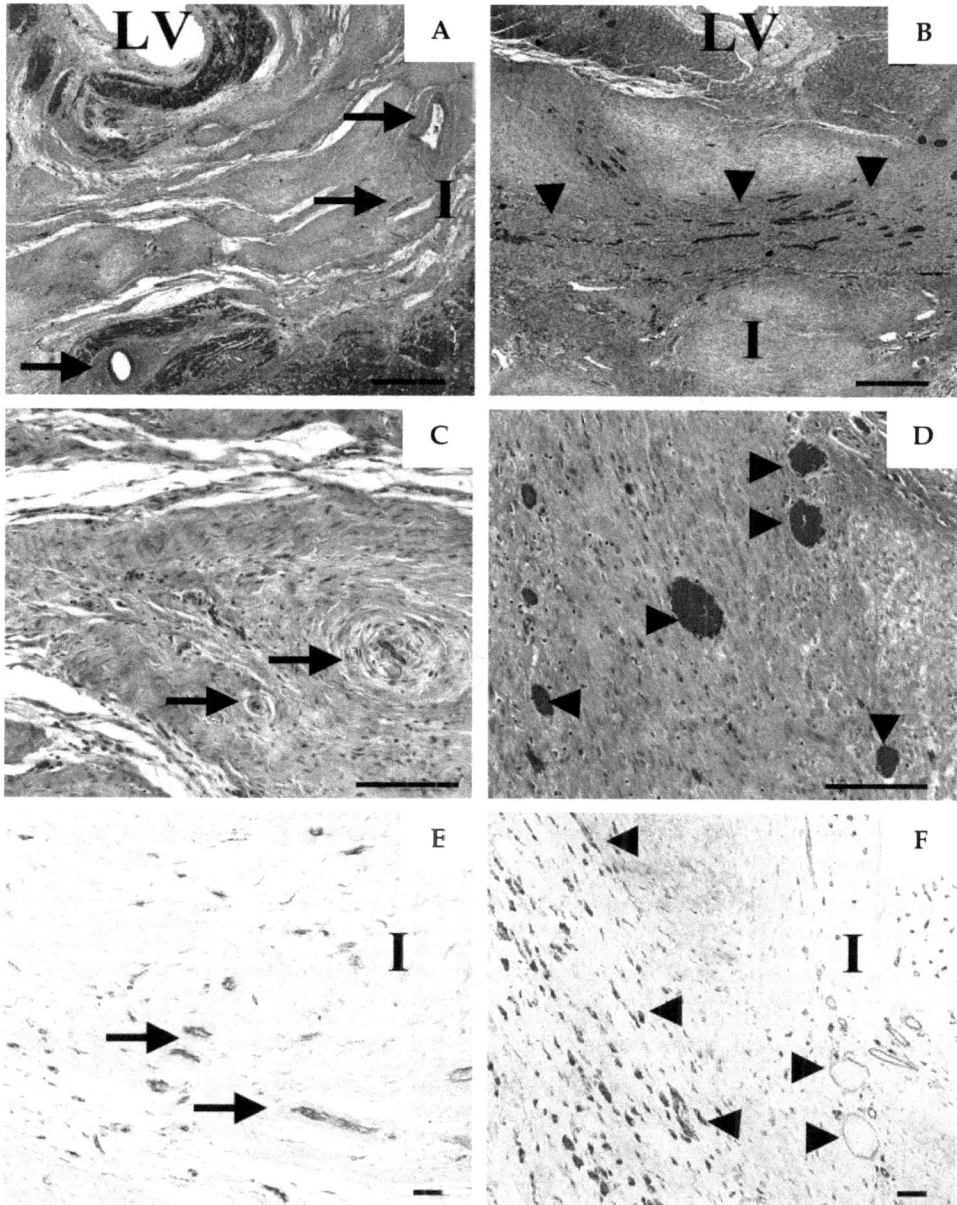

Figure 6: Histology of scar infarct in control (left) and VEGF gene–treated animals (right) 8 weeks after infarction. Sections A-D were stained with Masson trichrome stain, while E and F were stained with biotinylated isolectin B4. I = infarction in both groups which is comprised of homogeneous replacement fibrosis with a distinct boundary at the interface between scar and viable myocardium (M). Treated animal (right) contained numerous vessels (arrows), while control animal contained very few vessels. Biotinylated isolectin B4 localized vessels with brown reaction product, accentuating the neovascularity in VEGF gene–treated infarct animal compared with control animal. LV = left ventricle, calibration bars = 80 μm

MRI-guided coronary artery stent placement is a challenging interventional procedure because of the small size of the coronary arteries combined with incessant motion during the respiratory and cardiac cycles. These obstacles necessitate higher temporal and spatial resolution for real-time MR imaging techniques when compared with interventional peripheral MR angiography (Spuentrup et al., 2002b). Bock et al. (2008) described in detail the technical prerequisites for MR-guided endovascular interventions and addressed the safety aspects of this technique. The most common complications of coronary PCI are bleeding, hematoma, pseudoaneurysm, and arteriovenous fistulae at the access site.

6   MR-Guidance in Tissue Ablation

Ventricular tachycardia can lead to debilitating symptoms, hospital admissions, implantable cardioverter-defibrillator shocks and death. Radiofrequency catheter ablation of re-entrant circuits within myocardial scar is increasingly used in refractory cases with 50% success rate because of the limited depth of ablation. High-intensity focused ultrasound (HIFU) is an ablative energy source that can precisely penetrate deep into the targeted tissue without affecting surrounding tissues. This technique has been used in conjunction with MR-guidance to provide real-time anatomic and thermal mapping (Ellis et al., 2013). Clinical studies showed atrial scar on contrast enhanced MR imaging that results from RF ablation (McGann et al., 2008; Peters et al., 2007; Reddy et al., 2008). Other studies have demonstrated the association between infarct scar, border-zone and the risk of monomorphic ventricular tachycardia (Bello et al., 2005; Nazarian et al., 2005; Schmidt et al., 2007). Dong et al. (2006) found that 3D MR imaging is helpful for tailoring ablations to the variant pulmonary vein anatomy in 47% of patients with atrial fibrillation. They also noted that 3D images of the atria helped in localizing areas along the tissue ridge separating the left atrium from the pulmonary vein (Dong et al., 2006; Mansour et al., 2006). The ability of real-time MR imaging to visualize the needle tip in the inferior vena cava, atria, fossa ovalis, and surrounding vasculature during transseptal cardiac punctures has also been demonstrated (Arepally et al., 2005; Kenigsberg et al., 2007; Raval et al., 2006). The current interest is to develop a catheter based MRI-guided HIFU technique for ablation of ventricular arrhythmias, but this approach is limited due to the ribs block the energy of the HIFU system.

Recently, we successfully used MRI-guided HIFU in renal ablation and first pass perfusion and contrast enhanced MRI to assess the ablation. Figure 7 shows the perfusion deficits on first pass perfusion imaging of kidneys after ablation, while delayed contrast enhanced MR imaging shows the ablated lesion 10min after contrast administration (Figure 8).

7   Current Limitations and Future Potential

Currently, interventional MRI has several limitations. Installation and operation of MRI equipment is costly. Interventionists require knowledge on MRI and familiarity with the

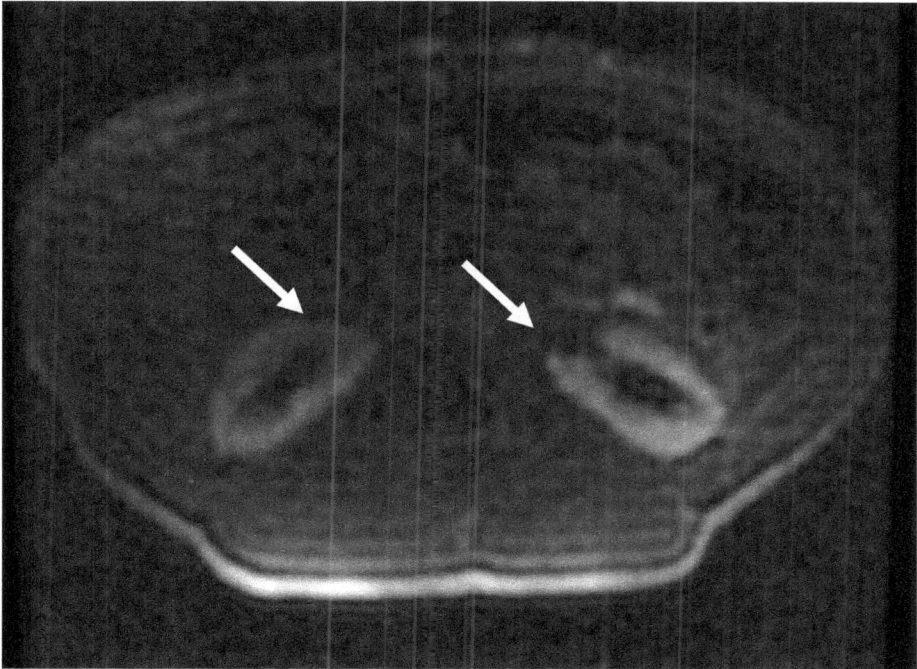

Figure 7: Renal ablation under MR-guided high intensity focused ultrasound (MRg-guided HIFU) using 2 sonication at energy of 4400J per site (left kidney) and 1 sonication per site at energy of 3300J. Perfusion MR images acquired in the first 2 min after bolus injection of 0.2 mmol/kg Gd-DTPA show regional ischemia (arrows). The ischemic lesion is larger on the left than the right kidney.

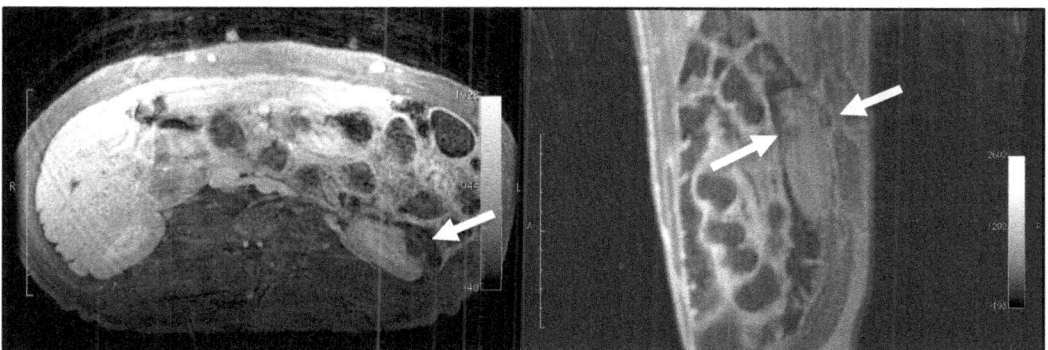

Figure 8: Axial (left) and sagittal (right) contrast enhanced MR images of renal ablation after MR-guided high intensity focused ultrasound (2 sonication showing the lesion in the left kidney (arrows). The deficits were visible for than 45min after contrast injection.

limited scanner bore, while patients must be cooperative during imaging. Transient bio-logical effects have been noted, such overheating due to alternating magnetic transmis-sions of the radiofrequency coils. At the present time, most medical and life support devices are MRI incompatible, therefore this technique is limited in acute settings. Thus, care must be taken for patients with aneurysm clips, intra-cranial or intra-ocular metal, shrapnel, cardiac pacemakers or pacemaker wires and cochlear implants. It is important to anticipate the side effects of MRI-guided procedures by using experimental animals before translation into routine clinical practice. Improving safety, spatial and temporal resolution of MRI enhances the feasibility of using interventional MRI in patients. Cur-rent, interventional MRI techniques are evolving at a dynamic pace in many centers in the United States and Europe. In the future, the use of contrast media during interven-tion must be reduced and 3D spatial resolution improved.

7.1   Cost Effectiveness

The potential of interventional MRI is great because as a single modality, it combines 3D anatomic imaging, device localization, hemodynamic/electrophysiologic information, tissue structure and function. The cost of x-ray suite is comparable with MRI suite, but the current costs of most interventional MRI procedures have yet to be reported. Marcy et al evaluated the benefit of performing certain MRI-guided interventional procedures, such as IVC filter placement, percutaneous placement of ureteral stents for obstructive uropathy and percutaneous gastrostomy tube placement. The procedures resolved the symptoms and improved quality of life in at least 80% of patients. The costs of the pro-cedures were relatively small based on the cost of hospitalization (0.85-11.3%) (Marcy et al., 1999). One might expect a negative financial impact, but increasing the utilization of interventional MRI can often result in significant economic benefit. Doubilet et al. (1986) reported that many medical decisions are influenced by factors that cannot be easily quantified or assigned a dollar value. While currently, insurance companies rarely re-imburse for these interventional MRI procedures, as they become more routine, they will be more affordable.

8   Conclusion

MR imaging provides 3D datasets, excellent soft-tissue contrast, multi-planar views, dynamic imaging and guidance of interventional vascular and cardiac procedures in a single imaging session. Non-enhanced MR imaging allows noninvasive monitoring of treatment success that is not available on X-ray fluoroscopy. Balloon dilation, stent placement, valvar replacement, atrial septal defect closure, radiofrequency ablation and local gene and cell delivery have been shown to be feasible on MR-guided imaging. It enables a substantially reduced level of invasiveness compared with open-chest sur-gery, potentially resulting in treatment on an outpatient basis, rapid patient recovery, eliminate radiation exposure and cost savings to the health care system. At present, car-diovascular interventions are addressed by utilizing multimodalities, such as multidetector computed tomography, X-ray fluoroscopy and echocardiography. Whether MR is suited to obviate the need for multimodality imaging is currently promising, butunclear. Translation of MR-guided interventions to routine clinical use has been very slow due to limited availability of MR-friendly equipment and funding by National Institute of Health and venders.

Reference

Allen KB, Dowling RD, Fudge TL, et al. (1999). Comparison of transmyocardial revascularization with medical therapy in patients with refractory angina. N Engl J Med 341(14):1029–1036

Amado LC, Saliaris AP, Schuleri KH, et al. (2005). Cardiac repair with intramyocardial injection of allogeneic mesenchymal stem cells after myocardial infarction. Proc Natl Acad Sci USA 102(32):11474–11479

Amado LC, Schuleri KH, Saliaris AP, et al. (2006). Multimodality noninvasive imaging demonstrates in vivo cardiac regeneration after mesenchymal stem cell therapy. J Am Coll Cardiol 48(10):2116–2124

Arai T, Kofidis T, Bulte JW, et al. (2006). Dual in vivo magnetic resonance evaluation of magnetically labeled mouse embryonic stem cells and cardiac function at 1.5 t. Magn Reson Med 55(1):203–209

Arbab AS, Yocum GT, Rad AM, et al. (2005). Labeling of cells with ferumoxides-protamine sulfate complexes does not inhibit function or differentiation capacity of hematopoietic or mesenchymal stem cells. NMR Biomed 18(8):553–559

Arepally A, Karmarkar PV, Weiss C, Atalar E (2006). Percutaneous MR imaging-guided transvascular access of mesenteric venous system: study in swine model. Radiology 238(1):113–118

Arepally A, Karmarkar PV, Weiss C, et al. (2005). Magnetic resonance image-guided trans-septal puncture in a swine heart. J Magn Reson Imaging 21(4):463–467

Assmus B, Honold J, Schachinger V, et al. (2006). Transcoronary transplantation of progenitor cells after myocardial infarction. N Engl J Med 355(12):1222–1232

Atalar E, Kraitchman DL, Carkhuff B, et al. (1998). Catheter-tracking FOV MR fluoroscopy. Magn Reson Med 40(6):865–872

Athanasoulis CA (2001). Vascular radiology: looking into the past to learn about the future. Radiology 218(2):317–322

Bakker CJ, Hoogeveen RM, Hurtak WF, et al. (1997). MR-guided endovascular interventions: susceptibility-based catheter and near-real-time imaging technique. Radiology 202(1):273–276

Bakker CJ, Smits HF, Bos C, et al. (1998). MR-guided balloon angioplasty: in vitro demonstration of the potential of MRI for guiding, monitoring, and evaluating endovascular interventions. J Magn Reson Imaging 8(1):245–250

Bartels LW, Smits HF, Bakker CJ, Viergever MA (2001). MR imaging of vascular stents: effects of susceptibility, flow, and radiofrequency eddy currents. J Vasc Interv Radiol 12(3):365–371

Bello D, Fieno DS, Kim RJ, et al. (2005). Infarct morphology identifies patients with substrate for sustained ventricular tachycardia. J Am Coll Cardiol 45(7):1104–1108

Bergvall E, Cain P, Arheden H, Sparr G (2006). A fast and highly automated approach to myocardial motion analysis using phase contrast magnetic resonance imaging. J Magn Reson Imaging 23(5):652–

661

Bernhardt A, Wilson MW, Settecase F, et al. (2011). *Steerable catheter microcoils for interventional MRI: reducing resistive heating. Acad Radiol. 18(3):270–276.*

Berrington de Gonzalez A, Darby S (2004). *Risk of cancer from diagnostic X-rays: estimates for the UK and 14 other countries. Lancet 363(9406):345–351*

Bock M, Muller S, Zuehlsdorff S, et al. (2006). *Active catheter tracking using parallel MRI and real-time image reconstruction. Magn Reson Med 55(6):1454–1459*

Bock M, Volz S, Zuhlsdorff S, et al. (2004). *MR-guided intravascular procedures: real-time parameter control and automated slice positioning with active tracking coils. J Magn Reson Imaging 19(5):580–589*

Bock M, Wacker FK (2008). *MR-guided intravascular interventions: techniques and applications. J Magn Reson Imaging. 27(2):326–38. doi: 10.1002/jmri.21271. PMID: 18219686.*

Boll DT, Lewin JS, Duerk JL, et al. (2004). *Assessment of automatic vessel tracking techniques in preoperative planning of transluminal aortic stent graft implantation. J Comput Assist Tomogr 28(2):278–285*

Bongartz G, Mayr M, Bilecen D (2008). *Magnetic resonance angiography (MRA) in renally impaired patients: when and how. Eur J Radiol 66(2):213–219*

Bucker A, Neuerburg JM, Adam GB, et al. (2001). *Real-time MR Guidance for inferior vena cava filter placement in an animal model. J Vasc Interv Radiol 12(6):753–756*

Budde MD, Frank JA (2009). *Magnetic tagging of therapeutic cells for MRI. J Nucl Med 50(2):171–174*

Buecker A, Adam GB, Neuerburg JM, et al. (2002a). *Simultaneous real-time visualization of the catheter tip and vascular anatomy for MR-guided PTA of iliac arteries in an animal model. J Magn Reson Imaging 16(2):201–208*

Buecker A, Neuerburg JM, Adam GB, et al. (2000). *Real-time MR fluoroscopy for MR-guided iliac artery stent placement. J Magn Reson Imaging 12(4):616–622*

Buecker A, Spuentrup E, Grabitz R, et al. (2002b). *Magnetic resonance-guided placement of atrial septal closure device in animal model of patent foramen ovale. Circulation 106(4):511–515*

Buecker A, Spuentrup E, Ruebben A, et al. (2004). *New metallic MR stents for artifact-free coronary MR angiography: feasibility study in a swine model. Invest Radiol 39(5):250–253*

Busse RF, Riederer SJ (2001). *Steady-state preparation for spoiled gradient echo imaging. Magn Reson Med 45(4):653–661*

Cahill KS, Germain S, Byrne BJ, Walter GA (2004). *Non-invasive analysis of myoblast transplants in rodent cardiac muscle. Int J Cardiovasc Imaging 20(6):593–598*

Carlsson M, Jablonowski R, Martin A, Ursell P, Saeed M (2011). *Impaired regional perfusion after coronary microembolization predicts long-term detrimental effects on regional left ventricular function. Scand Cardiovasc J 45(4):205–14.*

Carlsson M, Osman NF, Ursell PC, Martin AJ, Saeed M (2008). *Quantitative MR measurements of regional and global left ventricular function and strain after intramyocardial transfer of VM202 into infarcted swine myocardium. Am J Physiol Heart Circ Physiol 295(2):H522–H532*

Choudhury RP, Fuster V, Fayad ZA (2004). *Molecular, cellular and functional imaging of atherothrombosis. Nat Rev Drug Discov 3(11):913–925*

Chung YC, Duerk JL, Shankaranarayanan A, et al. (1999). Temperature measurement using echo-shifted FLASH at low field for interventional MRI. J Magn Reson Imaging 9(1):138–145

Cline HE, Hynynen K, Hardy CJ, et al. (1994). MR temperature mapping of focused ultrasound surgery. Magn Reson Med 31(6):628–636

Cline HE, Hynynen K, Watkins RD, et al. (1995). Focused US system for MR imaging-guided tumor ablation. Radiology 194(3):731–737

de Silva R, Gutierrez LF, Raval AN, et al. (2006). X-ray fused with magnetic resonance imaging (XFM) to target endomyocardial injections: validation in a swine model of myocardial infarction. Circulation 114(22):2342–2350

Dick AJ, Guttman MA, Raman VK, et al. (2003). Magnetic resonance fluoroscopy allows targeted delivery of mesenchymal stem cells to infarct borders in swine. Circulation 108(23):2899–2904

Dick AJ, Lederman RJ (2005). MRI-guided myocardial cell therapy. Int J Cardiovasc Interv 7(4):165–170

Dick AJ, Raman VK, Raval AN, et al. (2005). Invasive human magnetic resonance imaging: feasibility during revascularization in a combined XMR suite. Catheter Cardiovasc Interv 64(3):265–274

Dicks D, Saloner D, Martin A, et al. (2010). Cardiovascular magnetic resonance imaging for percutaneous transendocardial delivery and three dimensional left ventricular strain assessment of VEGF gene therapy in occlusive infarction. Int J Cardiol 143(3):255–263

Dicks DL, Carlsson M, Heiberg E, et al. (2009). Persistent decline in longitudinal and radial strain after coronary microembolization detected on velocity encoded phase contrast magnetic resonance imaging. J Magn Reson Imaging 30(1):69–76

Dion YM, Ben El Kadi H, Boudoux C, et al. (2000). Endovascular procedures under near-real-time magnetic resonance imaging guidance: an experimental feasibility study. J Vasc Surg 32(5):1006–1014

Dong J, Dickfeld T, Dalal D, et al. (2006). Initial experience in the use of integrated electroanatomic mapping with three-dimensional MR/CT images to guide catheter ablation of atrial fibrillation. J Cardiovasc Electrophysiol 17(5):459–466

Doubilet P, Weinstein MC, McNeil BJ (1986). Use and misuse of the term "cost effective" in medicine N Eng J Med. 314(4):253–6. PMID: 3079883.

Duerk JL, Lewin JS, Wendt M, Petersilge C (1998). Remember true FISP? A high SNR, near 1-second imaging method for T2-like contrast in interventional MRI at .2 T. J Magn Reson Imaging 8(1):203–208

Ebert SN, Taylor DG, Nguyen HL, et al. (2007). Noninvasive tracking of cardiac embryonic stem cells in vivo using magnetic resonance imaging techniques. Stem Cells 25(11):2936–2944

Elgort DR, Duerk JL (2005). A review of technical advances in interventional magnetic resonance imaging. Acad Radiol 12(9):1089–1099

Ellis S, Rieke V, Kohi M, Westphalen AC (2013). Clinical applications for magnetic resonance guided high intensity focused ultrasound (MRgHIFU): present and future. J Med Imaging Radiat Oncol. 57(4):391–393.

Freyman T, Polin G, Osman H, et al. (2006). A quantitative, randomized study evaluating three methods of mesenchymal stem cell delivery following myocardial infarction. Eur Heart J 27(9):1114–1122

Frush DP (2004). Review of radiation issues for computed tomography. Semin Ultrasound CT MR 25(1):17–24

Grauss RW, van Tuyn J, Steendijk P, et al. (2008). Forced myocardin expression enhances the therapeutic effect of human mesenchymal stem cells after transplantation in ischemic mouse hearts. Stem Cells 26(4):1083–1093

Hall WA, Liu H, Martin AJ, et al. (2000). Safety, efficacy, and functionality of high-field strength interventional magnetic resonance imaging for neurosurgery. Neurosurgery 46(3):632–641 (discussion 641–632)

Hamer OW, Borisch I, Paetzel C, et al. (2006). In vitro evaluation of stent patency and in-stent stenoses in 10 metallic stents using MR angiography. Br J Radiol 79(944):636–643

Hashemi SM, Ghods S, Kolodgie FD, et al. (2008). A placebo controlled, dose-ranging, safety study of allogenic mesenchymal stem cells injected by endomyocardial delivery after an acute myocardial infarction. Eur Heart J 29(2):251–259

Hill JM, Dick AJ, Raman VK, wt al (2003). Serial cardiac magnetic resonance imaging of injected mesenchymal stem cells. Circulation 108(8):1009–1014

Himes N, Min JY, Lee R, et al. (2004). In vivo MRI of embryonic stem cells in a mouse model of myocardial infarction. Magn Reson Med 52(5):1214–1219

Hsu L, Fried MP, Jolesz FA (1998). MR-guided endoscopic sinus surgery. AJNR Am J Neuroradiol 19(7):1235–1240

Hushek SG, Martin AJ, Steckner M, et al. (2008). MR systems for MRI-guided interventions. J Magn Reson Imaging 27(2):253–266

Hynynen K, Freund WR, Cline HE, et al. (1996). A clinical, noninvasive, MR imaging-monitored ultrasound surgery method. Radiographics 16(1):185–195

Jacquier A, Higgins CB, Martin AJ, et al. (2007). Injection of adeno-associated viral vector encoding vascular endothelial growth factor gene in infarcted swine myocardium: MR measurements of left ventricular function and strain. Radiology 245(1):196–205

Kenigsberg DN, Lee BP, Grizzard JD, Ellenbogen KA, Wood MA (2007). Accuracy of intracardiac echocardiography for assessing the esophageal course along the posterior left atrium: a comparison to magnetic resonance imaging. J Cardiovasc Electrophysiol 18(2):169–173

Kersting-Sommerhoff BA, Diethelm L, Stanger P, et al. (1990). Evaluation of complex congenital ventricular anomalies with magnetic resonance imaging. Am Heart J 120(1):133–142

Kleiman NS, Patel NC, Allen KB, et al. (2003). Evolving revascularization approaches for myocardial ischemia. Am J Cardiol 92(9B):9N–17N

Klein HM, Ghodsizad A, Marktanner R, et al. (2007). Intramyocardial implantation of CD133+ stem cells improved cardiac function without bypass surgery. Heart Surg Forum 10(1):E66–E69

Klemm T, Duda S, Machann J, et al. (2000). MR imaging in the presence of vascular stents: a systematic assessment of artifacts for various stent orientations, sequence types, and field strengths. J Magn Reson Imaging 12(4):606–615

Kocaturk O, Saikus CE, Guttman MA, et al. (2009). Whole shaft visibility and mechanical performance for active MR catheters using copper-nitinol braided polymer tubes. J Cardiovasc Magn Reson 11(1):29

Kos S, Huegli R, Hofmann E, et al. (2009). First magnetic resonance imaging-guided aortic stenting and cava filter placement using a polyetheretherketone-based magnetic resonance imaging-compatible guidewire in swine: proof of concept. Cardiovasc Intervent Radiol 32(3):514–521

Kraitchman DL, Heldman AW, Atalar E, et al. (2003). In vivo magnetic resonance imaging of mesenchymal stem cells in myocardial infarction. *Circulation* 107(18):2290–2293

Kramer CM, Budoff MJ, Fayad ZA, et al. (2007). *ACCF/AHA 2007 clinical competence statement on vascular imaging with computed tomography and magnetic resonance. Vasc Med 12(4):359–378*

Krueger JJ, Ewert P, Yilmaz S, et al. (2006). *Magnetic resonance imaging-guided balloon angioplasty of coarctation of the aorta: a pilot study. Circulation 113(8):1093–1100*

Krueger S, Schmitz S, Weiss S, et al. (2008). *An MR guidewire based on micropultruded fiber-reinforced material. Magn Reson Med 60(5):1190–1196*

Kuehne T, Saeed M, Higgins CB, et al. (2003). *Endovascular stents in pulmonary valve and artery in swine: feasibility study of MR imaging-guided deployment and postinterventional assessment. Radiology 226(2):475–481*

Kuehne T, Saeed M, Moore P, et al. (2002). *Influence of blood-pool contrast media on MR imaging and flow measurements in the presence of pulmonary arterial stents in swine. Radiology 223(2):439–445*

Kuehne T, Saeed M, Reddy G, et al. (2001). *Sequential magnetic resonance monitoring of pulmonary flow with endovascular stents placed across the pulmonary valve in growing Swine. Circulation 104(19):2363–2368*

Kuehne T, Yilmaz S, Meinus C, et al. (2004a). *Magnetic resonance imaging-guided transcatheter implantation of a prosthetic valve in aortic valve position: feasibility study in swine. J Am Coll Cardiol 44(11):2247–2249*

Kuehne T, Yilmaz S, Schulze-Neick I, et al. (2005). *Magnetic resonance imaging guided catheterisation for assessment of pulmonary vascular resistance: in vivo validation and clinical application in patients with pulmonary hypertension. Heart 91(8):1064–1069*

Kuehne T, Yilmaz S, Steendijk P, et al. (2004b). *Magnetic resonance imaging analysis of right ventricular pressure-volume loops: in vivo validation and clinical application in patients with pulmonary hypertension. Circulation 110(14):2010–2016*

Kuroda K, Mulkern RV, Oshio K, et al. (2000). *Temperature mapping using the water proton chemical shift: self-referenced method with echo-planar spectroscopic imaging. Magn Reson Med 43(2):220–225*

Kyriakos WE, Hoge WS, Mitsouras D (2006). *Generalized encoding through the use of selective excitation in accelerated parallel MRI. NMR Biomed 19(3):379–392*

Ladd ME, Zimmermann GG, McKinnon GC, et al. (1998). *Visualization of vascular guidewires using MR tracking. J Magn Reson Imaging 8(1):251–253*

Laham RJ, Sellke FW, Edelman ER, et al. (1999). *Local perivascular delivery of basic fibroblast growth factor in patients undergoing coronary bypass surgery: results of a phase I randomized, double-blind, placebo-controlled trial. Circulation 100(18):1865–1871*

Lakhan SE, Kaplan A, Laird C, Leiter Y (2009). *The interventionalism of medicine: interventional radiology, cardiology, and neuroradiology. Int Arch Med 2(1):27*

Leung DA, Debatin JF, Wildermuth S, et al. (1995). *Intravascular MR tracking catheter: preliminary experimental evaluation. AJR Am J Roentgenol 164(5):1265–1270*

Liu Y, Sun L, Huan Y, Zhao H, Deng J (2006). *Effects of basic fibroblast growth factor microspheres on angiogenesis in ischemic myocardium and cardiac function: analysis with dobutamine cardiovascular magnetic resonance tagging. Eur J Cardiothorac Surg 30(1):103–107*

Maes RM, Lewin JS, Duerk JL, Wacker FK (2005). *Combined use of the intravascular blood-pool agent, gadomer, and carbon dioxide: a novel type of double-contrast magnetic resonance angiography (MRA).*

J Magn Reson Imaging 21(5):645–649

Mahnken AH, Chalabi K, Jalali F, Gunther RW, Buecker A (2004). *Magnetic resonance-guided placement of aortic stents grafts: feasibility with real-time magnetic resonance fluoroscopy. J Vasc Interv Radiol 15(2 Pt 1):189–195*

Manke C, Nitz WR, Djavidani B, et al. (2001). *MR imaging-guided stent placement in iliac arterial stenoses: a feasibility study. Radiology 219(2):527–534*

Manke C, Nitz WR, Lenhart M, et al. (2000). *Stent angioplasty of pelvic artery stenosis with MRI control: initial clinical results. Rofo 172(1):92–97*

Mansour M, Refaat M, Heist EK, et al. (2006). *Three-dimensional anatomy of the left atrium by magnetic resonance angiography: implications for catheter ablation for atrial fibrillation. J Cardiovasc Electrophysiol 17(7):719–723*

Marcy PY, Chevallier P, Granon C, Falewee MN, Bleuse A, Bruneton JN (1999). *Cost-benefit analysis of percutaneous interventional radiological procedures in cancer patients. Supportive Care in Cancer 7(5):365-7. PMID: 10483824.*

Martin AJ, Hall WA, Liu H, et al. (2000). *Brain tumor resection: intraoperative monitoring with high-field-strength MR imaging-initial results. Radiology 215(1):221–228*

Martin AJ, Weber OM, Saeed M, Roberts TP (2003). *Steady-state imaging for visualization of endovascular interventions. Magn Reson Med 50(2):434–438*

McGann CJ, Kholmovski EG, Oakes RS, et al. (2008). *New magnetic resonance imaging-based method for defining the extent of left atrial wall injury after the ablation of atrial fibrillation. J Am Coll Cardiol 52(15):1263–1271*

McVeigh ER, Guttman MA, Lederman RJ, et al. (2006). *Real-time interactive MRI-guided cardiac surgery: aortic valve replacement using a direct apical approach. Magn Reson Med 56(5):958–964*

Mekle R, Zenge MO, Ladd ME, et al. (2009). *Initial in vivo studies with a polymer-based MR-compatible guide wire. J Vasc Interv Radiol 20(10):1384–1389*

Menasche P, Alfieri O, Janssens S, et al. (2008). *The myoblast autologous grafting in ischemic cardiomyopathy (MAGIC). trial: first randomized placebo-controlled study of myoblast transplantation. Circulation 117(9):1189–1200*

Moelker AD, Baks T, van den Bos EJ, et al. (2006). *Reduction in infarct size, but no functional improvement after bone marrow cell administration in a porcine model of reperfused myocardial infarction. Eur Heart J 27(24):3057–3064*

Narazaki G, Uosaki H, Teranishi M, et al. (2008). *Directed and systematic differentiation of cardiovascular cells from mouse induced pluripotent stem cells. Circulation 118(5):498–506*

Nazarian S, Bluemke DA, Lardo AC, et al. (2005). *Magnetic resonance assessment of the substrate for inducible ventricular tachycardia in nonischemic cardiomyopathy. Circulation 112(18):2821–2825*

Niendorf T, Sodickson DK (2006). *Parallel imaging in cardiovascular MRI: methods and applications. NMR Biomed 19(3):325–341*

Nitz WR, Oppelt A, Renz W, et al. (2001). *On the heating of linear conductive structures as guide wires and catheters in interventional MRI. J Magn Reson Imaging 13(1):105–114*

Omary RA, Frayne R, Unal O, et al. (2000). *MR-guided angioplasty of renal artery stenosis in a pig model: a feasibility study. J Vasc Interv Radiol 11(3):373–381*

Omeish A, Hijazi ZM (2001). Transcatheter closure of atrial septal defects in children & adults using the Amplatzer Septal Occluder. J Interv Cardiol 14(1):37–44

Paetzel C, Zorger N, Bachthaler M, et al (2005). Magnetic resonance-guided percutaneous angioplasty of femoral and popliteal artery stenoses using real-time imaging and intra-arterial contrast-enhanced magnetic resonance angiography. Invest Radiol 40(5):257–262

Park SM, Kamondetdacha R, Nyenhuis JA (2007). Calculation of MRI-induced heating of an implanted medical lead wire with an electric field transfer function. J Magn Reson Imaging 26(5):1278–1285

Pearlman JD, Laham RJ, Simons M (2000). Coronary angiogenesis: detection in vivo with MR imaging sensitive to collateral neocirculation–preliminary study in pigs. Radiology 214(3):801–807

Peters DC, Lederman RJ, Dick AJ, et al. (2003). Undersampled projection reconstruction for active catheter imaging with adaptable temporal resolution and catheter-only views. Magn Reson Med 49(2):216–222

Peters DC, Wylie JV, Hauser TH, et al. (2007). Detection of pulmonary vein and left atrial scar after catheter ablation with three-dimensional navigator-gated delayed enhancement MR imaging: initial experience. Radiology 243(3):690–695

Peters TM (2006). Image-guidance for surgical procedures. Phys Med Biol 51(14):R505–R540

Post MJ, Sato K, Murakami M, et al (2006). Adenoviral PR39 improves blood flow and myocardial function in a pig model of chronic myocardial ischemia by enhancing collateral formation. Am J Physiol Regul Integr Comp Physiol 290(3):R494–R500

Prasad KN, Cole WC, Hasse GM (2004). Health risks of low dose ionizing radiation in humans: a review. Exp Biol Med (Maywood) 229(5):378–382

Pruessmann KP, Weiger M, Scheidegger MB, Boesiger P (1999). SENSE: sensitivity encoding for fast MRI. Magn Reson Med 42(5):952–962

Quick HH, Kuehl H, Kaiser G, et al. (2002). Inductively coupled stent antennas in MRI. Magn Reson Med 48(5):781–790

Raman VK, Karmarkar PV, Guttman MA, et al. (2005). Real-time magnetic resonance-guided endovascular repair of experimental abdominal aortic aneurysm in swine. J Am Coll Cardiol 45(12):2069–2077

Rasche V, Holz D, Kohler J, Proksa R, Roschmann P (1997). Catheter tracking using continuous radial MRI. Magn Reson Med 37(6):963–968

Raval AN, Karmarkar PV, Guttman MA, et al. (2006). Real-time MRI guided atrial septal puncture and balloon septostomy in swine. Catheter Cardiovasc Interv 67(4):637–643

Raval AN, Telep JD, Guttman MA, et al. (2005). Real-time magnetic resonance imaging-guided stenting of aortic coarctation with commercially available catheter devices in swine. Circulation 112(5):699–706

Razavi R, Hill DL, Keevil SF, et al. (2003). Cardiac catheterisation guided by MRI in children and adults with congenital heart disease. Lancet 362(9399):1877–1882

Reddy VY, Schmidt EJ, Holmvang G, Fung M (2008). Arrhythmia recurrence after atrial fibrillation ablation: can magnetic resonance imaging identify gaps in atrial ablation lines? J Cardiovasc Electrophysiol 19(4):434–437

Rickers C, Jerosch-Herold M, Hu X, et al. (2003). Magnetic resonance image-guided transcatheter closure of atrial septal defects. Circulation 107(1):132–138

Ruel M, Laham RJ, Parker JA, et al. (2002). Long-term effects of surgical angiogenic therapy with fibroblast growth factor 2 protein. J Thorac Cardiovasc Surg 124(1):28–34

Sadowski EA, Bennett LK, Chan MR, et al. (2007). Nephrogenic systemic fibrosis: risk factors and incidence estimation. Radiology 243(1):148–157

Saeed M, Henk CB, Weber O, et al. (2006). Delivery and assessment of endovascular stents to repair aortic coarctation using MR and X-ray imaging. J Magn Reson Imaging 24(2):371–378

Saeed M, Martin A, Jacquier A, et al. (2008a). Permanent coronary artery occlusion: cardiovascular MR imaging is platform for percutaneous transendocardial delivery and assessment of gene therapy in canine model. Radiology 249(2):560–571

Saeed M, Martin A, Ursell P, et al. (2008b). MR assessment of myocardial perfusion, viability and function after intramyocardial transfer of VM202, a new plasmid human hepatocyte growth factor in ischemic swine myocardium. Radiology 249(1):107–118

Saeed M, Martin AJ, Lee RJ, et al. (2006). MR guidance of targeted injections into border and core of scarred myocardium in pigs. Radiology 240(2):419–426

Saeed M, Martin AJ, Saloner D, Do L, Wilson M (2010). Noninvasive MR characterization of structural and functional components of reperfused infarct. Acta Radiol 51(10):1093–1102

Saito T, Kuang JQ, Lin CC, Chiu RC (2003). Transcoronary implantation of bone marrow stromal cells ameliorates cardiac function after myocardial infarction. J Thorac Cardiovasc Surg 126(1):114–123

Samset E, Hirschberg H (1999). Neuronavigation in intraoperative MRI. Comput Aided Surg 4(4):200–207

Saybasili H, Faranesh AZ, Saikus CE, et al. (2010). Interventional MRI using multiple 3D angiography roadmaps with real-time imaging. J Magn Reson Imaging 31(4):1015–1019

Schalla S, Saeed M, Higgins CB, et al. (2005). Balloon sizing and transcatheter closure of acute atrial septal defects guided by magnetic resonance fluoroscopy: assessment and validation in a large animal model. J Magn Reson Imaging 21(3):204–211

Schalla S, Saeed M, Higgins CB, Martin A, Weber O, Moore P (2003). Magnetic resonance–guided cardiac catheterization in a swine model of atrial septal defect. Circulation 108(15):1865–1870

Schmidt A, Azevedo CF, Cheng A, et al. (2007). Infarct tissue heterogeneity by magnetic resonance imaging identifies enhanced cardiac arrhythmia susceptibility in patients with left ventricular dysfunction. Circulation 115(15):2006–2014

Schwartz RB, Hsu L, Wong TZ, et al. (1999). Intraoperative MR imaging guidance for intracranial neurosurgery: experience with the first 200 cases. Radiology 211(2):477–488

Settecase F, Hetts SW, Martin AJ, et al. (2011). RF heating of MRI-assisted catheter steering coils for interventional MRI. Acad Radiol. 18(3):277–85.

Shellock FG, Valencerina S (2005). Septal repair implants: evaluation of magnetic resonance imaging safety at 3 T. Magn Reson Imaging 23(10):1021–1025

Simonetti O, Lucarini G, Brancorsini D, et al. (2002). Immunohistochemical expression of vascular endothelial growth factor, matrix metalloproteinase 2, and matrix metalloproteinase 9 in cutaneous melanocytic lesions. Cancer 95(9):1963–1970

Simons M, Bonow RO, Chronos NA, et al. (2000). Clinical trials in coronary angiogenesis: issues, problems, consensus: an expert panel summary. Circulation 102(11):E73–E86

Smits HF, Bos C, van der Weide R, Bakker CJ (1998). *Endovascular interventional MR: balloon angioplasty in a hemodialysis access flow phantom.* J Vasc Interv Radiol 9(5):840–845

Sousa JE, Costa MA, Tuzcu EM, et al. (2005). *New frontiers in interventional cardiology.* Circulation 111(5):671–681

Spielman DM, Pauly JM, Meyer CH (1995). *Magnetic resonance fluoroscopy using spirals with variable sampling densities.* Magn Reson Med 34(3):388–394

Spuentrup E, Ruebben A, Schaeffter T, et al. (2002a). *Magnetic resonance–guided coronary artery stent placement in a swine model.* Circulation 105(7):874–879

Spuentrup E, Ruebben A, Schaeffter T, Manning WJ, Gunther RW, Buecker A (2002b). *Magnetic resonance—guided coronary artery stent placement in a swine model.* Circulation. 105(7):874–9. PMID: 11854130.

Stamm C, Kleine HD, Choi YH, et al. (2007). *Intramyocardial delivery of CD133+ bone marrow cells and coronary artery bypass grafting for chronic ischemic heart disease: safety and efficacy studies.* J Thorac Cardiovasc Surg 133(3):717–725

van der Weide R, Zuiderveld KJ, Bakker CJ, et al. (1998). *Image guidance of endovascular interventions on a clinical MR scanner.* IEEE Trans Med Imaging 17(5):779–785

Wacker FK, Hillenbrand C, Elgort DR, et al. (2005a). *MR imaging-guided percutaneous angioplasty and stent placement in a swine model comparison of open- and closed-bore scanners.* Acad Radiol 12(9):1085–1088

Wacker FK, Hillenbrand CM, Duerk JL, Lewin JS (2005b). *MR-guided endovascular interventions: device visualization, tracking, navigation, clinical applications, and safety aspects.* Magn Reson Imaging Clin N Am 13(3):431–439

Weber OM, Schalla S, Martin AJ, et al. (2003). *Interventional cardiac magnetic resonance imaging.* Semin Roentgenol 38(4):352–357

Wendt M, Wacker FK (2000). *Visualization, tracking, and navigation of instruments for magnetic resonance imaging-guided endovascular procedures.* Top Magn Reson Imaging 11(3):163–172

Yang X, Atalar E (2006). *MRI-guided gene therapy.* FEBS Lett 580(12):2958–2961

Yang X, Atalar E, Li D, et al. (2001). *Magnetic resonance imaging permits in vivo monitoring of catheter-based vascular gene delivery.* Circulation 104(14):1588–1590

Ziebart T, Yoon CH, Trepels T, et al. (2008). *Sustained persistence of transplanted proangiogenic cells contributes to neovascularization and cardiac function after ischemia.* Circ Res 103(11):1327–1334

Chapter 6

Treatment of Macroprolactinoma by Virtue of Phytotherapy

Ivo Trogrlić[1], Dragan Trogrlić[1], Zoran Trogrlić[1]

1 Introduction

Prolactinomas are the most common functional tumours of the pituitary gland, representing an approximate 45-percent share of the total hormone-releasing tumour pool (Horvath & Kovacs, 1992). Nearly 90% of prolactinomas are of the lactotrophic origin, while the remaining 10% are mixed tumours built up of both lactotrophic and somatotrophic cells characterised by enhanced prolactin and growth factor release (Scheithauer et al, 1986). Prolactinomas mutually differ in their size and secretion activity. Based on their size, they can be divided into micro-and macroprolactinomas. Microprolactiomas grow slowly, up to only a few millimetres in size and are usually distinctive and not prone to grow further (Mah & Webster, 2001; Guyton & Hall, 2003). In the majority of the diseased, macroprolactinomas grow over 10 mm in size; their growth is mostly rapid and expansive so that they infiltrate the adjacent anatomic structures and pressurise them, endangering thereby health and even life of the diseased (Mah and Webster, 2001). Of a particular note is the fact that the pituitary gland is seated next to the optical structures enables macroprolactinomas to pressurise the optical nerve and/or the optical chiasm, so that some patients may experience more or less pronounced visual field defects. The latter often represent the first symptom of a macroprolactinoma presence. As compared to macroprolactinomas, the secretion activity of microprolactinomas is by far lower. Due to the high level of prolactin they synthesise and release, macroprolactinomas are featured by a distinctive clinical presentation (Asa, 1998; Levy & Lightman, 1993). In order to treat them, contemporary medicine mostly resorts to dopamine agonists (DAs) as the first-line

[1] "DREN" Ltd, Žepče, Bosnia & Herzegovina.

pharmacotherapy. However, microprolactinomas and macroprolactinomas differ in their sensitivity to such treatment (Braucks et al, 2003). While microprolactinomas are only poorly responsive, a substantial reduction in prolactin level, but not in tumour size, can be seen in most patients diagnosed with macroprolactinomas and taking Das (Levy & Lightman, 1993). On top of dopamine agonists, contemporary medicine makes use of microsurgery and radiotherapy (Horvath & Kovacs, 1992, Braucks et al, 2003).

This study aims at demonstrating the efficiency of phytotherapy in macroprolactinoma downsizing and strives to prove that pharmacoactive ingredients present in remedial plant mixtures are ultimately capable of attaining tumour regression and consequently reducing the level of prolactin.

2   Subjects and Methods

The study was carried out within 2005 – 2010 timeframe and comprised a total of 32 patients, out of which 21 (65.6%) women and 11 (34.4%) men, all of them being the citizens of currently independent states occupying the territory of the former Yugoslavia (Bosnia and Herzegovina, Croatia, Serbia and Macedonia). The patients' age spanned from 16 to 78 (average age, 40.7). Prior to PT commencement, the patients submitted medical records revealing their diagnosis established based on the nuclear magnetic resonance imaging (NMRI) and/or computed tomography (CT) of the affected site, hormonal status and field-of-vision examination. These data served as the baseline for comparison and follow-up of the PT efficiency.

Throughout the study course, macroprolactinoma patients had been treated with three distinctive plant remedies (Preparations 1, 2 & 3). These preparations mutually differ in their composition and consist solely of pounded herbs lacking any additives whatsoever. The ingredients of the plant preparations are given in Tables 1, 2 and 3.

The constitutive plants are pounded to the standard degree (Lukić, 1993). Flowers, stalks and leaves were prepared using a number 6 sieve (rough cutting), roots and barks using a number 3 sieve, and seeds and fruits using a number 2 sieve (precise cutting) (Pekić, 1983; Kovačević, 2000). These plant preparations are prepared and drunk in form of tea and have to be used on an everyday basis in line with the following schedule: Preparation 1 at 7:00 am, Preparation 2 at 2:00 pm, and Preparation 3 at 7:00 pm. All of them are prepared in the same way, a single tea dose thereby calling for 1.5 g of the herbal mixture and 200 cm³ of water. Following the analysis of the PT efficiency in terms of tumour mass downsizing and the reduction of prolactin level carried out on the whole study sample level, the subjects were divided into two groups.

Group 1 (hereinafter referred to as: the PT only arm) consisted of 9 patients receiving only PT. Out of them, 8 (88.9%) were women and 1 (11.1%) was a man. They were aged 37.5 on the average (range, 20–70). Group 2 (hereinafter referred to as: the DA & PT arm) consisted of 23 patients, in specific, 10 men (43.47%) and 13 women (56.53%) receiving PT in addition to their regular DA medication. The group in reference was aged 41.9 on the average (range, 16–78).

Preparation 1				
Pharmaceutical Name	Botanical Name	Family	Part Used	Percentage Representation
Herba catariae	*Nepeta cataria* L.	Lamiaceae	Herba	20%
Melissae folium	*Melissa officinalis* L.	Lamiaceae	Folium	15%
Thymi herba	*Thymus vulgaris* L.	Lamiaceae	Herba	10%
Origani herba	*Origanum vulgare* L.	Lamiaceae	Herba	10%
Matricariae flos	*Matricaria chamomilla* L.	Asteraceae	Flos	10%
Lupuli strobili	*Humulus lupulus* L.	Cannabaceae	Storobili	10%
Rosmarini folium	*Rosmarinus officinalis* L.	Lamiaceae	Folium	5%
Calendulae flos	*Calendula officinalis* L.	Asteraceae	Flos	5%
Valerianae radix et rhzoma	*Valeriana officinalis* L.	Valerianaceae	Radix et Rhizoma	5%
Bursae pastoris herba	*Capsella bursa pastoris* L.	Brassicaceae	Herba	5%
Basilici herba	*Ocimmum basillicum* L.	Lamiaceae	Herba	5%

Table 1: Ingredients of preparation 1.

Preparation 2				
Pharmaceutical Name	Botanical Name	Family	Part Used	Percentage Representation
Althaeae radix	*Althaea officinalis* L.	Malvaceae	Radix	15%
Althaeae folium	*Althaea officinalis* L.	Malvaceae	Folium	15%
Betulae folium	*Betula pendula* Roth	Betulaceae	Folium	15%
Hyperici herba	*Hypericum perforatum* L.	Hypericaceae	Herba	15%
Menhtae piperitae folium	*Menhta piperita* L.	Lamiaceae	Folium	15%
Herba glechomae	*Glechoma hederacea* L.	Labiatae	Herba	15%
Cheliodonii herba	*Chelidonium majus* L.	Papaveraceae	Herba	10%

Table 2: Ingredients of preparation 2.

Preparation 3				
Pharmaceutical Name	Botanical Name	Family	Part Used	Percentage Representation
Herba catariae	*Nepeta cataria* L.	Lamiaceae	Herba	25%
Melissae folium	*Melissa officinalis* L.	Lamiaceae	Folium	20%
Thymi herba	*Thymus vulgaris* L.	Lamiaceae	Herba	15%
Matricariae flos	*Matricaria chamomilla* L.	Asteraceae	Flos	15%
Lupuli strobili	*Humulus lupulus* L.	Cannabaceae	Storobili	10%
Rosmarini folium	*Rosmarinus officinalis* L.	Lamiaceae	Folium	5%
Calendulae flos	*Calendula officinalis* L.	Asteraceae	Flos	5%
Bursae pastoris herba	*Capsella bursa pastoris* L.	Brassicaceae	Herba	5%

Table 3: Ingredients of preparation 3.

Our next goal was to determine the manner in which the length of previous DA therapy affects PT outcomes. To that end, the members of the DA & PT arm were further subdivided into two subgroups based on the length of their pre-PT DA therapy. Subgroup 2A embraced the patients previously treated with DAs for 8–26 months and consisted of 19 patients, out of which 12 (63.1%) were women and 7 (36.9%) were men. The patients were aged 41.4 on the average, the youngest among them being 16 and the oldest one being 78. Prior to the PT launch, 4 of our study patients had been treated with DAs for over 36 months (Subgroup 2B). This subgroup embraced 3 (75%) men and one (25%) woman at the average age of 44.7 (range, 22–59).

Out of the entire study pool, 15 (46.8%) patients had experienced more or less severe pre-PT visual symptoms arising on the grounds of compression of optical structures exerted by macroprolactinoma. Out of those, 8 (53.3%) were of a female and 7(46.7%) of a male gender. These patients were aged 40 on the average (range, 18–59). Within the frame of the statistical analysis and outcome reporting, this patient subgroup was processed and presented separately.

The comparison between the pre-PT and post-PT health statuses carried out throughout the follow-up period made use of the following key endpoint measures:

1   Data on tumour size

2   Prolactin levels

3   Data on PT length and side-effects

4   Data on the state of the field-of-vision of the patients suffering from pre-PT visual field defects;

Data on the parameters detailed above posed as the baseline for mathematical-statistical analysis aimed at corroborating or rejecting certain hypotheses on PT outcomes. In order to reach as reliable conclusions as possible, the analysis of changes in PRLs established prior to and following PT was preceded by the analysis of baseline data credibility. Nevertheless, the primary goal of the analyses completed within this frame was to verify PT efficiency. To that effect, the hypothesis on the existence of significant differences in pre- and post-PT PRLs was tested at the significance levels of 5%, 1%, and 0.1% (exceptionally also at the significance level above 5% in cases where information on PT efficiency was short). To the aforementioned goal, not only standard, but also non-parametric statistical methods were used. Namely, the sample size and the statistical parameters obtained (central values, ranges and metric output dispersion) clearly indicated that parametric, i.e. "classical" statistical methods would be an inappropriate choice. Therefore, statistical evaluation primarily made use of non-parametric methods capable of accurately testing the hypothesis independent of data distribution. The following tests were employed:

- Wilcoxon matched-pairs signed-rank test

- Kruskal-Wallis test

- Wilcoxon signed-rank test

- Mann-Whitney U test (rank-sum test)

The results obtained by virtue of the statistical methods quoted above, were further verified using the program package IBM SPSS Statistics 18 (test version), as well as using the free software environment R Statistics, version 2.11.1, that serves the purposes of statistical computing and graphics. The results of the hypothesis accuracy testing shall be given not only in form of figures, but in form of graphs as well.

3   Results

As pointed out previously, data on the efficiency of the pituitary gland tumour phytotherapy (PT) came as a result of a five-year follow-up of relevant endpoint measures obtained across the sample of 32 macroprolactinoma patients. In the pertaining diagrams and tables, the patients were assigned ordinal numbers spanning from 1 to 32 — their sequence thereby matching the order of their applications. Within this particular study frame, the efficiency analyses were focused on changes in tumour size.

3.1   Tumour Size

The first analysis of PT influence on tumour size was conducted in all 32 patients. The patients had afterwards been divided in groups relative to their DA pre-treatment length and whether they were treated with DA at all. This was done due to existing assumption that DA pre-treatment influences the results of PT and needed to be confirmed through a statistical analysis.

3.1.1   Analysis of Changes in Tumour Size Following PT (as Compared to the Pre-PT Status) on the Entire Patient Sample

The basic tumour size indicators obtained by virtue of descriptive statistics revealed significant changes in the mean tumour size prior to and following PT.

Prior to PT, the mean tumour size equalled to 22.00 mm; following PT, it decreased to 9.72 mm. This is to say that a 56%-tumour downsizing was achieved. Based on the latter result, the assumed PT efficiency in tumour downsizing was corroborated at the level of significance of 1%. The same was obtained using the 0.1%-significance merit. Graphical display of the results descriptive of differences in tumour sizes prior to and following PT, obtained on the entire sample level, is given in Figure 1.

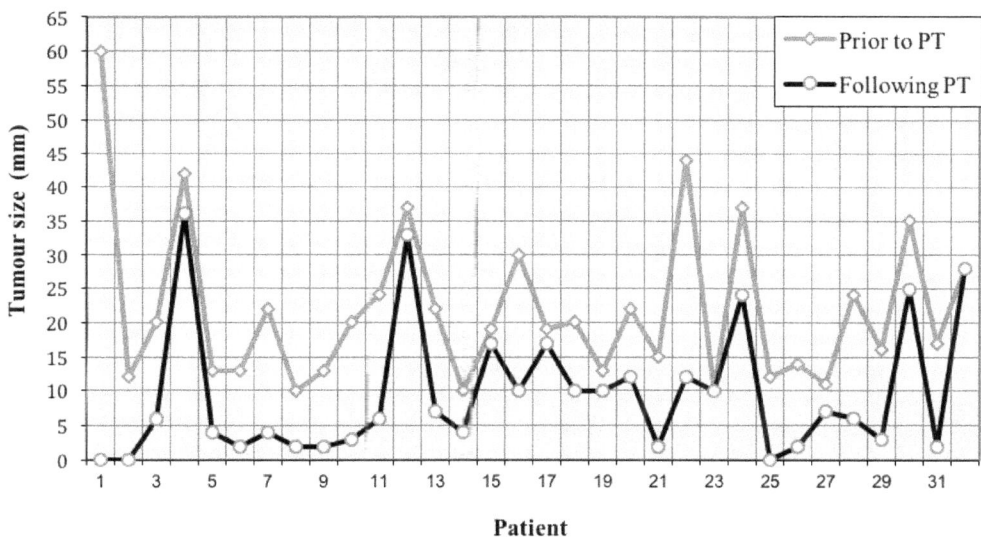

Figure 1: Tumour size prior to and following PT; during the course of PT female patients number 19 and 23 managed to conceive due to the decrease in prolactin levels, so the data on their tumour size are lacking. Therefore, these patients were excluded from the statistical analysis. For the sake of further data processing, the sizes of their tumours were deemed to be equal to the mean tumour size seen across their respective study groups (see Figure 1, 3 and 4).

3.1.2   Group 1: DA & PT Arm

Following the analysis of changes in tumour size witnessed across the entire study sample, the patients were divided into 2 groups: DA & PT arm (Group 1) and the PT only (Group 2). The analyses of changes in tumour size were then separately run across these two groups.

DA & PT arm was constituted of 23 patients simultaneously receiving phytotherapy and dopamine agonists. In this patient group, the basic parameters, descriptive of tumour size and obtained by virtue of descriptive statistics, also revealed a significant difference in the mean tumour size prior to and following PT. The mean pre- and post-PT tumour sizes registered across these patients were 22.74 mm and 11.93 mm, respectively (Figure 2); in other words, a 48%-tumour downsizing was achieved. The statistical significance of the difference in tumour size prior to and post the combined treatment was corroborated both at the level of significance of 1% and at the level of significance of 0.1 %.

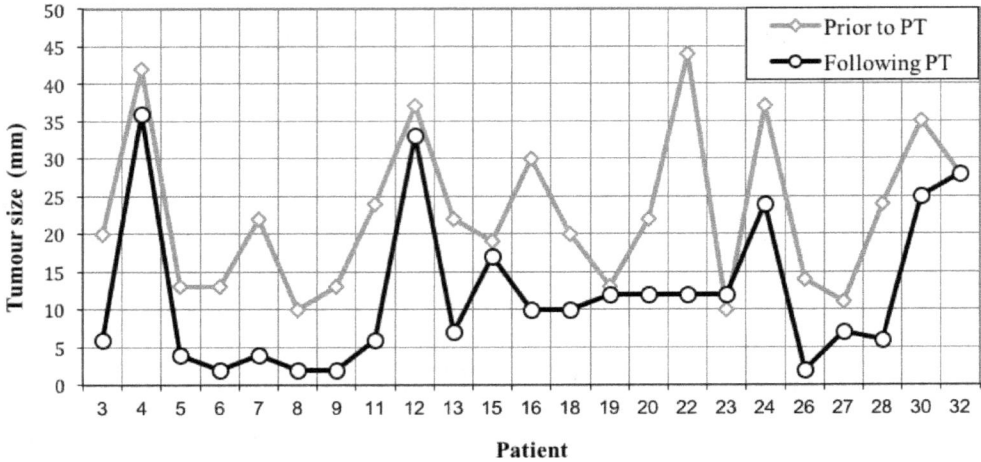

Figure 2: DA & PT arm.

3.1.3   Group 2: PT only Arm

Out of 32 participating patients, 9 gave up on DAs prior to PT and continued taking herbal remedies only (PT only arm). The basic parameters descriptive of the tumour size, obtained by virtue of descriptive statistics, revealed a significant difference in the mean tumour size prior to and following PT. Prior to PT, the mean tumour size equalled to 20.11 mm; following PT, the mean tumour size decreased to 3.4 mm, meaning that an 83%-tumour downsizing ultimately managed to be attained (Figure 3). The statistical significance of the tumour mass downsizing seen following PT, as compared to the pre-PT state, was corroborated at the level of significance of 5%. However, if tested at the significance level of 1%, the difference in pre- and post-PT tumour sizes became statistically insignificant.

3.1.4   The Comparison of Tumour Downsizing Attained in Group 1 vs. Group 2

Based on the data on mean tumour sizes and other statistical indicators, a comparative analysis of data on tumour sizes registered in DA & PT arms and PT only arm has been

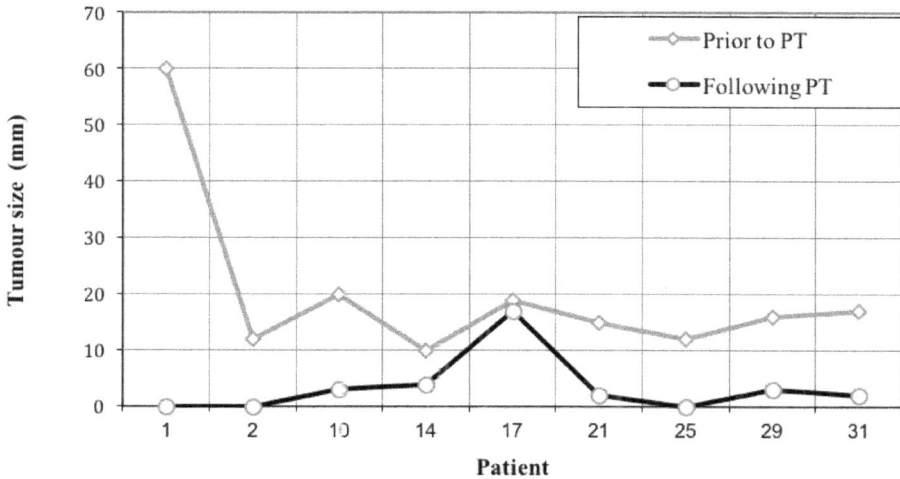

Figure 3: PT only arm.

carried out. This analysis aimed at comparing the outcomes of the two different treatments. When tested for their individual significance at 5%-significance level, the differences in mean tumour sizes were proven to be insignificant. Comparative analysis of mean tumour sizes registered following the concomitant DA and PT and following PT only treatment confirmed the anticipated efficiency of both treatment modalities. The testing that ran at the 5% significance level revealed the phyto-monotherapy, as well as DA & PT combination therapy, to be capable of reducing the size of the tumour in statistically significant manner, which is a finding justifiable by PT administration. Nevertheless, the same failed to be proven at the significance level of 1%, suggesting that a more reliable comparative analysis would call for larger patient samples.

3.1.5   Subgroup 2A: DA & PT Arm: Patients Previously Receiving DAs for 8–26 Months

The next step taken during the course of the study was to verify the impact of previous DA treatment on PT outcomes. To that goal, the total of 23 DA & PT patients was divided into two subgroups: Subgroup 2A, consisting of 19 patients previously receiving DAs for 8 to 26 months, and Subgroup 2B, consisting of 4 patients previously receiving DAs longer than 36 months.

In Subgroup 2A (whose members had received DAs for 8 to 26 months prior to the PT launch) statistically significant differences were revealed in mean tumour sizes prior to and following the combined therapy. Prior to the PT commencement, the mean tumour size seen across these patients equalled to 19.9 mm, as compared to 8.9 mm measured following the PT completion, indicating a 56%-downsizing of the tumour mass. The difference in pre-PT and post-PT mean tumour sizes remained significant at 5%-, 1%-, and 0.1%-significance levels. The results are graphically represented by Figure 4.

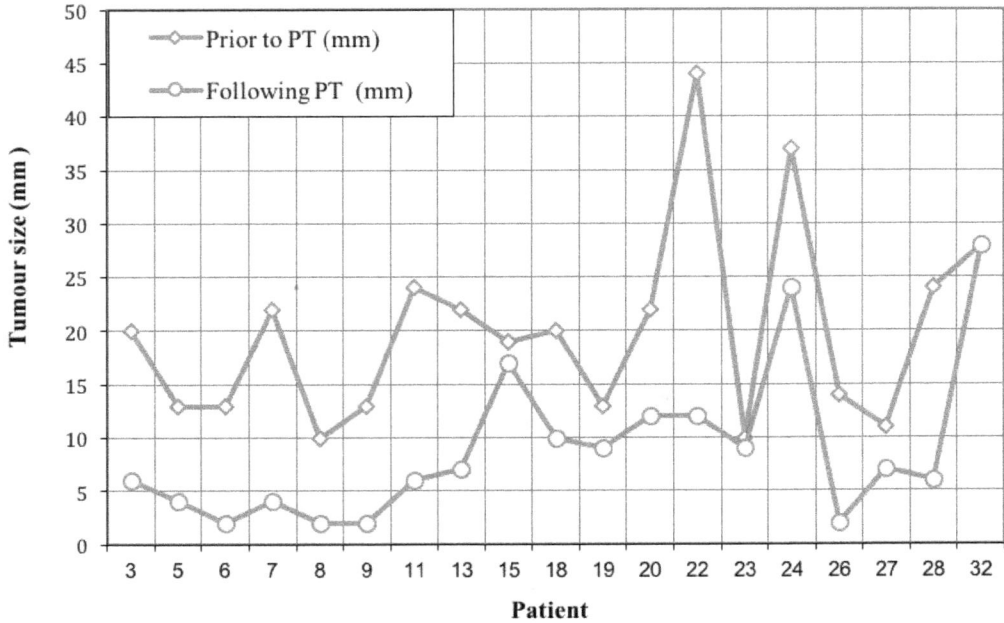

Figure 4: Patients previously receiving DAs for 8-26 months.

3.1.6 Subgroup 2B: DA & PT Arm: Patients Previously Receiving DAs > 36 Months

Prior to the PT commencement, 4 of the study subjects had taken DAs for longer than 36 months. Prior to the PT implementation, the mean size of the tumour equalled to 36.0 mm; following the combined DA & PT therapy, the mean size of the tumour was reduced to 26.0 mm (Figure 5), hence by 28%. Statistical indicators corroborated that certain changes in tumour size did occur, but the difference in tumour sizes prior to and following the combined therapy lacked statistical significance, at least at the level of significance of 5%.

The results obtained in this patient subgroup might be indicative of an unfavourable impact of a multiyear DA therapy reflecting in the PT efficiency hindrance. However, given the fact that the subgroup in reference was composed of no more than 4 patients, one should not jump to conclusions, but rather provide for a more representative future patient sample. Nevertheless, it is to be reiterated that, even though insignificant, certain tumour regression was noted in these cases as well.

3.2 Prolactin Analysis

The analysis of the prolactin (PRL) level changes has been performed in all patients by replicating the manner of analysing the effect of PT on tumour size. Patients had later been divided into groups depending on the length and amount of DA pre-treatment.

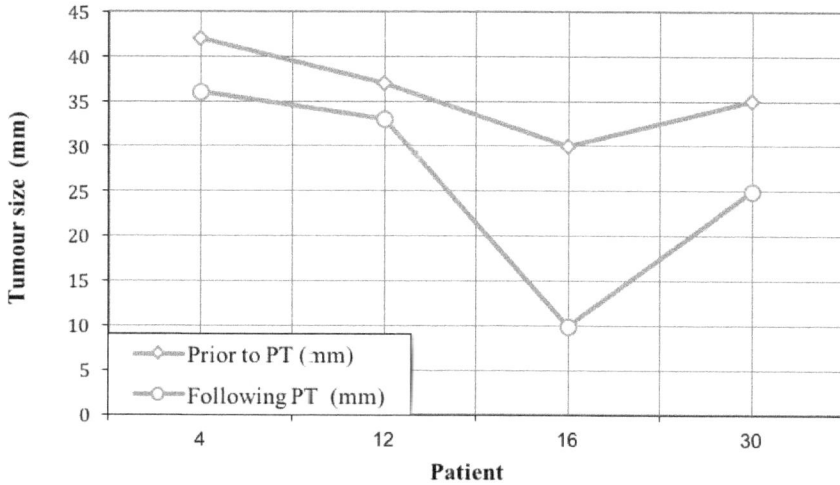

Figure 5: Patients previously receiving DAs > 36 months.

3.2.1   Analysis of PRL Changes Witnessed Prior to and Following PT (the Entire Patient Sample)

In order to assess the PT efficiency, PRL changes were first analysed in all study patients. Prior to PT commencement, the levels of this hormone were increased in 31 patients, while the remaining male patient had his PRLs within normal boundaries; however, he decided to undergo PT due to other tumour-induced symptoms. Primary PRL indicators, obtained using descriptive statistics, point towards significant differences in PRL means registered prior to and following PT. The mean PRL recorded in the entire patient sample prior to PT commencement equalled to 245.1, while the one seen following PT equalled to 30.5 ng/mL. Expressed as an absolute number, the difference in pre- and post- PT PRLs equals to 214.6 ng/mL, suggesting an 87.6% decrease in value of the parameter under observation. However, the difference in the mean PRLs recorded prior to and following PT calls for corroboration of its statistical significance, as well as for the ascertainment of the level of significance at which the aforementioned difference had been witnessed. Variance and other statistical indicators (standard error, median, etc.) also corroborate the existence of significant differences between pre- and post-PT PRLs attributable to PT. For visual display of differences in PRL prior to and following PT, please refer to Box-Whisker diagrams (Figures 6 and 7).

Prior to and following phytotherapy, PRLs ranged from 14.2 to 1,398.0 and from 3.2 to 102.7, respectively. Correspondent differences in PRLs witnessed prior to and following PT spanned from [– 4.7 to 1,359.6]. PRL confidence intervals seen *prior to* and *following* PT, as well as the difference between pre-PT and post-PT PR values, provide a solid ground for estimation of ranges within which PRLs are likely to span. These intervals were shown in Table 4. Calculation of p-values that pose as complementary statistical indicators, corroborate the validity of confidence intervals displayed in Table 4 (reference intervals: female population, 2-30 ng/mL; male population, 2-20 ng/mL).

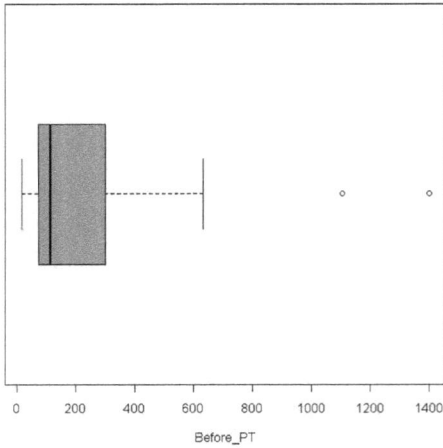

Figure 6: Box-Whisker prior PT.

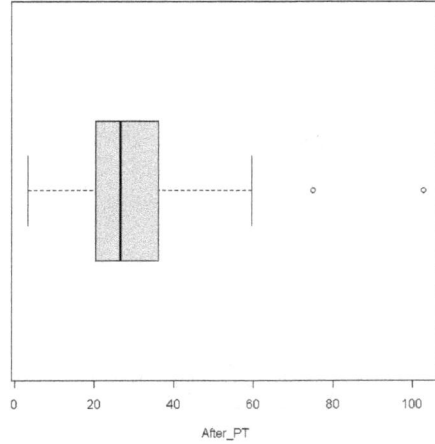

Figure 7: Box-Whisker following PT.

Confidence interval	Prior to PT	Following PT	Mutual difference
95%	[121.2; 369.0]	[22.3; 38.7]	[92.0; 337.0]
99%	[77.7; 412.5]	[19.4; 41.6]	[49.1; 379.9]

Table 4: Confidence interval for prolactin in all patients.

The assumed PT efficiency was corroborated by testing the hypothesis on PRL means prior to and following PT, done at the significance levels of 5% and 1%. Namely, the differences in PRLs seen prior to and following PT, reveal a significant decrease in PRLs determined following the PT completion. More precisely, it can be stated with 95% and even 99% certainty (and the pertaining risk of error of 5% and 1%, respectively) that the mean PRLs seen in the PT arm following PT completion are significantly lower as compared to those registered *prior to* PT commencement. It can be easily proven that the above statement applies also for 0.1%-significance level, as corroborated by an adequate hypothesis testing. For visual display of the results discussed above, please see reference intervals in Figure 8.

3.2.2   Group 1: Changes in PRLs Seen in the DA & PT Arm

At the PT launch point, a total of 23 patients had already been administered with pharmacotherapy (in form of dopamine agonists, DAs); the patients in reference continued to use these drugs as prescribed throughout the PT period. PRL means obtained by virtue of descriptive statistics prior to and following PT, viewed as the primary outcome measure, revealed statistically significant changes in PRL means seen following the PT completion. Prior to PT commencement, the PRL mean of 189.4 ng/mL was registered, while the correspondent value registered following PT completion equalled to 27.5 ng/mL. The

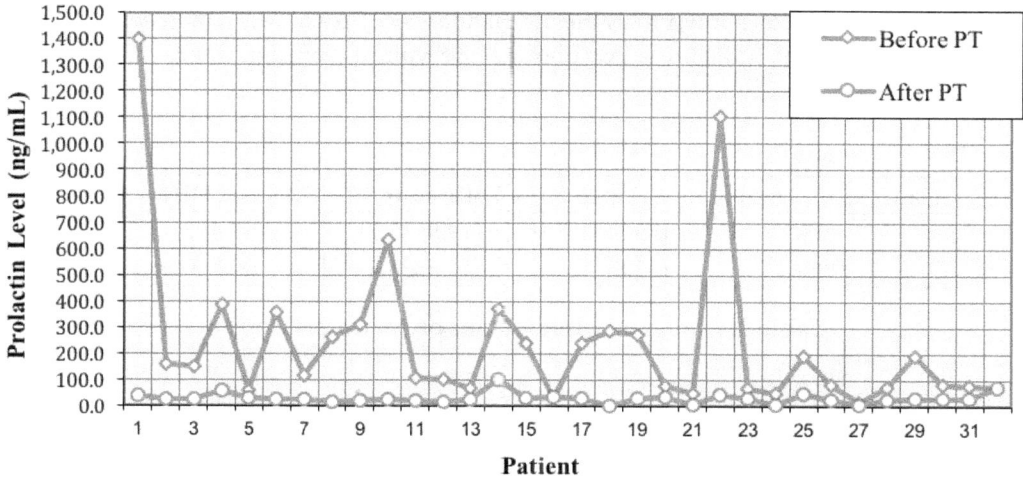

Figure 8: Prolactin Level Analysis.

difference in pre- and post-PT PRL means equals to 161.9 ng/mL, disclosing an 85.5%-PRL decrease illustrated by Box-Whisker diagrams displayed below (Figures 9 and 10). Computing of variance and other statistical parameters corroborated the favourable impact of PT on PRL decrease.

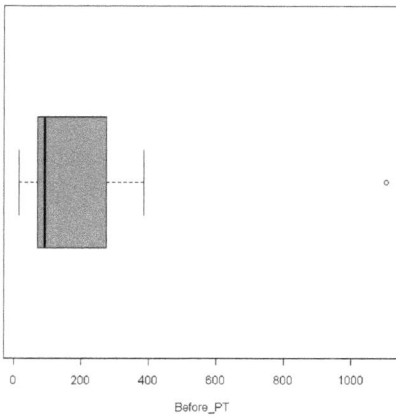

Figure 9: Box-Whisker prior PT.

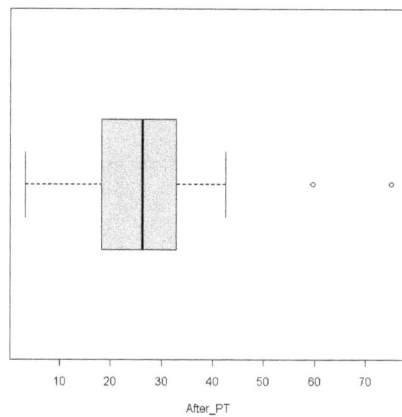

Figure 10: Box-Whisker following PT.

Prior to PT commencement, PRLs spanned from 14.2 to 1,104.0, while the values ranging from 3.2 to 75.0 were seen following its completion. The corresponding differences fell into the interval spanning from [-4.7 to 1,089.8]. PRL confidence intervals seen *prior to* and *following* PT, as well as the difference between pre-PT and post-PT PR values, provide a solid ground for estimation of ranges within which PRLs are likely to span.

These intervals were as shown in Table 5. Calculation of p-values, which serve as complementary statistical indicators, corroborate the validity of confidence intervals displayed in Table 5.

Confidence Interval	Prior to PT	Following PT	Mutual Difference
95%	[75.5; 303.3]	[19.5; 35.5]	[49.4; 274.2]
99%	[33.8; 345.0]	[16.6; 38.4]	[8.2; 315.4]

Table 5: Confidence interval for prolactin in Group 1.

The assumed PT efficiency was corroborated by testing the hypothesis on PRL means prior to and following PT, done at the significance levels of 5% and 1%. The above statement applies also for 0.1%-significance level, as corroborated by an adequate hypothesis testing. For visual display of the results obtained with both lines of treatment (DA and PT), please refer to Figure 11.

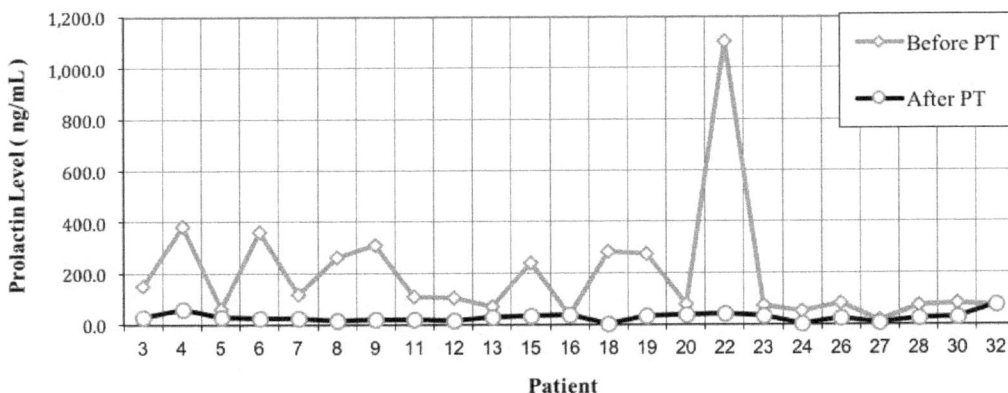

Figure 11: DA & PT arm;

3.2.3   Group 2: PRL Changes Witnessed in the PT Arm

Out of the 32-patient pool, 9 were unable to tolerate side-effects arising on the grounds of DA treatment, so that after a short trial period they ceased taking the prescribed medication and resorted to PT only. Prior to the PT launch, some of the patients in this arm had the highest PRLs of them all, so that the decrease in PRLs seen following phytotherapy was far more striking than in the remaining study patients. PRL decrease witnessed following PT only (illustrated by Figures 12, 13, and 14) proves, without a shred of doubt, the efficiency of herbal remedies in diminishing macroprolactinoma secretory potential. In 7 of these patients, PRL fell beyond 50 ng/mL, while in one female patient (designated as patient No 14), who chose to undergo PT until the pre-scheduled surgery term, a 4 month-lasting PT resulted in PRL drop from 373.0 to 102.0 ng/mL.

In this arm as well, descriptive statistics pointed towards significant differences in pre- and post-PT PRL means, viewed as the primary outcome measure. Prior to PT commencement, the PRL mean of 384.3 ng/mL was registered, while following PT completion the value in reference equalled to 38.0 ng/mL. The difference in pre- and post-PT PRL means equals to 346.3 ng/mL, disclosing a 90.1%-PRL decrease illustrated by Box-Whisker diagrams displayed below (Figures 12 and 13). Computing of variance and other statistical parameters further corroborated the favourable impact of PT on PRL decrease.

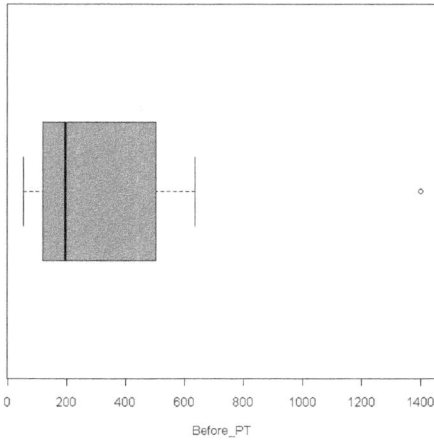

Figure 6: Box-Whisker prior PT.   Figure 7: Box-Whisker following PT.

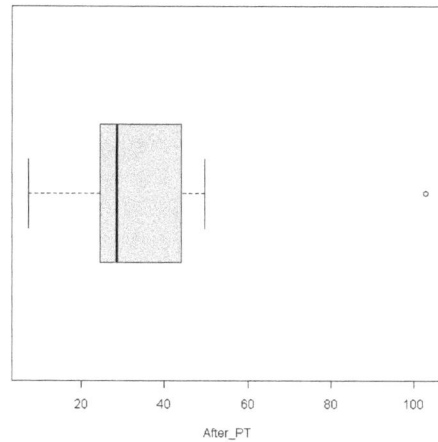

Prior to PT commencement, PRLs spanned from 51.2 to 1,398.0, while following its completion the values ranging from 7.3 to 102.7 had been seen. The corresponding differences fell into the interval spanning from [43.9 to 1,359.6]. PRL confidence intervals seen *prior to* and *following* PT, as well as the difference between pre-PT and post-PT PR values, provide a solid ground for estimation of ranges within which PRLs are likely to span. These intervals were as shown in Table 6. Calculation of p-values that pose as complementary statistical indicators, corroborate the validity of confidence intervals displayed in Table 6.

Confidence interval	Prior to PT	Following PT	Mutual difference
95%	[7.8; 760.8]	[13.9; 62.1]	[27.9; 720.5]
99%	[33.8; 345.0]	[16.6; 38.4]	[207.4; 900.0]

Table 6: Confidence interval for prolactin in Group 2.

The assumed PT efficiency was corroborated by testing the hypothesis on PRL means prior to and following PT, done at the significance level of 5%. The above statement applies also for 1%-significance level, as corroborated by an adequate hypothesis testing. For visual display of the results discussed above, please refer to Figure 14.

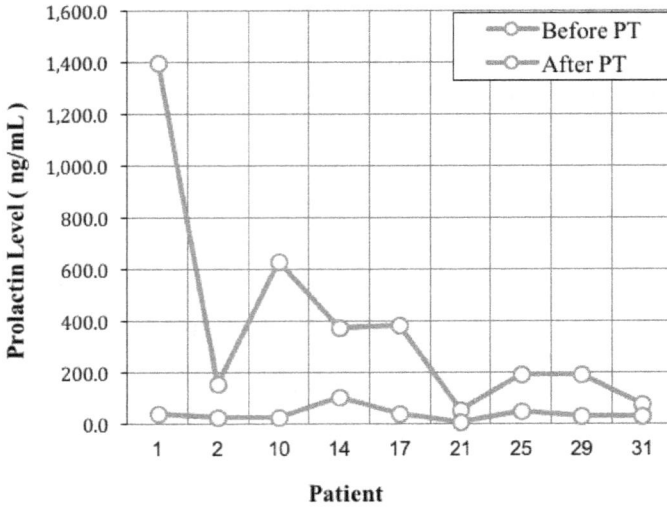

Figure 14: PT arm.

3.2.4   Comparison of PRLs Registered in DA & PT vs. PT Arm

Comparative analysis of PRLs registered in the patients constituting the DA & PT versus those registered in the patients constituting the PT arm, aims at comparing the outcomes of these two distinctive lines of treatment. Testing of hypotheses on differences in PRL means completed at 5%-significance level, failed to reveal any statistically significant changes in pre-treatment PRL means registered in these two arms. In other words, it can be stated with a 95%-certainty (and a risk of error of 5%) that the PRL means seen across these two patient arms prior to treatment did not significantly differ from each other. From the statistical standpoint, this means that both patient arms had even "starting positions" allowing therefore for a substantiated evaluation of efficiency of different therapeutic modalities.

However, comparative analysis of mean PRLs seen in PT vs. DA & PT arm, corroborate the hypothesised efficiency of both treatment modalities. By virtue of testing the hypothesis on differences in PRL means, done at 5%-significance level, it was proven that a statistically significant difference in PRLs obtained across the PT arm and those obtained across the DA & PT arm is virtually non-existent. To rephrase, one can be 95% certain (risk of error = 5%) that mean PRLs obtained across these two distinctively treated arms following treatment completion, do not differ to a statistically significant extent.

Given the small number of PT arm members (n=9 only), one should not jump into conclusions on the sole virtue of this line of treatment, but rather strive to repeat the analysis once a more substantial, i.e. a statistically more representative number of patients/data are at hand.

3.2.5   Subgroup 2A: DA & PT Arm (Previously Receiving DAs 8–26 Months)

The basic statistical indicators of the prolactin level in 23 patients treated with PT and DA, who were also treated prior to phytotherapy in the period of 8 to 26 months, imply that there is a statistical significance in the mean values of prolactin levels before and after the treatment. The mean value of prolactin level before and after the therapy equalled to 196. 2 ng/mL and 25. 6 ng/mL, respectively. This suggests an 87% decrease in the mean value of prolactin level after the treatment. The variance values and the remaining statistics as well confirm the existence of significant differences i.e. the positive effect of the treatment with the above mentioned methods.

By testing the hypotheses on the mean values of prolactin levels before and after the treatment, the assumption about the effectiveness of this therapy has been confirmed on 5% and 1% - levels of significance, which further means that the mean value of the prolactin level after the treatment with PT and DA is significantly less than the corresponding value before the therapy with probability of 95% (5% risk level) and even 99% (1% risk level). However, this claim is not valid for the 0. 1% level of significance; hence, it cannot be confirmed with 99.9% probability of being correct (risk level 0. 1%). The graphical interpretation of the prolactin levels before and after the conducted therapy (Figure 15) illustrates the tested hypotheses.

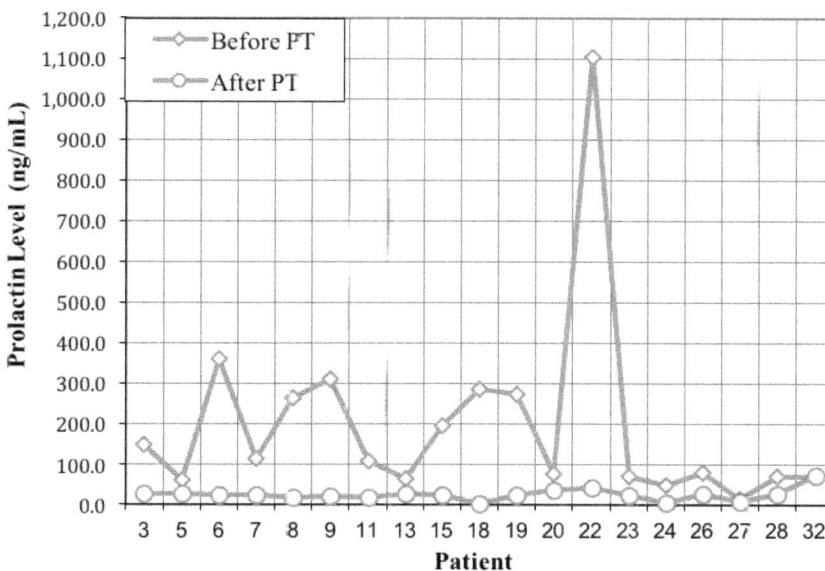

Figure 15: Patients previously receiving DAs for 8-26 months.

3.2.6   Subgroup 2B: DA & PT Arm (Previously Receiving DAs for > 36 Months)

Basic statistic indicators of the prolactin level in patients treated with PT and DA (previously receiving DAs for > 36 months) reveal the existence of differences between the mean values of prolactin levels before and after the treatment in this case. The mean value of prolactin level before and after the therapy equalled to 149. 9 ng/mL and 35. 4 ng/mL, respectively. This indicates a 76% reduction in the prolactin level after the therapy. The variance values and the remaining statistics also confirm the existence of differences, i.e. a certain effect of this kind of treatment.

The hypotheses testing on the significance levels of 5% and 10% did not confirm the assumption about the effectiveness of this therapy, meaning that it can be claimed with 95% (risk level 5%) and 90% (risk level 10%) probability that the mean values of prolactin levels before and after this treatment do not differ significantly. The reasons for this claim could be the small number of patients who were treated more than 36 months before the PH-DA treatment was introduced. The graphical interpretation (Figure 16) of the prolactin levels before and after the conducted therapy illustrates the tested hypotheses.

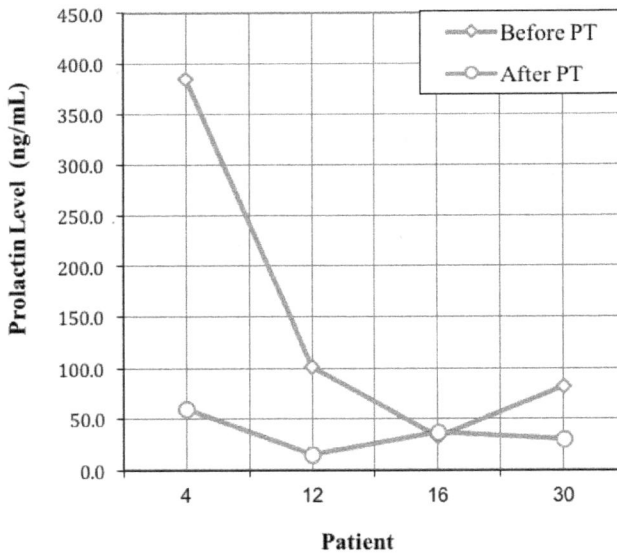

Figure 16: Patients previously receiving DAs>36 months.

Except for the analysis on the reduction of the prolactin level caused by differing methods of treatment within the mentioned groups, hypotheses testing on eventual differences in the mean values of prolactin levels, after the conducted therapies and among the individual groups, have been undertaken. The results have been compared across different groups: group 2 & 2A, group 2 & 2B and group 2A & 2B. It can be claimed with 95% certainty (5% significance level) that the mean values of prolactin levels after the conducted therapies do not differ. Nevertheless, there are indications that the results of prolactin level reduction in PT-only treatment deserve particular attention. In order to make a suitable conclusion with a high level of certainty, i.e. with the lowest possible risk, it is necessary to collect more data on the treatment of patients under the stated circumstances.

3.3   Tumour Size and PT Duration

The next step in our data analysis was to determine whether the functional relationship exists between the reduction in tumour size and PT length and, if yes, how to express the relationship in terms of appropriate mathematical-statistical or regression models. Whenever some strong functional relationship exists, it makes sense to talk about the correlation between the reduction in tumour size and therapy duration. In this case, the main goal is to establish relationship i.e. regression model which make it possible to predict reductions of tumour size in terms of the therapy duration. Effects of tumour size reductions are expressed in percentages (%) and are represented in two ways:

a)   Decrease of tumour size prior to the PT

b)   Residual value of tumour size after PT

To model relationships between the aforementioned characteristic, available computer software has been used and appropriate regression models have been built up. The reduction in tumour size versus therapy duration (a) could be described by the following regression models:

$$y = 26.719 \, \text{Ln}(x) + 12.561,$$
$$R^2 = 0.6561, R = 0.8100, \tag{1}$$

$$y = 0.1782 \times 3 - 4.6116 \times 2 + 37.888x - 30,$$
$$R^2 = 0.7928, R = 0.8904, \tag{2}$$

$$y = -26.719 \, \text{Ln}(x) + 87.439,$$
$$R^2 = 0.6561, R = 0.8100, \tag{3}$$

$$y = -0.1782 \times 3 + 4.6116 \times 2 - 37.888x + 130.718,$$
$$R^2 = 0.7928, R = 0.3904, \tag{4}$$

where x = length of phytotherapy (in months); y = reduction and / or residual value, tumour size (%); R^2 = coefficient of determination and R = coefficient of correlation.

The evaluation of regression models in this study indicated that the residual logarithmic regression model was appropriate for practical application. Namely, this model is best suited for the mathematical modelling approach of tumour size reduction versus therapy duration. However, polynomial regression models are not good enough to be used for practical purposes, although they show better characteristics.

A graphical representation of the logarithmic model (Figure 17) confirms a relatively high degree of correlation between the observed and expected values of tumour size reductions.

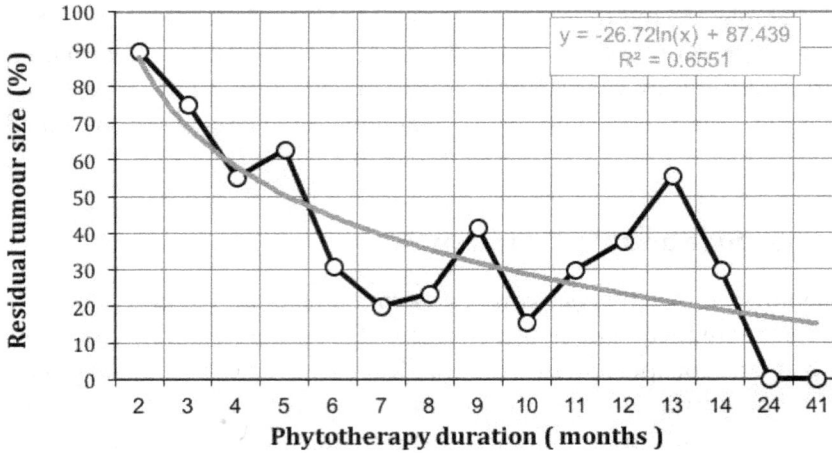

Figure 17: Residual Tumour Size Chart.

3.3.1   The Link between the Tumour Size and PT Duration (< or ≥ 10 Months)

In patients undergoing PT for less than 10 and/or longer than 10 months, basic indicators of tumour size obtained by virtue of descriptive statistical analysis reveal the difference in mean tumour sizes. In case of a PT shorter than 10 months, the tumour size averages to 49.7 %, as oppose to 21.8 % established with longer treatments. A 56% - tumour downsizing obtained with treatments lasting over 10 months or longer, as compared to tumour downsizing achieved with treatments shorter than 10 months, advocate the efficiency of PT treatment. However, when drawing conclusions on the treatment outcome, one should by all means verify the statistical significance of the obtained findings and the degree of possible pertaining risk. Variances and other statistical parameters also point toward the difference arising on the ground of PT length. In the cases elaborated above, the ranges within which the tumour dimensions had spanned (expressed in mm) were [20; 89] and [0; 55], respectively.

Testing of the hypothesis on mean sizes of tumours typical of therapies shorter than 10 and/or longer than 10 months, corroborated the hypothesized influence of PT duration on tumour downsizing at the level of significance of 5%. In other words, it can be claimed with 95%-certainty that, with a 10-month-PT or longer, the mean size of the tumour will significantly decrease as compared to the decrease gained by PTs shorter than 10 months.

Nevertheless, the same cannot be claimed at 1% significance level, as corroborated by testing of the appropriate mean value hypotheses.

3.3.2   PT Duration < 10 Months

The relationship between the decrease in tumour size and the length of therapy on the one side and the PT duration of less than 10 months on the other can be represented with an accurate statistic-mathematical model. As similar to the previous example, the usage of available program support produced several regression models which can have different analytical forms based on the given value sets. In the concrete case brunt of the models produced through the analysis and validation was directed at the models with the determination coefficient larger than 60 ($R^2 > 60$). Accordingly, the subject of the analysis was cubic and logarithmic model for residual tumour values. The evaluation of the obtained regression models indicates that residual logarithmic model is better for practical usage than it is the case with cubic. Graphical interpretation of the model (Figure 18) shows a high level of correlation ($R=0.8965$) between the real calculated values and the reduction in tumour size.

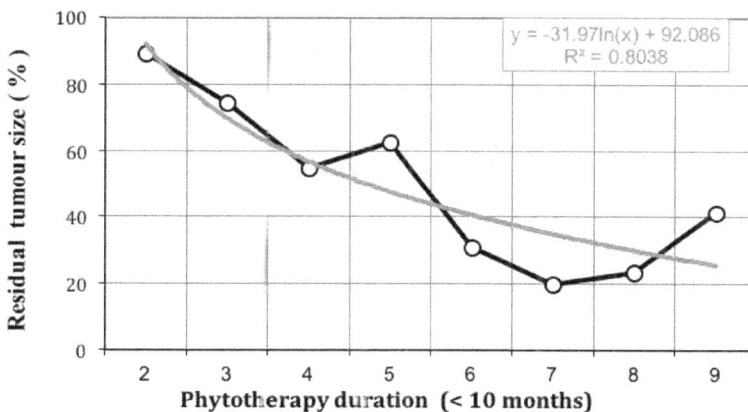

Figure 18: Residual Tumour Size Chart (<10 months).

3.3.3   PT Duration Longer or Equal to 10 Months

The relationship between the reduction in tumour size and the duration of the therapy that equals to or longer than 10 months can be represented with a statistic-mathematical model.

The usage of available program support enabled the creation of several regression models which can have different analytical forms based on their value sets. The subject of the analysis was cubic model for residual tumour values. Graphical interpretation of the model (Figure 19) indicates a high level of correlation ($R = 0.7939$) between real calculated values and the decrease in tumour size.

3.4   Visual Field Defect (VFD) and the Size of the Tumour

VFD comes as a result of tumour compression exerted on optical structures. The results displayed below prove the favourable impact of phytotherapy on tumour downsizing. The impact of PT on VFD was not analysed in all of the 32 patients, but only in those 15 that had experienced vision problems prior to the PT commencement (Table 7).

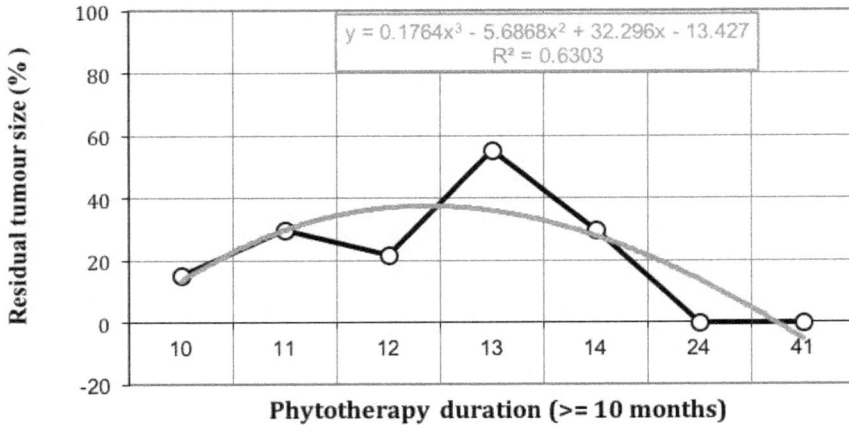

$$y = 0.1764x^3 - 5.6868x^2 + 32.296x - 13.427$$
$$R^2 = 0.6303$$

Figure 19: Residual Tumour Size Chart (≥ 10 months).

Patient's Ordinal Number	VFD Prior to PT	VFD Following PT
1	+	−
3	+	−
4	+	+*
10	+	−
11	+	−
12	+	+*
16	+	−
17	+	+
20	+	−
22	+	−
24	+	+
26	+	−
29	+	−
30	+	+
32	+	+

Table 7: VFD status prior to and following PT (PT: phytotherapy; VFD: visual field defect; +: VFD present; −: VFD lacking; +*: permanent VFD).

Following PT, in 9 (60%) out of these 15 patients, the vision was restored to normal. The reduction of tumour size following PT spanned from 45% to 100% in these patients. In 6 (40%) patients in whom a VFD persisted despite of PT, the attained tumour down-sizing ranged from 0 % to 35% (marked with black dots in Figure 20). As can be seen from the data, in patients lacking a VFD following PT, the reduction in tumour size was far greater than in those having a persistent, PT-irresponsive VFD (statistical significance of the difference in tumour downsizing proven at the level of significance of 5%, but not at the level of significance of 1%).

Statistical analyses proved a close correlation between the tumour downsizing and the VFD status. Duly chosen tests examining the interrelation between these two variables ran at the level of significance of 0.1%, definitely proving their interdependence.

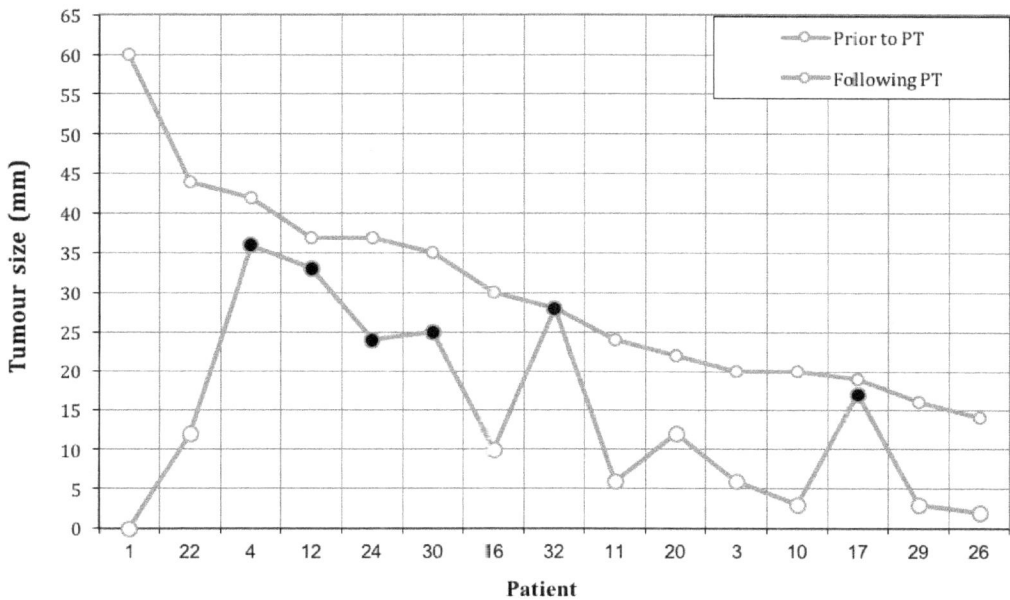

Figure 20: Tumour downsizing seen in patients presenting with VFDs.

4   Discussion

Roughly 70% of raw materials utilised by pharmaceutical industry are of biological, i.e. natural origin; the vast majority of them thereby being isolated from plants (Kovačević, 2000; Pekić, 1983). Contemporary medicine stemmed from the traditional, folk medicine, but its huge development witnessed throughout the 20th century had eventually led to a marked loss of interest in herbal preparations, so that their production had been pursued only within narrow circles of laymen heavily dependent on tradition, old ways and recipes passed across generations. Lack of medical knowledge among herbal remedy manufacturers and disregard shown by medical profession are the reasons why, until recently, the studies of the therapeutic efficiency of herbal remedies had been so scarce and rare. In the last twenty years, major changes in these views and attitudes have been witnessed, resulting in a re-evoked interest in plant-based preparations. Within this context, not only laymen, but medical profession as well, have decided to review their standpoints and attitudes towards this line of treatment. As a result, a more thorough and more in-depth research of therapeutic potentials of certain remedial plants and plant mixtures has been performed. Especially in the last few years, an ever-growing number of studies has proven that remedial plants deserve to be considered as a valid therapeutic option in a number of conditions (Block &Mead, 2003; Kanowski & Hoerr, 2003; Yale & Liu, 2004). The fact that our study patients had previously been treated in ward specialised healthcare facilities, gives an additional rise to the significance of our results.

4.1   The Impact of PT on Macroprolactinoma Size

The subjects included into this study had unanimously started their macroprolactinoma treatments with the most commonly employed dopamine agonist bromocriptine. Nowadays, medical research is designed in a way so as to provide the intention-to-treat population with the "gold standard" therapy for the condition under investigation (Geddes & Cipriani, 2004). Respecting that principle, our DA-treated patients also continued taking DAs concurrently with PT. Mono-PT was administered only to patients forced to give up on DAs due to severe side-effects. Any other approach to this study would jeopardise its ethics and integrity. Nevertheless, this line of approach had a substantial impact on our study design and resulted in the formation of several study groups/subgroups. Based on the aforementioned, the researchers were given the opportunity not only to observe the impact of PT on tumour size across the entire (32-patient) sample, but to compare the results obtained with PT only (9-patient) arm and DA & PT (23-patient) arm.

On top of medication, a total of 15 study patients had surgery prior to the PT commencement. The surgery allowed for the removal of almost the entire tumour mass, as well as for the subsequent depressurisation of the adjacent structures and temporary alleviation of macroprolactinoma-related symptoms. However, none of the patients had his/her tumour totally removed, so that in time the residual tumour cells served as the grounds for macroprolactinoma re-formation. In four of the operated patients, the surgery failed even twice. Medical records obtained prior to the PT commencement clearly showed that each and every study subject had an optimal treatment delivered by their attending healthcare facilities, so that, as far as contemporary medicine is concerned, the best possible care had been provided.

The herbal remedy efficiency analysis carried out on the entire sample level and particularly the results obtained across the PT only arm have clearly demonstrated the favourable impact of herbal remedies on tumour mass reduction. The results attained across the PT only arm represent the most important outcome of this study, since they showed beyond any doubt that tumour mass reduction and even restoration to health (patients no. 1, 2, and 25) can be achieved in those suffering from macroprolactinomas solely by virtue of herbal remedy use, allowing for the possibility of PT implementation as the first-line macroprolactinoma treatment. A substantial, however less striking effect in terms of tumour mass reduction was also achieved in the DA & PT arm. Given that the statistical analysis revealed no significant pre-PT differences between the mean sizes of the tumours seen in patients who gave up on their medication as compared to those still taking DAs, it became obvious that pharmacotherapy had no significant impact on tumour size, so that the substantial tumour downsizing can mostly be attributed to PT implementation.

Far better results obtained with the FT only arm (average tumour downsizing of 83%) as compared to the DA & PT arm (average tumour downsizing of 48%), suggest that, when it comes to tumour mass reduction, earlier DA treatment might decrease the PT efficiency. Further analysis of the results obtained in DA-treated patients (subgroups 2A and 2B) led to a conclusion that therapeutic effectiveness of herbal remedies weakens as DA administration goes on, so that the poorest results were obtained in patients treated with DAs for longer than 3 years; the average tumour mass reduction seen across these patients (56% in subgroup 2A and 28% in subgroup 2B) supports this standing. The analysis of the study data indicated that prior DA treatment interferes with signalling paths utilised by pharmacoactive plant ingredients, so that the PT efficiency declines with DA treatment duration.

The analysis of the study data indicated that prior DA treatment interferes with signalling paths utilised by pharmacoactive plant ingredients, so that the PT efficiency declines with DA treatment duration. Based on the aforementioned, it can also be clearly understood that tumour downsizing, coming as a result of the pharmacoactive plant ingredients' administration, is not mediated by D2 receptors.

4.2   The Influence of PT on Prolactin Level (PRL)

The introduction of bromocriptine in modern medicine has generated weak results in the regulation of the prolactin level. The results of DA treatment had been poor and, except for one patient, boiled down to a modest PRL decrease. As a rule, in case of resistance to therapy or in case of a poor response, treating physicians decide to switch their patients to cabergoline. However, it should be noted that our study sample consisted of patients coming from the former Yugoslavia (most of them from B&H and Croatia, two from Serbia and one from Macedonia). Throughout the study period (2005-late 2009), the only DA authorised for market release in these countries was bromocriptine, while other DAs could be obtained exclusively from abroad and had to be paid out of the patients' pockets. Therefore, only 3 of our patients got to be treated with cabergoline, which might explain the poor results of pharmacotherapy administered to our study group prior to, or concurrently with, phytotherapy. In addition to pharmacotherapy, 15 patients included into this study underwent surgery, 4 of them even twice. However, due to various reasons, not a single patient had his/her tumour fully removed, so that, over time, tumour residual had re-grown into a macroprolactinoma. Facing such unsatisfactory results, the patients in reference decided to make PT arrangements.

The results achieved in the DA & PT arm as well as those obtained in the PT arm, demonstrate, beyond doubt, a favourable effect of herbal remedies on macroprolactinoma secretory potential in terms of its putdown. A special attention should be paid, and a special credit given to, the results achieved in 9 patients undergoing PT only, since they pose as a role model for the efficiency analysis of PT chosen to be not merely an adjuvant, but the "number one" macroprolactinoma therapy. The results obtained within this frame suggest that in some macroprolactinoma patients satisfactory PRL regulation can be achieved by virtue of herbal remedies as the first choice treatment. Following the PT completion, a similar percentage of PRL decrease was seen across the DA & PT arm as well.

Comparison of PRL means registered prior to and following PT failed to reveal any statistically significant differences in the aforementioned outcome measure between the PT and the DA & PT arm. It should be noted, however, that the decrease in PRLs that DAs should be given credit for, seen across the DA & PT arm, was only modest, the prescribed DA dose thereby being more in function of maintenance of the achieved PRL levels then in function of their further diminishment. Truth is that DAs had succeeded in their mission and had prevented PRLs from further rise, but had never managed to reduce them beyond the values displayed on Figure 11, so that further decrease in PRLs, seen across this arm post treatment, should apparently be attributed to the PT introduced later on.

Concurrent PT and DA administration failed to reveal any synergy between the two. The action mechanism of pharmacoactive plant ingredients remains unclear; however, possible mediation of this suppression of PR secretion by D2 receptors can definitely be ruled out.

This article brings the report on favourable effects of herbal preparation administration. Nevertheless, the identification of individual pharmacologically active components is associated with a number of problems.

The majority of plants composing the herbal preparations administered to macroprolactinoma patients are aromatic plants basically composed of ethereal oils; it has been shown without a shred of doubt that the pharmacoactivity of these oils gives rise to PT efficiency. However, given that these herbal preparations come in form of infusions, one should take into account that only some of their hydrophobic ingredients get to pass into the water solution, together with a number of other secondary metabolites. In line with the foregoing, it is reasonable to assume that pharmacological activity of aromatic plants does not depend solely on the presence and efficiency of ethereal oils, but also on the activity of other ingredients constituting the plant mixtures; for that matter, the possibility of their synergistic effect cannot be ruled out.

One can also expect to come across a number of difficulties when trying to identify active ingredients of ethereal oils, since the activity of the latter actually represents a "combined effort" of all ingredients. Therefore, the pharmacoactivity of aromatic plants differs from that of ethereal oils isolated from such plants (Kovačević, 2000). Due to the aforementioned, the pharmacological activity of ethereal oils is commonly defined for the oil "in toto" rather than for its individual components whose pharmacokinetics and metabolism are often very hard or virtually impossible to track. Consequently, most studies akin to our actually report on the effects of PT administration and make ex iuvantibus judgements.

Elucidation of the exact action mechanism through which active substances present in herbal mixtures used within this study take their course of action and eventually manage to downsize the tumour shall contribute to better understanding of the development of tumours of neurohormonal aetiology.

Noteworthy, data on PT impact on macroprolactinoma secretory potential presented herein, are genuine and the very first in these parts and, to the best of our knowledge, in the world as well. The available literature offers no similar studies, so that the comparison to the experience of other authors is rendered virtually impossible.

4.3   Contraindications and the Length of PT

DA-treated patients are forced to a multiyear therapy, but the use of DA drugs has its limitations. Subsequent to a multiyear follow-up of patients taking DAs for a prolonged period of time, on June 26th 2008 the European Medicines Agency (EMEA) released the announcement that communicates new warnings and contraindications for DA use, in specific an increased risk of fibrosis, especially heart fibrosis, attributed to a chronic ergot alkaloid (DA derivative) use (Pehaček & Sajdl, 1990). The revision in reference addressed two most commonly used DAs, i.e. bromocriptine and cabergoline, as well. In line with the EMEA recommendations, the maximal daily cabergoline dose is restricted to 3 mg, while that of bromocriptine should not surpass 30 mg (EMEA, 2014). The highest daily bromocriptine dose used by one of our patients equalled to 40 mg.

The length of PT pursued by our patients spanned from 2 to 41 months, while 9 of them had been treated for 10 months or longer. Regardless of treatment duration, the patients had no contraindications for PT at all, nor did they experience any symptoms potentially attributable to phytotherapy. The earliest benefits of PT-induced PRL put-down were witnessed by female patients of childbearing age, in whom ovulation and normal menstrual cycle had been restored.

What the authors find most encouraging and intriguing about their results is the fact that two female patients (number 19 and 23) got pregnant while on PT and eventually gave birth to healthy children. Though counted into the study sample, data on these two patients were not included into the statistical analysis since PRL data were lacking due to pregnancy that occurred during the course of PT. Nevertheless, PR levels in these two patients must have been somewhere within the reference boundaries or just slightly above the upper normal; otherwise, getting pregnant would be virtually impossible. Therefore, we attributed them the mean value of prolactin levels obtained from all patients who were previously treated with PT (30. 5 ng/mL). Prior to the PT commencement, both patients were treated with DAs. Once they got pregnant, the patients ceased to take DAs but continued PT throughout pregnancy. PT continuation throughout pregnancy was recommended for preventative reasons, since it is well known that oestrogens, whose levels rise during pregnancy, play an important role in tumour development and growth by means of stimulating lactotrophic cell hyperplasia. This goes especially for large, rapidly-growing tumours, known to be more prone to estrogenic stimulation (Mah & Webster, 2001). Nevertheless, having regard to the fact that our experience in this matter currently boils down to two female patients only, additional data on the impact of herbal remedies during pregnancy should be gathered on a fairly large, more representative sample, so as to be able to obtain more reliable and substantiated results on the effectiveness and safety of phytotherapy during pregnancy.

The ultimate PT length, needed for the reduction of prolactin level, is not precisely defined; the same applies also for the optimal length of PT administration. To our knowledge, PT duration needed for its benefits to become apparent, is dependent on pre-PT prolactin levels, but the first therapeutic results should be expected 3-5 months following the PT commencement. The statistical analysis has clearly demonstrated that the best results in tumour reduction occur in patients whose PT lasted more than 10 months.

This is an important fact since one group of the patients, who received positive results after phytotherapy, used the preparations for less than 10 months. The most common reason for treatment disruption was the acceptance of operative procedure suggested to patients by their doctors. This was enabled through the reduction in tumour size caused by the phytotherapeutic treatment which ultimately increased the chances of successful operative procedure.

4.4   PT Impact on Visual Field Defect (VFD)

In 15 study participants, the size of the tumour and the direction of its growth finally caused a visual field defect (VFD). The subjects had been subjected to occasional MRI or CT controls, most often scheduled every 6 months; in those who experienced tumour regression, clearance of sight symptoms posed as the first sign of tumour downsizing, later corroborated by virtue of the pituitary gland diagnostic imaging. In addition to optical structures' depressurisation, a smaller degree of sinus involvement was established in patients having their tumours penetrated into the cavernous sinuses. The macroprolactinoma invasion into the cavernous sinuses speaks of its aggressiveness, forecasts a poor prognosis and makes the tumour virtually inoperable (Asa, 1998). In patients whose tumours became substantially smaller, full cavernous sinus riddance from the tumour was noted, making the chances for a successful surgery markedly higher. In these patients, vision recovery took place within 6 months of the PT commencement. Of note, even prior to PT, two of our patients had been diagnosed with a permanent visual field defect, so that much could not be done anyway.

The results brought by this article demonstrate the efficiency of PT in macroprolactinoma downsizing, therefore opening the prospects for the following:

- Non-surgical treatment and consequential avoidance of risks associated with surgical procedures;

- Adjuvant therapy, to be administered to those whose tumour is inoperable either due to its size or due to the position of its seat, as well as to those who refuse to undergo surgery or cannot have it due to contraindications;

- Administration of phytotherapy to the effect of preoperative tumour downsizing, allowing for the possibility of a more effective subsequent surgery;

- The possibility of a preventative PT, to be carried out in pregnant women suffering from macroprolactinoma and refusing DAs during pregnancy.

- The possibility of combined PT + DA treatment;

- The possibility of using PT as the first choice therapy for macroprolactinoma in carefully selected patients;

5   Conclusion

The results of this five-year study suggest the possibility of phytotherapeutic treatment of macroprolactinoma patients to the effect of hyperprolactinemia regulation and tumour size reduction. This line of treatment had proven itself worthy of being not merely an adjuvant, but, in some patients, the first choice macroprolactinoma therapy. This claim is particularly based on the encouraging results obtained across our PT arm. Future research should attempt to demonstrate the efficiency of PT as the first choice therapy capable of downsizing macroprolactinoma-induced prolactin hyper-secretion, while the results obtained with this line of research should be compared against the current notions on DA efficiency.

Acknowledgement

We are most indebted to all of our patients for putting their trust in us and confiding us with their health. Without their faith in phytotherapeutic benefits and potentials, this study wouldn't be possible. The research has been financed by the family business "DREN" DOO Žepče, whose founders create and distribute the herbal remedies used for the treatments.

References

Asa, S.L. (2007). Atlas of tumor pathology: Tumours of the Pituitary Gland. 3rd series, Fascicle 22. Washington:Armed Forces Institute of Pathology.

Block, K.I. & Mead, M.N. (2003). Immune System Effects of Echinacea, Ginseng, and Astragalus: A Review. Integrative Cancer Therapies. 247–267.

Braucks, G.R., Naliato, E.C., Tabet, A.L., Gadelha, M.R. & Violante, A.H. (2003). Clinical and therapeutic aspects of prolactinoma in men. Arq. Neuropsiquiatr. 1004–1110.

European Medicines Agency. (2014). EMEA recommends new warnings and contraindications for ergot-derived dopamine agonists. EMEA, 2014. Web. 22 August 2014. http://www.ema.europa.eu/docs/ en_GB/document_library/Maximun_Residue_Limits_-_Report/2014/08/WC500171572.pdf.

Geddes, J.R. & Cipriani, A. (2004). Selective serotonin reuptake inhibitors. BMJ. 809–810.

Guyton, A.C. & Hall, J. E. (2003). Textbook of Medical Physiology. Pennsylvania: W.B. Saunders Company.

Horvath, E. & Kovacs, K. (1992). Ultrastructural diagnosis of human pituitary adenomas. Microscopy Research and Technique. 107–135.

Kanowski, S. & Hoerr, R. (2003). Ginkgo biloba extract EGb 761 in dementia: intent-to-treat analyses of a 24-week, multi-centre, double-blind, placebo-controlled, randomized trial. Pharmacopsychiatry. 97–303.

Kovačević, N. (2000). Pharmacognostic basics. Belgrade: Faculty of Pharmacy University of Belgrade.

Levy, A & Lightman, S.L. (1993). The pathogenesis of pituitary adenoma. Clinical Endocrinology. 559–570.

Lukić, P.B. (1993). Pharmacognostics. Belgrade: Faculty of Pharmacy University of Belgrade.

Mah, P.M. & Webster, J. (2001). Hyperprolactinaemia: aetiology, diagnosis and management. Thieme Medical Publishers. 365–374.

Pehaček, Z. & Sajdl, P. (1990). *Ergot alkaloids: Chemistry, biological effects, biotechnology. Prague. Prague Academy.* 1–42.

Pekić, B. (1983). *Chemistry and technology of pharmaceutical products – alkaloids and ether oils. Novi Sad. Faculty of Technology University of Novi Sad.*

Scheithauer, B.W., Horvath, E., Kovacs K., Laws, E.R.Jr., Randall, R.V. & Ryan, N. (1986). *Plurihormonal pituitary adenomas. Semin Diagn Pathology.* 69–82.

Yale, S.H. & Liu, K. (2004). *Echinacea purpurea Therapy for the Treatment of the Common Cold: A Randomized, Double-blind, Placebo-Controlled Clinical Trial. Archives of Internal Medicine.* 1237–1241.

Chapter 7

Cerebral Calcifications as a Differential Diagnosis of Psychiatric Disorders

Amir Mufaddel[1], Ossama T. Osman[2], Ghanem Al Hassani[1]

1 Introduction

It is of vital importance to differentiate psychiatric symptoms secondary to organic causes from primary psychiatric disorders. Early diagnosis of the primary organic etiology is necessary for early intervention and for avoiding side effects of using long term psychotropic medications. This will be particularly helpful if the underlying cause is treatable and its treatment can lead to improvement in psychiatric symptoms. Organic psychiatric disorders are more likely if the patient is presenting with first episode of psychiatric symptoms, prominent cognitive symptoms or with clinical features that are not typical for functional psychiatric disorder. Several physical causes can contribute to the etiology of organic psychiatric disorders. Examples of such conditions include neurological conditions, infectious diseases, constipation, dehydration, pain and vascular causes.

Organic psychiatric disorders can present with different pictures including:

1. Delirium

2. Dementia

3. Other organic mental disorders: those are classified in ICD-10 as organic hallucinosis, organic catatonic disorder, organic delusional or schizophrenia-like disorder, organic mood disorder, organic anxiety disorder and organic personality disorder (Mufaddel et al., 2014b).

---

[1] Behavioral Sciences Institute, Al Ain Hospital, Al Ain, United Arab Emirates.
[2] Department of Psychiatry, College of Medicine and Health Sciences, United Arab Emirates University, Al Ain, United Arab Emirates.

Table 1 summarizes the differential diagnosis of psychiatric symptoms that can occur due to organic conditions. The table includes organic conditions that can lead to cerebral calcifications. It is important to consider that there are many other organic conditions that can present with psychiatric symptoms, but this chapter discusses only those associated with cerebral calcification.

Psychiatric Condition	Possible Etiological Conditions with Cerebral Calcification
Mood changes/ Depression	**Intra-axial:** Temporal lobe tumors Parietal lobe tumors Thalamic lesions Craniopharyngioma Infections (brucellosis, toxoplasmosis) Hypoparathyroidism Fahr's disease Tuberous sclerosis **Extra-axial calcifications:** Frontal lobe meningioma Gorlin –Goltz syndrome
Psychotic symptoms	**Intra-axial:** Hypoparathyroidism Fahr's disease Infections (influenza virus, HSV-1, congenital rubella) **Extra-axial calcifications:** Frontal lobe meningioma Gorlin –Goltz syndrome
Personality changes	Extra-axial calcifications (Frontal lobe tumors such as meningioma)
Autism spectrum disorders	Tuberous sclerosis Infections (congenital rubella,
ADHD	Sturge-Weber syndrome Neurofibromatosis
Mental retardation	Tuberous sclerosis Sturge-Weber syndrome Neurofibromatosis Craniopharyngioma. Infections: Congenital toxoplasmosis, CMV infection
Dementia	Vascular lesions Hypoparathyroidism

Table1: Differential diagnosis of psychiatric conditions that can be associated with calcified cerebral lesions.

Radiological investigations are useful tools to exclude organic pathology in patients presenting with psychiatric symptoms. One of the possible radiological findings that can indicate presence of current or previous organic pathology contributing to the clinical psychiatric presentation is the presence of cerebral calcifications which can occur in a wide range of conditions with different etiologies. Calcifications can occur as physiologic, dystrophic, congenital or vascular calcifications. For psychiatric patients who present with cerebral calcifications, the location of calcification and the clinical psychiatric and systemic presentations are important in establishing a final diagnosis (Mufaddel & Al Hassani, 2014b).

Intracranial calcifications are frequent findings on radiological brain examinations. It is sometimes difficult to conclude whether such calcifications are of clinical significance or are just incidental findings particularly when the lesions are not clearly explaining the clinical picture. This is particularly applied when the presenting complaint is of only psychopathological nature.

In this chapter, the differential diagnosis of brain calcifications will be discussed in relation to the possible psychiatric presentations reported in the literature.

Based on their location, cerebral calcifications can be divided into extra-axial and intra-axial calcifications (Table 2). Intra-axial calcifications occur within the brain parenchyma; and extra-axial calcifications are external to the brain parenchyma. Examples of structures involved in extra-axial calcifications are: falxcerebri and the pineal gland. Intraventricualr calcifications are discussed as intra-axial calcifications but they are sometimes considered as a third type of cerebral calcification. Structures commonly involved in intra-axial clarifications are the basal ganglia and the cerebellum. Causes of intra-axial calcifications include neoplasms (e.g. oligodendrogliomas and astrocytomas), vascular causes (e.g. angiomatous malformations and aneurysms), Infectious (e.g. congenital childhood infections, and parasitic infections such as neurocysticercosis and cerebral hydatid cyst disease), congenital causes (e.g. tuberous sclerosis); and endocrine/metabolic causes (e.g. hypoparathyroidism, and hyperparathyroidism) (Celzo et al., 2013; Makariou & Patsalides, 2009).

Both acquired and congenital infections can lead to intracranial calcifications. Example of infections causing calcifications includes TORCH infections (toxoplasmosis, other, rubella, cytomegalovirus, herpes simplex virus). Metabolic disorders that affect calcium homeostasis can lead to calcifications predominantly involving the basal ganglia. Inflammatory lesions, such as sarcoidosis and tumors, may also lead to cerebral calcifications (Celzo et al., 2013; Makariou & Patsalides, 2009).

The basal ganglia calcifications are usually seen in the globus pallidus, the head of the caudate nucleus, and the putamen and they commonly occur in middle-aged and the elderly subjects. Brain calcifications are interpreted as incidental findings of no significance by some clinicians. However, individuals with brain calcifications, particularly those below the age of 30 years, should be carefully evaluated for underlying etiologies (Celzo et al., 2013; Makariou & Patsalides, 2009)

Extra-axial Calcifications	Intra-axial Calcifications
Structures Involved:	**Structures involved:**
Falxcerebri	Basal ganglia
The pineal gland	Cerebellum
Choroid plexus	
Habenula	**Causes:**
Dura and arachnoid	Neoplastic
Tentorium cerebelli	• Oligodendrogliomas
Superior sagittal sinus	• Astrocytomas
Petroclinoid and interclinoid ligaments	• Medulloblastomas
Arachnoid granulations	• Other primary brain tumours.
	• Metastasic tumours
Causes:	Vascular
Meningiomas	• Angiomatous malformations
Dural osteomas	• Arteriovenous malformations
Calcifying tumours	• Dystrophic calcification in chronic infarction
Exaggerated physiological calcifications	• Chronic vasculitis
	• Aneurysms
	Infectious
	• Congenital childhood infections, particularly the 'TORCH'
	• Tuberculosis
	• Parasitic infections such as neuro-cysticercosis and cerebral hydatid cyst disease
	Congenital:
	• Sturge-Weber syndrome
	• Tuberous sclerosis
	• Lipomas
	• Neurofibromatosis
	Endocrine/metabolic
	• Diabetes mellitus
	• Hypoparathyroidism
	• Pseudohypoparathyroidism
	• Hyperparathyroidism
	Idiopathic/genetic:
	• Familial idiopathic basal ganglia calcification.

Table 2: Differential diagnosis of extra- and intra-axial cerebral calcifications.

2   Extra-axial Calcifications:

Extra-axial cerebral calcifications are commonly caused by meningiomas, dural osteomas, calcifying tumours, and physiological calcifications (Celzo et al., 2013). Some rare conditions with multi-system involvement can also be associated with extra-axial calcifications such as that occurring in Gorlin-Goltz syndrome with characteristic falx-cerebri calcification (Mufaddel et al., 2014a). Anatomical locations for extra-axial calcifications are shown in Figure 1.

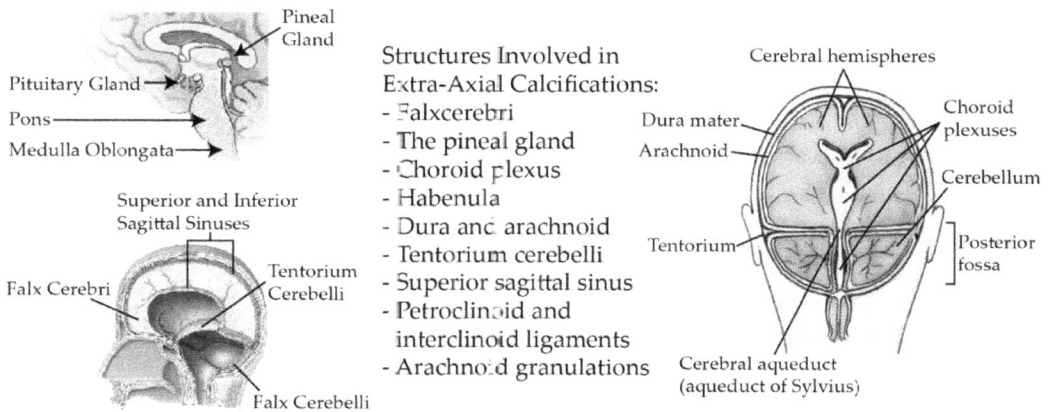

Structures Involved in Extra-Axial Calcifications:
- Falxcerebri
- The pineal gland
- Choroid plexus
- Habenula
- Dura and arachnoid
- Tentorium cerebelli
- Superior sagittal sinus
- Petroclinoid and interclinoid ligaments
- Arachnoid granulations

Figure 1: Anatomical locations for extra-axial calcifications.

Based on etiology, the differential diagnosis of extra-axial calcification in relation to psychiatric presentations is discussed below.

2.1   Extra-axial Neoplasm

Frontal meningiomas can compress the frontal lobes externally, and if they are large in size they can lead to personality and intellectual changes. They are sometimes seen by psychiatrists before the diagnosis of meningioma is established due to the nature of their psychiatric symptoms. Delayed diagnosis of frontal meningiomas presenting with psychiatric features has been reported in several cases presenting with longstanding history of visual hallucinations and personality change. Other presenting symptoms can occur such as headache and visual loss; and such patients are sometimes misdiagnosed as conversion disorder (Panzer et al., 1991). Some patients may suffer from headache preceding or during the psychiatric symptoms and others may later develop epilepsy. Other psychiatric presentations of frontal meningiomas include symptoms resembling depression, anxiety, hypomania, and schizophrenia. Surgical treatment was associated with improvement of symptoms and even improved level of functioning in some cases.

Severe psychiatric symptoms and epilepsy have also been reported as presenting symptoms in patients with huge osteoma in the anterior cranial fossa (Hudolin et al.,1961).

2.2   Gorlin-Goltz Syndrome

Gorlin-Goltz syndrome is an autosomal dominant syndrome with multiple and diverse clinical features that involve the nervous system, skin, eyes, endocrine system, and bones. In 1960, Gorlin and Goltz reported the triad that characterized the diagnosis of Gorlin-Goltz syndrome, the triad included the presence of nevoid basal cell carcinoma, kerato-cystic odontogenic tumors in the jaws, and bifid ribs. There are several other clinical features of this syndrome including calcification of the falx cerebri, facial milia, palmar and plantar epidermal pits, spine and rib anomalies, relative macrocephaly, medulloblasto-mas, frontal bossing, cleft lip and/or palate, ocular malformation, and developmental malformations (Gorlin & Goltz, 1960; Casaroto et al., 2011). Gorlin-Goltz syndrome is di-agnosed by the presence of either two major criteria or one major and two minor criteria. The major criteria:

1.   Multiple (>2) basal cell carcinomas (or one if under 20 years of age).

2.   Odontogenic keratocysts of the jaws proven by histopathology.

3.   Three or more palmar or plantar pits.

4.   Bilamellar calcification of the falx cerebri.

5.   Bifid, fused or markedly splayed ribs.

6.   First-degree relatives with nevoid basal cell carcinoma.

The minor criteria:

1.   Macrocephay

2.   Frontal bossing, cleft lip/palate, pectus, and syndactyly of digits.

3.   Sprengel deformity, pectus, and syndactyly of digits.

4.   Radiology abnormalities: bridging of sella turcica, hemivertebrae, and flame-shaped radiolucencies.

5.   Ovarian fibroma

6.   Medulloplastoma

Cases with complicated multiple clinical presentations have been reported with history of pleomorphic psychiatric features, basal cell carcinoma, low vitamin-D level, high parathroid hormone levels, and extensive calcification along falx cerebri and around the cerebellar vermis. Possible presenting psychiatric symptoms include irritability, ag-gressive behavior, labile mood, hallucinations, paranoid delusions, and transient cogni-tive impairment (Mufaddel et al., 2014a). Figures 2, 3 & 4: show palmar pits, falx cerebri calcification, & cerebellar vermis calcifications in a patient with Gorlin-Goltz syndrome who presented with psychiatric symptoms.

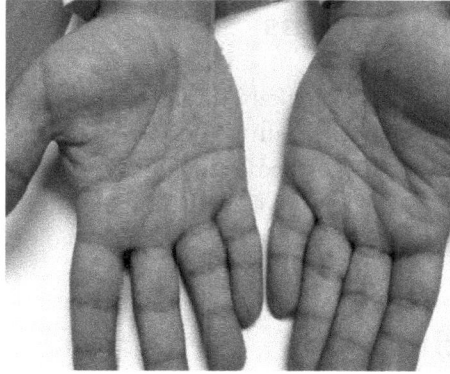

Figure 2: Palmar pits in a patient with Gorlin-Goltz syndrome (Mufaddel et al., 2014a).

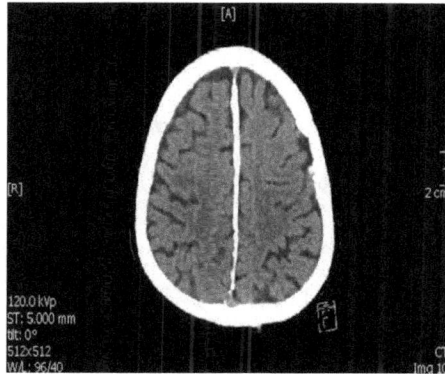

Figure 3: falx cerebri calcification in a patient with Gorlin-Goltz syndrome (Mufaddel et al., 2014a).

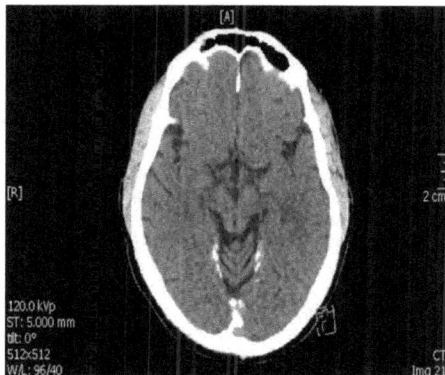

Figure 4: ceberllar calcification in a patient with Gorlin-Goltz syndrome (Mufaddel et al., 2014a).

3   Physiologic calcifications

Physiologic cerebral calcifications are likely if they are not associated with any evidence of disease and have no demonstrable pathological cause. They most commonly occur in the pineal gland, habenula, choroid plexus, basal ganglia, falx, tentorium, petroclinoid ligaments and sagittal sinus. The size of calcification and age at presentation should be considered before concluding that the calcification is physiologic (Kıroğlu et al., 2010).

4   Intra-axial calcifications

Intra-axial calcifications have several etiologies including neoplasm, vascular causes, infections, congenital disorders, and endocrine/ metabolic causes. They could also be idiopathic such as that occurring in Fahr's disease. Anatomical locations for intra-axial calcifications are shown in Figure 5. Based on etiology, the differential diagnosis of intra-axial calcification in relation to psychiatric presentations is discussed below.

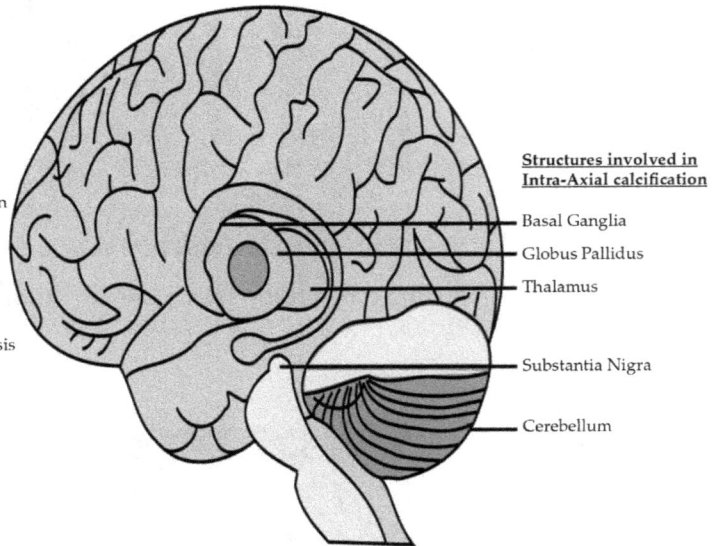

Causes
Neoplastic:
Oilgodendrogliomas
Astrocytomas
Medulloblastomas
Other primary brain tumours
Metastasictumours
Vascular:
Angiomatous malformations
Arteriovenous malformations
Dystrophic calcification in chronic infraction
Chronic vasculitis
Aneurysms
Infectious:
Congenital chilhood infections, particularly the 'TORCH'
Tuberculosis
Parasitic infections such as neurocysticercosis and cerebral hydatid cyst disease
Congential:
Sturge-Weber sydrome
Tuberous sclerosis
Lipomas
Neurofibromatosis
Endocrine/metabolic:
Diabetes melitus
Hypoparathyroidism,
Pseudohypoparathyroidism
Hyperparathyroidism
Idiopathic/genetic:
Familial idiopathic basal ganglia calcification

Structures involved in Intra-Axial calcification
Basal Ganglia
Globus Pallidus
Thalamus
Substantia Nigra
Cerebellum

Figure 5: Anatomical locations and causes of intra-axial calcifications.

4.1   Neoplastic Causes

Tumors that are commonly associated with intracranial calcifications include oligodendrogliomas, astrocytomas, craniopharyngiomas, meningiomas, pineal gland tumors and ependymomas. In some instances, the presence of calcification and its pattern can be path-ognomonic in some tumors such as oligodendrogliomas and craniopharyngiomas (Ma-kariou & Patsalides, 2009; Celzo et al., 2013).

In some cases, psychiatric symptoms can be the first presenting symptoms of brain tumours in the absence of neurological signs. For example, incidental MRI findings of thalamic tumor have been reported in patients presenting only with psychiatric symp-toms. Patients may present with mood change, psychotic symptoms, panic attacks, per-sonality changes, or memory problems. (Moise & Madhusoodanan ,2006). In other cases, neurological signs can be minimal and the psychiatric symptoms are more prominent. Example of these is parietal lobe tumors which can present with depression accompanied by minimal neurological. (Madhusoodanan et al., 2004). Therefore, radiological investi-gations are necessary for early detection of possible brain tumors in individuals present-ing with psychiatric symptoms particularly in those presenting with new symptoms, atypical presentation or treatment-resistant psychiatric symptoms.

No clear association could currently be confirmed between the nature of psychiat-ric symptoms and the location of tumor or its histological type (Madhusoodanan et al., 2007). However, mood disorders and schizophrenia-like conditions can be related to right and left hemispheres dysfunctions, respectively. Lesions located in the temporal lobes are commonly associated with depression (Uribe, 1986).

Craniopharyngiomas are locally invasive and are frequently recurrent and they are associated with neurological and endocrinological dysfunction. Most studies regarding psychiatric sequale of craniopharyngiomas were conducted in patients who have been treated for the tumor. Children treated prior to the age of 18 years had an overall neuro-behavioral dysfunction in 57% of cases including social impairment (41%), school dys-function (35%), and emotional/affective dysfunction with primarily depressive symp-toms (40%) (Zada et al., 2013).

4.2   Vascular Disorders

Vascular calcification can be due to atherosclerosis, aneurysm, arteriovenous malfor-mation or cavernous malformation. Atherosclerotic calcifications could be related to cog-nitive dysfunction and to brain changes on MRI examination. Larger volumes of calcifi-cation are associated with lower cognitive scores and smaller total brain volumes (Bos et al., 2012).

Vascular disorders are associated with developing neurodegenerative conditions such as Alzheimer's disease, multiple sclerosis and Huntington's. Cerebrovascular dis-ease may also lead to vascular type of dementia which is the second commonest cause of dementia. It usually occurs in the seventh and eighth decades with a relatively acute onset and it might follow stroke. It may be difficult to establish a clear diagnosis of vascular dementia in the absence of history of stroke or localizing neurological signs.

High risk of dementia is associated with larger calcification volume in all vessels, except in the coronary vessels. Also extra-cranial calcification of carotid artery is signifi-cantly associated with a higher risk of dementia. Similarly, this finding remains also sig-nificant for Alzheimer's disease (Bos et al., 2014).

Alzheimer's disease is primarily related to the hippocampus as brain tissue develops neuro-degeneration with characteristic tau and amyloid protein deposits. Clinical features of Alzheimer's disease are memory impairment with gradual onset and continuing decline. Aphasia, apraxia, agnosia and disturbances in executive functioning may occur. Findings on CT or MRI characteristically show hippocampal atrophy and ventricular enlargement. Microscopic neuropathological features of neurofibrillary tangles and senile plaques (amyloid plaques) are cardinal diagnositic features.

One of the hypotheses aimed to explaining the pathological changes in Alzheimer's disease suggest possible breakdown of blood brain barrier (BBB) following traumatic brain injury. BBB leakage can occur secondarily to abnormal brain activity with associated increase in the number of endothelial caveolae, leading totranscytosis of plasma proteins andreductionof tight junction proteins (Franzblau et al., 2013).

4.3   Infections

Both acquired and congenital infections can be associated with cerebral calcifications as well as psychiatric symptoms which can be either acute or chronic symptoms. Psychiatric symptoms can be the initial clinical presentation of systemic and central nervous system infections, and they can occur in the absence of neurological symptoms in some disorders as in some cases of viral encephalitis. Mood symptoms can occur secondary to brucellosis or toxoplasmosis. Late-onset neuropsychiatric complications, occurring several years following the infection, have also been reported such as in the case of subacute sclerosing panencephalitis due to measles. Some Infectious diseases are thought to have possible etiological role for major psychiatric disorders such as schizophrenia (e.g. Influenza virus and HSV-1), (Mufaddel et al., 2014b).

The most common acquired intracranial infections that are typically associated with intracranial calcifications include: cysticercosis, tuberculosis, HIV and cryptococcus infections (Makariou & Patsalides, 2009).

Congential anomalies are caused by perinatal infectionsin 2% to 3% of cases. TORCH (Toxoplasmosis, Other, Rubella, Cytomegalovirus (CMV), and Herpes infections), are among the most common infections that can lead to congenital anomalies (Stegmann & Carey, 2002).

Congenial toxoplasmosis usually presents with the classic triad of chorioretinitis, hydrocephalus, and intracranial calcifications. Other variety of symptoms can also occur and systemic manifestations may include fever, hepatomegaly, splenomegaly, jaundice, lymphadenopathy, anemia and abnormal spinal fluid (Halonen & Weis, 2013). Congenital toxoplasmosis can lead to brain and eye tissues abnormalities including destruction or remodeling of the white substance and blockade of the aqueduct of Sylvius by infected necrotized foci which may further calcify. Sequelae of congenital toxoplasmosis include mental retardation, psychomotor abnormalities, seizures, deafness, microcephalus, and hydrocephalus (Robert-Gangneux & Dardé, 2012).

Congenital cytomegalovirus (CMV) infection is one of the most common viral causes of congenital infections with incidence that varies between 0.15% and 2.0% (Gaytant et al., 2002). CMV infection can be associated with mental retardation, cerebral palsy, psychomotor retardation and sensorineural hearing loss. These complications are often irreversible even with antiviral treatment. Abnormal CT findings were reported in 70% of symptomatic children with CMV with intracerebral calcifications being the most common finding. Most of those who had abnormal CT scan findings during neonatal period (90%) developed at least one long-term sequel. About 50% of children with CT abnormalities had an IQ < 50, (Boppana et al., 1997). Other radiological features include enlarged ventricles, white matter abnormalities, polymicrogyria, cysts, structural changes, and extensive encephalopathy (Cheeran et al., 2009).

Few studies have been conducted to investigate psychiatric manifestations in individuals with congenital rubella. There are conflicting results and views regarding the association between congenital rubella and developing autism and mental retardation (Chess, 1971). Congenital rubella is commonly associated with CNS manifestations including hearing loss and psychomotor retardation. Psychiatric manifestations have been reported in up to 50% of cases (Rorke, 1973). One study investigated the radiological findings in adult deaf patients with schizophrenia-like symptoms and documented prenatal rubella virus infection and compared them with controls. The study concluded that there are abnormal white matter lesions which may correspond to neurovascular lesions but they do not appear to be directly related to schizophrenia-like symptoms (Lane et al., 1996). Calcifications due to congenital rubella are commonly located in the periventricular white matter, basal ganglia, and brain stem (Kıroğlu et al., 2010).

Neonatal herpes simplex encephalitis is accompanied by early rapid atrophic changes which may be evident in the 3d week. Late findings may include cortical atrophy and calcification with variety of distributions ranging from punctate to an extensive gyral pattern with possible involvement of the cerebellum (Noorbehesht et al., 1987). Case control studies suggest a significant association between presence of maternal antibodies to HSV2 glycoprotein gG2 and developing subsequent psychotic illness (Buka et al., 2001).

4.4   Congenital Disorders

Cerebral calcification in congenital disorders is frequently seen in Sturge-Weber syndrome, tuberous sclerosis, neurofibromatosis, intracranial lipoma, Cockayne and Gorlin syndromes.

4.4.1   Tuberous sclerosis

Tuberous sclerosis is an autosomal dominant condition that presents with adenoma sebaceum, epilepsy, retinal Phakomas, subungualfibromata, white skin patches, shagreenskin and cognitive impairment. It can be associated with multiple tumours in kidneys, spleen and lungs. Cognitive impairment is often severe and learning disability occurs in 38%-64% of cases (Gelder et al., 2004; Gillberg et al. 1994; Kumar et al., 2005; Webb et al., 1991).

Autism and broadly-defined features of pervasive developmental disorders are common in patients with tuberous sclerosis. One study suggested a prevalence of 24% and 19% respectively. Autistic features were found more common in females than males with tuberous sclerosis (Hunt & Shephred, 1993).

Epidemiological studies have shown that individuals with tuberous sclerosis complex had mental retardation and autistic-like pervasive developmental disorders with a prevalence of 50-60% and 43-86% respectively. On the other hand, children with autism have tuberous sclerosis complex existing in 1% of cases (Harrison & Bolton, 1997).

There are few established medical causes of autism spectrum disorder. One of these causes is tuberous sclerosis which is a unique neurogenetic model for investigating the brain basis of the syndrome (Bolton et al., 2002).

Factors that may have greater likelihood of developing an autism spectrum disorder in children with tuberous sclerosis include: mutation in the TSC2, early-onset infantile and presence of an epileptiform focus in the temporal lobes (Bolton, 2004).

Other psychiatric symptoms include psychosis, anxiety and depression. Childhood-onset mood disorders were also reported in some cases (Chopra et al., 2006).

4.4.2   Sturge-Weber syndrome

Sturge-Weber Syndrome (encephalofacialangiomatosis) is a congenital disorder with exceptional familial occurrence. There is capillary malformations involving the skin, eye and the brain. Skin involvement usually presents with port-wine naevus involving one side of the face in the distribution of a fifth nerve division. Brain involvement presents withleptomeningealangioma which tends to involve the parietal and occipital lobes (Kumar et al., 2005). Eye involvement may lead to glaucoma. Computed tomography and contrast-enhance MRI are helpful in the diagnosis of brain involvement. Radiological features are common in patients with Sturge-Weber syndrome who have facial involvement. These are commonly involving the frontal and parietal lobes and less commonly occipital lobe brain involvement. When the port-wine nevus is bilateral, there will be a greater risk of brain involvement (Crosley & Binet, 1978; Taly et al., 1987) .

Neuropsychiatric features that are commonly associated with Sturge-Weber syndrome include epilepsy, cognitive symptoms, attention deficit hyperkinetic disorders, headache, hemiparesis, and visual field defects (Lo et al. 2012).

Small study including 16 patients with Sturge-Weber syndrome has shown that they have psychiatric diagnoses including mood disorder (31%), disruptive behaviour (25%), and adjustment disorder (25%). Substance-related disorders were most frequently found in adults (67%), (Turin et al., 2010).

Epilepsy, hemiparesis, mental retardation and ocular problems were found the most common and the most severe presentations in one series of 55 patients with Sturge-Weber syndrome. Cerebral lesions were associated a progressive course during childhood. Surgical treatment has shown benefits in controlling seizures but it has poor benefits in hemiparesis and intellectual deficits (Pascual-Castroviejo et al., 2008).

4.4.3   Neurofibromatosis (NF)

Neurofibromatosis (Von Recklinghausen's disease) was described in 1882 by Friedrich

Daniel Von Recklinghausen. It is characterized by multiple skin neurofibromas and pigmentation due to neuroectodermal abnormality. It has several clinical symptoms involving the skin, nervous system, bones, eyes and other sites. There are two clinical types of NF including peripheral type (NF1) and central type (NF2) (Kumar et al., 2005).

NF1 is more frequent than NF2 and presents as subcutaneous, soft, and sometimes pedunculated tumors which increase in number. The gene responsible for NF1 is located on the long arm of chromosome 17 (17q11.2) which encodes a protein called neurofibromin which is expressed in neurons, Schwann cells, oligodendrocytes and astrocytes. Learning disabilities may occur due to NF1 mutation (Antônio et al., 2013).

Recent studies suggest slight increase in the frequency of mental retardation in children with NF1 (North et al., 2002).

Psychiatric and cognitive disorders are more often encountered in patients with NF1 than NF2. Specific learning disabilities exist in only 20% of children with NF1; and their neuropsychological profile indicates deficits in perceptual skills (visuospatial and visuoperceptual), executive functioning, and attention (sustained and switching). Difficulties in sustained attention were present in 63% of children with NF1, with 38% fulfilling criteria for attention deficit-hyperactivity disorder (Hyman et al., 2005).

The abnormal gene responsible for NF2 is located on chromosome 22(q122), and the abnormal protein is merlin or schwarnomin which is a cytoskeletal protein. Several tumors may occur in NF2 such as meningioma, acoustic neuroma, lexiform neuroma, glioma and cutaneous neurofibroma (Evans et al., 2000).

4.5   Metabolic Causes

Basal ganglia and subcortical calcifications may occur in patients with chronic renal failure and secondary hyperparathyroidism. Calcification due to hypoparathyroidism typically involve the basal ganglia, thalami, and the cerebellum. Cerebral calcifications are more common pseudohypoparathyroidism than idiopathic hypopharatyroidism. Hypothyroidism can be associated with basal ganglia and cerebellar calcifications (Makariou & Patsalides, 2009). Psychiatric features in hypoparathyroidism include depression, anxiety, emotional lability, confusion, and psychosis (Hossain, 1970).

Cognitive deficits commonly occur in patients with chronic hypoparathyroidism with positive correlation between symptoms of cognitive dysfunction and the presence of cerebral calcification (Kowdley et al., 1999). Neuropsychological dysfunctions were in 35.5 % of patients with idiopathic hypoparathyroidism; and they correlated with illness duration, female gender, and serum calcium but not with intracranial calcifications (Aggarwal et al., 2013).

Elderly patients with hypoparathyroidism and associated calcifications can be misdiagnosed as cases of senile dementia. Symptoms of dementia that occur due to hypoparathyroidism are treatable and should be considered in the differential diagnosis of dementia (Katsidzira et al., 2010).

4.6   Familial Idiopathic Basal Ganglia Calcification (Fahr's disease)

Fahr's disease is a rare neurodegenerative disorder which is characterized by the presence of symmetrical and bilateral calcification of the basal ganglia. Calcifications were also reported in other brain regions such as dentate nucleus, thalamus and cerebral cortex. Familial and non-familial cases of the disease have been reported, with predominantly autosomal-dominant fashion. Neuropsychiatric features and movement disorders are the common presenting clinical features (Mufaddel & Al Hassani, 2014). The clinical features of Fahr's disease are shown in Table 3, and the criteria for the diagnosis are shown in Figure 6.

Psychiatric Features	Cognitive deterioration: dementia, delirium, confusion. Psychotic symptoms: hallucinations, delusions. Catatonia. Mood disorders: depression, manic symptoms. Anxiety. Irritability. Aggression.
Somatic Symptoms	Parkinsonism and movement disorders. Seizures. Headache. Vertigo. Paresis. Stroke. Syncope. Ataxia. Dysarthria. Tremor. Orthostatic hypotension.
Radiological Findings	Bilateral symmetrical calcifications of basal ganglia and dentate nucleus. Other sites of calcifications: thalamus, Centrum semi-ovale, cerebellum and cerebral white matter.

Table 3: Clinical presentations of Fahr's disease (Mufaddel & Al-Hassani, 2014).

References

Aggarwal, S., Kailash, S., Sagar, R., Tripathi, M., Sreenivas, V., Sharma, R., Gupta, N., et al. (2013). Neuropsychological dysfunction in idiopathic hypoparathyroidism and its relationship with intracranial calcification and serum total calcium. Eur J Endocrinol. 168 (6): 895–903.

Antônio, J.R., Goloni-Bertollo, E.M., Trídico, L.A. (2013). Neurofibromatosis: chronological history and current issues. An Bras Dermatol. 88 (3): 329–43.

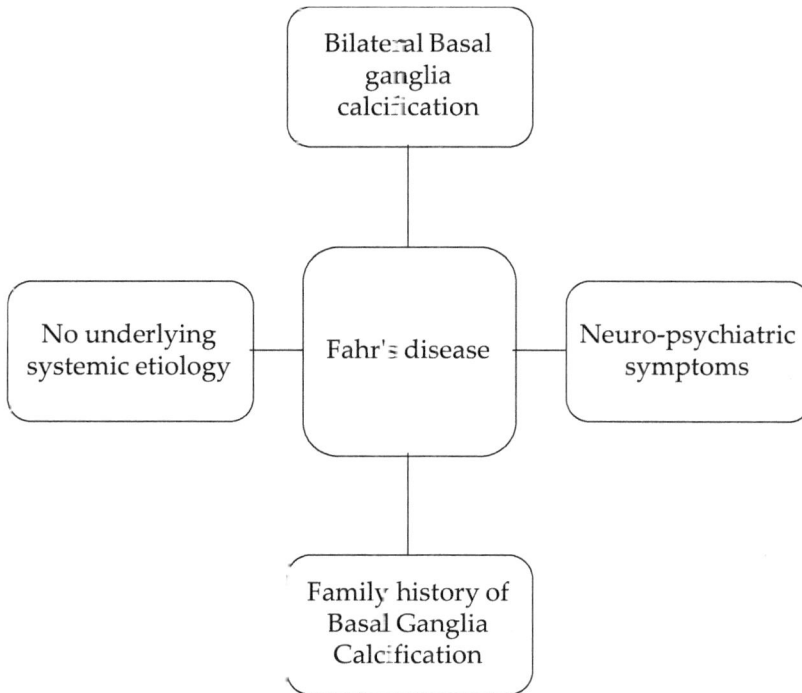

Figure 6: Criteria for the diagnosis of Fahr's disease (Mufaddel & Hassani, 2014).

Bolton, P.F. (2004). Neuroepileptic correlates of autistic symptomatology in tuberous sclerosis.Ment Retard Dev Disabil Res Rev. 10 (2): 126–31.

Bolton, P.F., Park, R.J., Higgins, J.N., Griffiths, P.D., Pickles, A. (2002). Neuro-epileptic determinants of autism spectrum disorders in tuberous sclerosis complex. Brain. 125 (6): 1247–55.

Boppana, S.B., Fowler, K.B., Vaid, Y., Hedlund, G., Stagno, S., Britt, W.J. et al. (1997). Neuroradiographic findings in the newborn period and long-term outcome in children with symptomatic congenital cytomegalovirus infection. Pediatrics. 99 (3): 409–14.

Bos, D., Vernooij, M.W., de Bruijn, R.F., Koudstaal, P.G., Hofman, A., et al. (2014). Atherosclerotic calcification is related to a higher risk of dementia and cognitive decline. Alzheimers Dement

Bos, D., Vernooij, M.W., Elias-Smale, S.E., Verhaaren, B.F., Vrooman, H.A., Hofman, A., et al. (2012). Atherosclerotic calcification relates to cognitive function and to brain changes on magnetic resonance imaging. Alzheimers Dement. 8 (5 Suppl): S104–11.

Buka, S.L., Tsuang, M.T., Torrey, E.F., Klebanoff, M.A., Bernstein, D., Yolken, R.H. (2001). Maternal Infectionsand Subsequent Psychosis among Offspring.Archives of General Psychiatry. 58: 1032–1037.

Casaroto, A.R., Rocha Loures, D.C.N., Moreschi, E., et al. (2011). Early diagnosis of Gorlin-Goltz syndrome: case report. Head and Face Medicine. 7.

Celzo, F.G., Venstermans, C., De Belder, F., van Goethem, J., van den Hauwe, L., et al. (2013). Brain stones revisited-between a rock and a hard place. Insights Imaging. 4 (5): 625–635.

Cheeran, M.C., Lokensgard, J.R., Schleiss, M.R. (2009). Neuropathogenesis of congenital cytomegalovirus infection: disease mechanisms and prospects for intervention. ClinMicrobiol Rev. 22 (1): 99–126.

Chess, S. (1971). Autism in children with congenital rubella.Journal of autism and childhood schizophrenia 1 (1): 33–47

Chopra, V.K., Cintury, Y., Sinha, V.K. (2006). Bipolar disorder associated with tuberous sclerosis: Chance association or aetiological relationship? Indian J Psychiatry. 48 (1): 66–8.

Crosley, C.J., Binet, E.F. (1978). Sturge-Weber Syndrome: presentation as a focal seizure disorder without nevus flammeus. ClinPediatr (Phila) 17: 606–9.

Evans, D., Sainio, M., Baser, M. (2000). Neurofibromatosis type 2. J Med Genet. 37 (12): 897–904.

Franzblau, M., Gonzales-Portillo, C., Gonzales-Portillo, G.S., Diamandis, T., Borlongan, M.C., Tajiri, N., et al. (2013). Vascular damage: a persisting pathology common to Alzheimer's disease and traumatic brain injury. Med Hypotheses. 81 (5): 842–5.

Gaytant, M.A., Steegers, E.A., Semmekrot, B.A., Merkus, H.M., Galama, J.M. (2002). Congenital cytomegalovirus infection: review of the epidemiology and outcome. Obstet Gynecol Surv. 57 (4): 245–56.

Gelder, M., Harrison, P. and Cowen, P., Eds. (2004) Shorter Oxford Textbook of Psychiatry, 5th Edition, Oxford University Press, Oxford, 321–357.

Gillberg, I.C., Gillberg, C., Ahlsen, G. (1994). Autistic behaviour and attention deficits in tuberous sclerosis.A population-based study. Dev Med Child Neurol. 36: 50–6.

Gorlin, R.J., Goltz, R.W. (1960). Multiple nevoid basal-cell epithelioma, jaw cysts and bifid rib. A syndrome. The New England journal of medicine. 262: 908–912.

Halonen, S.K., Weiss, L.M. (2013). Toxoplasmosis.HandbClin Neurol. 114: 125–45.

Harrison, J.E., Bolton, P.F. (1997). Annotation: tuberous sclerosis. J Child Psychol Psychiatry 38: 603–614.

Hossain, M. (1970). Neurological and psychiatric manifestations in idiopathic hypoparathyroidism: response to treatment. J. Neurol. Neurosurg.Psychiatry 33 (2): 153–156

Hudolin, V.I., Riessener, D., Kadrnka, S., Knezevic, M. (1961). A huge osteoma in the anterior cranial fossa. J Neurol Neurosurg Psychiatry. 24: 80–83.

Hunt, A., Shepherd, C.A. (1993). prevalence study of autism in tuberous sclerosis. J Autism Dev Disord. 23 (2): 323–39.

Hyman, S.L., Shores, A., North, K.N. (2005). The nature and frequency of cognitive deficits in children with neurofibromatosis type 1. Neurology. 65 (7): 1037–44.

Katsidzira, L., Machiridza, T., Ndlovu, A. (2010). A potentially treatable cause of dementia. Cent Afr J Med. 56 (5–8): 41–4.

Kıroğlu, Y., Çallı, C., Karabulut, N., Öncel, C. (2010). Intracranial calcifications on CT. Diagn Interv Radiol 16: 263–269.

Kowdley, K.V., Coull, B.M., Orwoll, E.S. (1999). Cognitive impairment and intracranial calcification in chronic hypoparathyroidism.Am J Med Sci. 317 (5): 273–7.

Kumar, P., Clark, M. Eds. (2005) Clinical Medicine. 6th Edition, Chapter 2, Elsevier Saunders, Pheladeliphia, 19–152.

Lane, B., Sullivan, E.V., Lim, K.O., Beal, D.M., et al. (1996). White Matter MR Hyperintensities in Adult Patients withCongenital Rubella.AJNR Am J Neuroradiol. 17: 99–103.

Lo, W., Marchuk, D.A., Ball, K.L., Juhász, C., Jordan L.C., et al. (2012). Updates and future horizons on the understanding, diagnosis, and treatment of Sturge-Weber syndrome brain involvement. Dev Med Child Neurol. 54 (3): 214–23.

Madhusoodanan, S., Danan, D., Brenner, R., Bogunovic, O. (2004). Brain tumor and psychiatric manifestations: a case report and brief review. Ann Clin Psychiatry 16 (2): 111–3.

Madhusoodanan, S., Danan, D., Moise, D. (2007). Psychiatric manifestations of brain tumors: diagnostic implications. Expert Rev Neurother. 7 (4): 343–9.

Makariou, E., Patsalides, A.D. (2009). Intracranial calcifications. Applied Radiology. 38 (11): 48–60.

Moise, D., Madhusoodanan, S. (2006). Psychiatric symptoms associated with brain tumors: a clinical enigma.CNS Spectr. 11 (1): 28–31.

Mufaddel, A., Al-Hassani GA. (2014). Familial idiopathic basal ganglia calcification (Fahr`s disease). Neurosciences (Riyadh). 19 (3): 171–7.

Mufaddel, A., AlSabousi, M., Salih, B., AlHassani, G., Osman, O.T. (2014a). A Case of Gorlin-Goltz Syndrome Presented with Psychiatric Features. Behav Neurol. 830874.

Mufaddel, A., Omer, A., Salem, M. (2014b). Psychiatric Aspects of Infectious Diseases. Open Journal of Psychiatry. 4: 202–217.

Noorbehesht, B., Enzmann, D.R., Sullender, W., Bradley, J.S., Arvin, A.M. (1987). Neonatal herpes simplex encephalitis: correlation of clinical and CT findings. Radiology. 162 (3): 813–9.

North, K., Hyman, S., Barton, B. (2002). Cognitive deficits in neurofibromatosis 1. J Child Neurol. 17 (8): 605–12; discussion 627–9, 646–51.

Panzer, M.J., DeQuardo, J.R., Abelson, J.L. (1991) Delayed Diagnosis of a Frontal Meningioma. 3 (3): 259–262.

Pascual-Castroviejo, I., Pascual-Pascual, S.I., Velazquez-Fragua, R., Viaño, J. (2008). Sturge-Weber syndrome: study of 55 patients. Can J Neurol Sci. 35 (3): 301–7.

Robert-Gargneux, F., Dardé, M.L. (2012). Epidemiology of and diagnostic strategies for toxoplasmosis. ClinMicrobiol Rev. 25 (2): 264–96.

Rorke, L.B. (1973). Nervous system lesions in the congenital rubella syndrome.Arch Otolaryngol. 98: 249–251.

Stegmann, B.J., Carey, J.C. (2002). TORCH Infections.Toxoplasmosis, Other (syphilis, varicella-zoster, parvovirus B19), Rubella, Cytomegalovirus (CMV), and Herpes infections.CurrWomens Health Rep. 2 (4): 253–8.

Taly, A.B., Nagaraja, D., Das, S., Shankar, S.K., Pratibha, N.G. (1987). Sturge-Weber-Dimitri disease without facial nevus.Neurology. 37: 1063–4

Turin, E., Grados, M.A., Tierney, E., Ferenc, L.M, Zabel, A., Comi, A.M. (2010). Behavioral and psychiatric features of Sturge-Weber syndrome. J NervMent Dis. 198 (12): 905–13.

Uribe, V.M. (1986). Psychiatric symptoms and brain tumor.Am Fam Physician. 34 (2): 95–8.

Webb, D.W., Fryer, A.E., Osborne, J.P. (1991). On the incidence of fits and mental retardation in tuberous sclerosis.J Med Genet. 28: 395–7.

Zada, G., Kintz, N., Pulido, M., Amezcua, L. (2013). Prevalence of neurobehavioral, social, and emotional dysfunction in patients treated for childhood craniopharyngioma: a systematic literature review. PLoS One. 8 (11): e76562.

Chapter 8

Incorrect Diagnosis by Positioning Errors in Panoramic Radiographs

Glauce Crivelaro Nascimento[1], Yamba Carla Lara Pereira[1],
Rafael Rondon[2]

1 Introduction

The "strange phenomenon", discovered by Wilhelm Conrad Röntgen in the nineteenth century, that sensitized barium platinocyanide plates at the time of their studies on cathode rays in the gas tube, were called Ray X. The discovery of these new rays with singular characteristics gave greater clinical and practical insight into dentistry. This new form of energy gave rise to imaging obtained from the record of an image made by x-irradiation, which in passing through an object reaches a radiographic senssor producing a latent image that is capable of processing. The importance of this examination has been established since its discovery (Sewell et al., 2001). The risks of using ionizing radiation for diagnostic purposes emerged some time later. Therefore, measures such as the improvement of apparatuses, the use of faster image receptors, and the selection of the most appropriate technique are increasingly in evidence (Muhammed et al., 1982). The deleterious effects of X-radiation on living organisms emerged after its intensified use in the field of radiology, which resulted in chronic dermatitis and caused even lethal changes. Providing necessary information is essential to presenting an image of quality; otherwise, the diagnosis may be harmed. Furthermore, quality radiographic images are fundamental to a conservation file, being of great value in legal issues.

---

[1] Department of Morphology, Physiology and Basic Pathology, School of Dentistry of Ribeirão Preto, University of São Paulo, Brazil.
[2] Stomatology and Oral Diagnostic Program, Scholl of Dentistry of São Paulo, University of São Paulo, Brazil.

The two-dimensional image, obtained by a radiography of a three-dimensional structure, is one of the limitations to overcome. Aiming to overcome this difficulty, several researchers have over the years developed specific radiographic techniques to increase the security of diagnosis. A radiographic examination is an important resource for obtaining the diagnosis of lesions of the complex jaw. One of the complementary exams more often performed by the dentist is the radiographic examination, which is important for the auxiliary diagnostic in oral problems (Sewell et al., 2001).

Panoramic radiographs are a type of radiographs obtained from equipment and senssor located outside the patient's mouth; they are therefore, extraoral. In this type of examination, the head and the doorframe rotate around the patient's head, giving the professional a final exam that allows a broader view of the anatomical regions, although less rich in detail and accuracy of information compared with the intraoral technique. In contrast, the radiographic examination of the dentoalveolar region and its adjacent structures in a single image receptor has become a key point in clinical practicality, highlighting its role in the diagnosis. In this sense, quality control in dental radiology has been wrongly understood as only in how to control the equipment, such as X-ray apparatuses and processors (Zubeldia et al., 2003). However, another fundamental parameter that influences the quality service provided is the training of professionals who perform radiographs, the quality of which must kept control of in order to provide security for the exams.

Therefore, professionals who perform radiographs in dental clinics have a responsibility to perform them with a high diagnostic quality. They must be competent in the execution of techniques and in the management and processing of i, since unsatisfactory quality of radiographs may result in mistakes in diagnosis and, consequently, in treatment (Langland & Langlais, 2002; Freitas & Becker, 2000). Obtaining better image quality becomes an important factor to be considered. The image quality, without blur, is determined by the distance of the tube, the focal plane, film, and the rotation of the tube. It is known that the epicenter of rotation changes as the image receptor or sensor revolves in an elliptical way around the dental arches format.

Currently, the most commonly extraoral examination performed is panoramic radiography. Radiographs commonly used are the conventional Panoramic (Standard), the Panoramic for purposes of implant, the Panoramic for temporomandibular joint, including ascending branches of right and left sides, and the Panoramic for paranasal sinuses. The evolution of this test is related to the improvement in image quality obtained with a decreased radiation dose at the lowest cost to the patient; increasing the dose, thus, has indications. In this radiographic technique, the patient's position is critical how in focus the teeth and bones are in the image (Dhilon et al., 2012).

So, in the execution of a panoramic radiograph, care with positioning of the patient and the following procedures is essential (Kaviani et al., 2008). Passler and Visser (2006) reported in their work that to obtain a panoramic radiograph with an appropriate standard, the technician must observe the following rules: positioning the patient upright with an elongated neck, shoulders down, back straight, and feet together; Frankfurt plane parallel to the ground and the median sagittal plane perpendicular to the ground; mental supported in the chincup support of the frontal region and the tongue

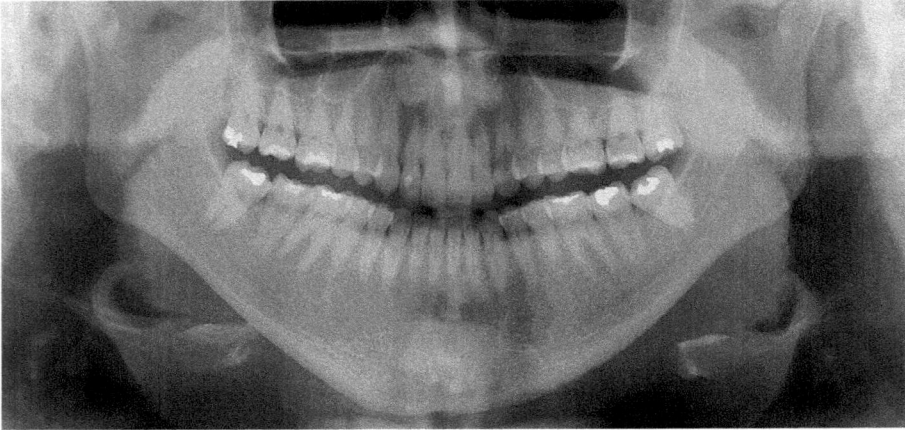

Figure 1: Panoramic Radiograph with high standard, within the normal range.

against the palate (Figure 1).

Thus, properly positioning the patient in the machine is the most important factor in preventing a cascade of errors, since multiple mistakes may follow automatically from the first mistake. Given the importance of this type of error, the aim of this study discusses what the literature offers to evaluate common positioning errors associated with the panoramic radiographs. Whereas it is not always obvious to the operator that an error has been made, this work will approach errors based on problems seen in radiography that injure their diagnostic quality. This study emphasized the most important factor for obtaining panoramic radiographs with good quality is by properly positioning the patient in the machine. This issue has been continually of interest since panoramic radiography was first invented.

2   The Panoramic Radiograph

The first panoramic radiograph happened in 1934 (Ramesh et al., 2001). This radiograph is an imaging of the mouth, which allows better visualization of the maxillomandibular complex in just one radiograph (Alkurt et al., 2007). It consists of a single incidence of the maxilla and mandible (Maloney et al., 2001), which permits an easy visualization of all dental elements and their anatomical structures for the dentist, and there is a low dose of emitted radiation for the patient (Devlin & Yuan, 2013). For a perfect visualization of anatomical structures, panoramic radiography should be performed in an extraoral radiographic unit and with a high standard of quality in both the technical procedure as well as in the revelation process (Alkurt et al., 2007).

The panoramic radiography should be achieved by following all manufacturer's recommendations, and the patient should have to remain perfectly positioned while the X-ray tube and the image receptor simultaneously revolve around the him head (Gallimidi et al., 1989). About the radiation exposure, the mean of kilovoltage (kVp) and/or regulation of milliamperes (mA) as recommended by the manufacturer had varied from patient to patient due to size, teeth, color of skin, muscles, and bone structure, among others. On panoramic radiographs, the exposure time is set to allow the device to complete a full turn around for the patient (White & Pharaoh, 2004 and 2014).

The image receptor in an extraoral radiography is a combination of two intensifying screens with a sensor between them. Each intensifying screen has a layer of phosphor that fluoresces when activated by X- radiation, which penetrates the patient and the cassette, which is a compartment where radiographic films are accommodated at the time of radiography (Ludlow & Platin). This fluorescent glow sensitizes the image receptor. This receptor used in panoramic radiography is 10-60 times more sensitive than the fluorescence X-radiation and as the X-ray tube and image receptor surround the patient, the image is recorded on in vertical increments, which are restricted by narrowing the X-ray tube and the collimator (Van Ongeval, 2007).

This examination is indicated in dental practice for allowing a panoramic view of many general anatomical structures of interest to the dentist, and is the dental radiography that facilitates "radiographic findings" in the diagnosis of pathologies (Ramesh et al., 2001).

Panoramic radiography is already part of the routine; for example, the prosthetic planning, whether for diagnosing maxillary changes, the presence of root fragments, foreign bodies, bony ridge height. can also be used for evaluation of systemic conditions (Friedlander et al., 2002). It was found that a significant correlation between changes in the trabecular bone viewed on panoramic radiographs and radiographs of the wrist (carpal) with osteoporosis in the spine and femur detected by bone densitometry (Ciftci et al., 2005). This allows an approach prior to the establishment of complications that can debilitate the quality of life for patients (Taguchi et al., 2006). This imaging test has disadvantages, too, since it is a two-dimensional image and presents distortions that interfere with surgical planning (Correa et al., 2013).

Panoramic radiography is considered useful and practical to complement the clinical examination in the diagnosis of diseases of the teeth, such as endodontic diseases, and diseases of the bones of the face (Rushton & Horner, 1996). Through this examination, the dentist can see all the teeth at once, even those that have not yet erupted. Thus, tooth fractures, infections, or other diseases of the bones that support the teeth can be viewed and often diagnosed (Royal College of Radiologists, 1994). It is possible to search through this exam, situations of bone resorption, and radicular cysts, tumors, inflammations, post-accident fractures, temporomandibular joint disorders and sinusitis. It is common to request it also as a preoperative examination in surgery of the teeth and bones, although Ohman et al. have been considering it insufficient for this analysis (Ohman et al., 2006).

The pediatric dentist can monitor the teeth before they erupt into the oral cavity and can analyze their location, shape, angle and the presence of teeth in excess of the normal number, or agenesis that is missing a tooth germ, and thus prevent or attenuate future aesthetic problems (Peretz et al., 2012).

The main indications of panoramic radiography are the general survey and oral health; provide best subsidies for surgical procedures; initial and progressive evaluation for orthodontic treatment; information on growth and development in children; reviews about chronological dental eruptions and axes of eruptions of permanent teeth; cystic lesions or neoplastic views; dimensional measurements for implantology; historical documentation of the patients; evaluation of the temporomandibular joint and to detect the presence of foreign bodies (Mahl & Fontanella, 2008).

As we can note, nowadays, with the large amount of supply, radiographic examination are of great importance in the diagnosis of oral alterations, because it allows the professional to gain evidences, together with the clinical examination, a quantity of information that become solid for the process of diagnostics. Therefore, it is essential that professionals perform radiographs surrounded care technicians, starting from the storage of radiographic films, through the processing of these tests, until you reach the stage of interpretation (Choi et al., 2012). Failures during the taking of these tests can lead to erroneous conclusions, causing unnecessary exposure to patients by increasing the need for repeats (Akarslan et al., 2003).

To interpret panoramic radiograph is necessary prior knowledge of anatomy. There are a number of variations, which are shown within the normal range and should be examined carefully before the erroneously determine the presence of anomalies (Ono et al., 2005). Therefore, the radiographic images should be considered carefully.

There are four anatomical plans used for proper patient positioning. The plan or line Atar-tragal, the plan or line orbit/meatus (Frankfurt plan), the plan or line canine/meatus and the median sagittal plan. Devices for head positioning and support for chin are also important for precise positioning. It is a necessary time and explanation to the patient of the purpose and operation of the equipment to a proper position of the patient. It is important instruct the patient to bite the bite block, close the lips, and put the tongue against the roof of the mouth (Narhi et al., 2000). The patient should always use lead aprons covering them.

3   Radiographic Errors of Positioning

Radiographs are considered technically good and those that possess good quality were those presented the following criteria: presence of sharpness or detail, minimal distortion, correct framing sensor in the region, lack of artifacts, density and adequate contrast (Ezoddini et al., 2011). The examinations that don't present these characteristics demonstrate that some mistake occurred in the moment of the radiographic or during its processing.

The difficulty in the interpretation of radiographs is often correlated to errors in obtaining and interpreting the image. The anatomy of the oral area is rich in features that represent the bone and tooth structures, and these traits are distributed in various directions, forming images that give illusions and overlaps. Coupled to this, there is the inherent technical error. The main errors that may occur in relation to panoramic radiographs are associated with technical errors or processing. In this way, in execution of this radiograph, the care with the positioning of the patient and the processing of steps are essential. Studies indicate that the errors more observed in oral radiology institutes are positioning errors (Kaviani et al., 2008); meanwhile, those related to exposure factors, errors related to the presence of artifacts and technical errors, in that order.

In this way, positioning errors of patients are most common and a critical factor in the possibility of errors is patient positioning being controlled by the operator (Dhillon et al., 2012).

Between the presentation of mistakes by the operator at the time of positioning patients and handling the film, a common error that can occur is the patient that positions your head in front with the plane of focus. This produces an image in a radiograph with the dental arches, especially the front teeth, located out of focus, with a blurred aspect, shortened and narrowed. Besides that, the premolars overlap and may cause an overlap of the columns on the ramus of the mandible (Choi et al., 2012).

In this another to context, it was shown that incorrect positioning of the patient's head was responsible for most of the repetitions: the patient's head was on the front of the plane of focus in 21.15% of cases, turned to the right or left at 24.84 %, inclined forward in 21.21% and positioned behind the plane of focus in 20.30%. When the patient's head positioned behind the plane of focus, the dental arches, especially the anterior teeth are located outside of focus, looking blurred experiences in expanding along a horizontal direction. The condyles can be designed to the side edges of the image receptor (Passler & Vesser, 2006; Langland & Langlais, 2002). Now, when the patient's head tilted back, the occlusal plane is flattened or with reverse curve. The apexes of the upper incisors are out of focus. The condyles can be projected out of the imaged area due to an increase in the intercondylar distance.

In this way, it's possible to observe the occlusal plane with an excessive curvature in panoramic radiographs when patient's head leaning forward. About this problem, the apex of the lower incisors is out of focus too and there are an overlap image of the hyoid bone in the anterior mandible. The upper region of the condyles may not appear and there is a narrowing of the intercondylar distance (Passler & Vesser, 2006; Langland & Langlais, 2002).

It is very common for the patient to incline or turn the head to the right or left (Dhillon et al., 2012). In the first case, it's possible to observe the radiographic image in an asymmetric structure (the side to which was the slope seems to have reduced in size compared to the opposite side) and occurs marked overlapping in the proximal surfaces (Figure 2). In the second case, in the other hand, the teeth on one side of the midline appear to have extended and to overlapped the sharp proximal surfaces; whereas, the teeth on the opposite side are shown shortened. The branch from one side of the mandible appears much larger than the other one, and the condyles differ in size.

The chin of the patient and the occlusal plane must be positioned correctly so that distortions are avoided (Ezoddini et al., 2011) (Figure 3). The occlusal plane should be aligned so that it is lower above, angled 20 to 30 degrees below the horizontal plane. One way to position the chin is to place the patient so that the line connecting the tragus of the ear to the outer corner of the eye is parallel to the ground. If the chin is elevated, the occlusal plane on the radiograph appears flattened or inverted, and it creates a distorted image of the jaw. Furthermore, the shadow radiopaque palate bone overlaps the roots of the maxillary teeth. Conversely, if the chin is low, the teeth are too overlapping

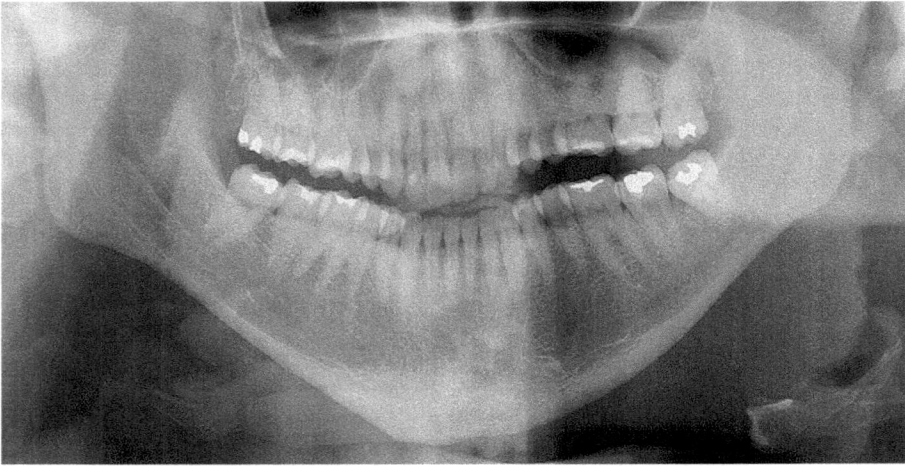

Figure 2: Panoramic Radiograph with inclination of patient's head to right.

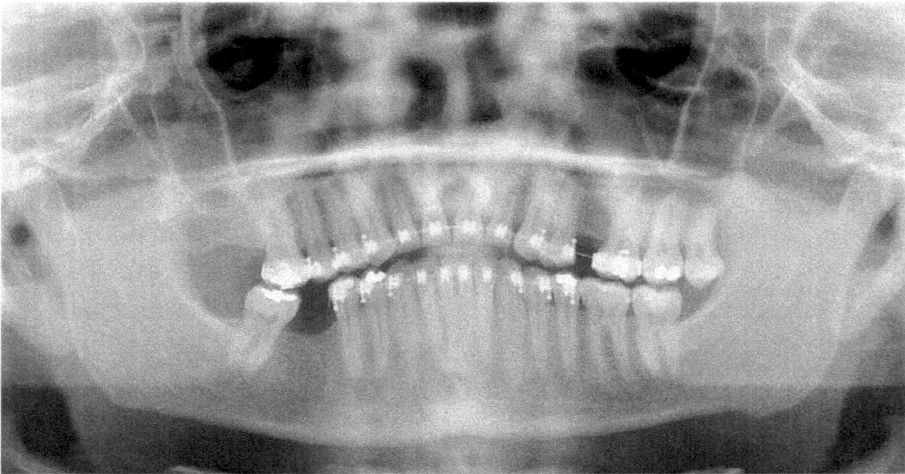

Figure 3: Panoramic Radiograph with patient's chin elevated.

region and the symphysis may be out of the jaw radiography, in addition, both mandibular condyles can be projected out of the upper edge of the image (Sewerin, 1990).

The position of the tongue also has a great influence on the quality of the radiographic image (Akarslan et al., 2003). The absence of tongue contact with the palate is identified by the visualization of a radiolucent band designed at the height of the apex of the upper teeth in a panoramic radiograph. Also, if the tongue is not on the palate (Figure 4) or the lips are open (Figure 5); the air between the parted lips obscures the crowns of the upper and lower teeth. The apical region of the maxillary teeth is obscured by dark air space between the dorsum of the tongue and the hard and soft palates (palatoglossal air spaces). To avoid confusion and compromise our ability to reset

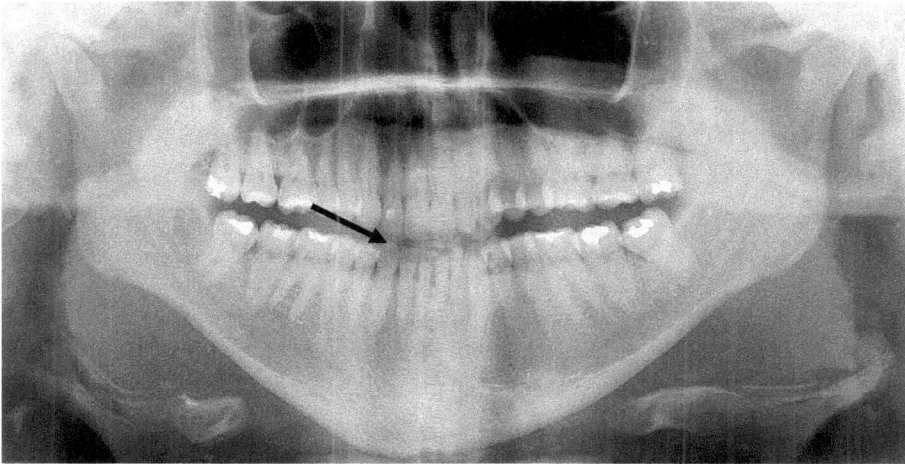

Figure 4: Panoramic Radiograph with positioning error of the tongue.

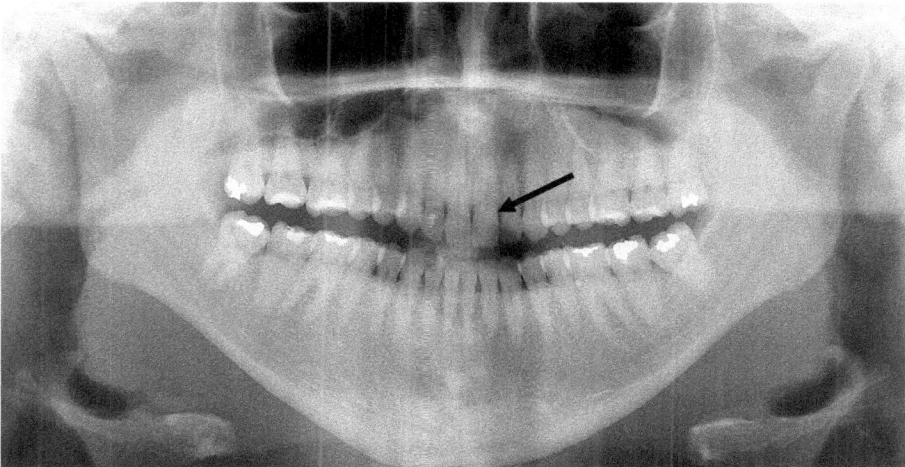

Figure 5: Panoramic Radiograph with positioning error of the lips (open lips).

after an analysis above the apices of the central incisors; it's necessary to ask the patient throughout the radiography that it remains positioned with the tongue stuck to the palate (roof of the mouth) and do not swallow the saliva to prevent movement during radiography (Schiff et al., 1986).

Regarding the posture of the patient, the incorrect column positioned and movement during radiography, can produce a "ghost image" in radiopaque area in the center of the radiography, in the region of the incisors, as well as blurred portions in radiograph and large step defects in inferior border of mandible (Dhillon et al., 2012). A summary of positioning errors and their consequences for the radiographic image can be seen in Table 1.

Common Positioning Errors	Description of the Radiographic Obtained Image
Head positioned behind the plane of focus	Increased and blurred image of the anterior teeth and bone structures of the region, as well as condyles at edge of the film.
Head positioned forward of the plane of focus	Narrowed and blurred anterior teeth and bone structures of this region plus an overlay image of the spine, visible bilaterally.
Chin pointing upward	Flattening of the occulsal plane, blurred imaging of the roots of the maxillary anterior teeth, hard palate appears superimposed on the roots of these same teeth and the distance between the condyles is increased on the obtained image.
Chin pointing down	Roots of the lower anterior teeth appear blurry, there is excessive curvature of the occulsal plane.
Patient's head tilted to the left of right	The image appears tilted, so there is unequal distance between the right and left bottom edges and the bottom edge of the film and consequently, the condyles can e loss on top of the film. There is a significant overlap between the approximal surfaces of teeth and structures are asymmetrical, since the side to which the patient has bent the head present smaller structures in the image.
Patient's head turned to the left of right	The teeth near the film will appear shortened, while the teeth near the X-ray will be wider and longer on an image like this. The nasal structures are not clear and the left and right mandibular branches as well as condyles differ in size.
Absence of contact between tongue and palate	Radiolucent shadow projected on the height of the apex of the upper teeth due to palatoglossal airspace.
Open lips	Radiolucent area in the coronal part of the maxillary and mandibular anterior teeth.
Incorrect positioning of the patient's spine	This usually occurs because a low positioning of the patient. It is possible identify a radiopaque area projected on the radiographic central area that protrudes in the region of incicivos.
Patient movement during exposure	There are distortions of irregularities in all structures, and the image presents a blurred appearance.

Table 1: Summary of the positioning errors more common during radiographic technique and their consequences in the image

Radiographic images distorted caused by anatomical structures or objects positioned outside the focal zone is known by several names: reverse shadows, secondary images, pictures attached, double images, triple pictures, shadows, ghosts earrings (cysts), contralateral and ghosting images (Sewerin, 1990). These images, found only on rotational panoramic radiographs, are anatomical structures such as vertebrae, the rami, or the hyoid bone, artificial objects, such as metallic material, dental crowns, wires, plates containment, earrings, necklaces, and machine parts, among others. Therefore, the appearance of ghost images is complex, since the anatomical structures or artificial objects can form multiple images.

3.1   Implications of Positioning Errors in Diagnosis

The Panoramic image is a complex projection due to its size and the wide range of anatomic areas. Thus, this technique allows for multiple radiographic distortions and overlapping, which can be exacerbated by technical errors during image acquisition. Furthermore, the wide range of areas can be seen in this x-ray, creating additional challenges for interpretation.

In the field of dentistry, since hard tissues such as teeth and bony structures are mainly targeted in the treatment, a radiographic diagnosis has been widespread and has become a form of routine.

Radiographic examination is an important complement in obtaining a diagnosis of soft and hard tissue lesions, and sometimes becomes the sole means to detect possible residual changes; however, the radiographic interpretation may be impaired when faults are introduced during a radiographic processing (Zubeldia et al., 2003). The protection against unnecessary exposure to X-radiation, also called radiation protection, should be a main concern in order to avoid unnecessary use of radiation, which in practice, also means avoiding the repetition of exposure to radiographs (Moreno, 2011).

The main role of imaging is to evaluate the presence or absence of a disease, its location, and the monitoring of disease's progression, making the imaging exam an indispensable method in planning the guidelines treatment and assessing its effects. However, images do not always accurately show the condition, nor do they allow total denial of its existence. Therefore, if the disease is diagnosed only by radiographic imaging, there is a possibility of reaching an erroneous diagnosis. On the other hand, by dwelling too much on the clinical view, there is a danger of losing the important aspect of an image. In this way, during the interpretation of an image, it is necessarily a good understanding of the characteristics of each of the methods assessment, in addition to being aware of the limitations of an exam imaging.

A good knowledge of normal anatomy can be quite useful to compare both sides of the image to make a decision that the finding is normal, since the bilateral structures appear are typically anatomic. This comparison between left and right sides also allows recognition of asymmetries that may be indicative of an established pathology or one in development.

There are several restrictions regarding the use of this image as an auxiliary diagnosis. In this sense, it is important to note that for assessing the presence of care, panoramic radiography has no good definition and increased real size. It is because of this fact that the direction of the X-ray source is not adjustable in relation to the teeth, so, a proximal area may overlap the adjacent tooth and dis allow a visualization of the region. There is also a contraindication to the use this type of radiography for periodontal diagnosis, since there is a distortion caused by the projection angle and little definition, not allowing easy visualization of smaller structures, such as the periodontal ligament and lamina dura, bone crest, and salivary calculi.

Panoramic radiography is commonly used for the evaluation of third molars and the temporomandibular joint (TMJ). In the latter case, it has some limitations, since their two-dimensional vision has the easy possibility to present distortions to avoid a detailed analysis of this region. However, there are still other abnormalities of medium to large proportions in TMJs who may be identified in this overview. Still, the panoramic image is so important in checking the edges of an existing lesion, as this enables the vision of all limits of a neoplasm. Thus, the shape, correct location, and conditions of neighboring structures are identifiable characteristics in a panoramic radiograph when detecting pathology.

For specialties in pathology and oral surgery, this tool becomes very important, because the overall configuration of the oral region offered by a dental panoramic radiograph allows you to view apical lesions, impacted or uninterrupted supernumerary teeth, apical fragments, dental cysts, degree of bone resorption, malignant and benign tumors, osteosclerosis, calcification of ligaments estilohióids, ectopic calcification, bone defects, fracture lines, severity of injury and repair of osteopathy (Larheim and Westesson, 2006). The panoramic radiograph is well used in children because has an extra oral examination and is well accepted by them. It becomes possible to identify in these patients the process of eruption and resorption of tooth germs, and the presence of mesiodens, agenesis and odontoids, that could not appear in periapical radiographs. Furthermore, radiography is valuable for an orthodontics examination, since through it, is the possible to compare the positions of all the teeth at different times during the treatment, as well as overall the quality of the teeth against mechanical forces.

Ghost images are very common and happen when errors occurs during the execution of radiographic technique. The structures appear blurred and changed in size, and the professional must be careful not to confuse them with pathological conditions. In this sense, a panoramic radiograph is an important complementary diagnostic test that may be affected by the errors of radiographic positioning as quoted in this chapter. Many of these mistakes generate blurred images, and they can be wrongly diagnosed as a disorder. Moreover, these errors can camouflage the real presence of pathologic features, making it clinically impossible to identify them. The main danger in the presence of these errors is the mishandling of the case and the incorrect treatment decision for the patient. Thus, a radiopaque image caused by overlapping teeth in an incorrect positioning of the patient's head in radiography can lead to a clinical misdiagnosis of the presence of mesiodens. This same case can cause severe radiolucent jaw, which can be confused with a kind of cyst. In addition, this type of error can cause a large overlap of all structures of the maxillofacial region and you may notice a buildup of radiolucent images in the region appear as paranasal sinuses. In both misinterpretations, driving the treatment plan can be altered and cause great harm to the patient.

Among the positioning errors during a panoramic radiograph, the wrong positioning of the patient's head is critical. In this case, it is important to note that the operator can have greater responsibility for this error than the patient himself. This fact may occur due to lack of guidance for the patient and the lack of knowledge of the perfect head position by the professional.

The time spent by the professional in positioning the patient correctly before performing radiography is essential for obtaining an image of suitable quality. Also, instructing the patient regarding the movement of the machine during an application of the method makes it is important to prevent him or her from moving during the procedure for alarm and consequently to avoid positioning errors.

According to previous studies (Oro et al., 2005) some errors are inevitable for some patients due to his physical stature, facial asymmetry or by not following the instructions correctly (Figure 6). So, changes in the image are not always related to distortion or poor positioning of the patient, but rather the presence of asymmetry. According to Ono et al. (Ono et al., 2005), anatomical variations may determinedly different using paper grade radiographic images and, according to Gianni et al. (Gianni et al., 2002), the professional must have this knowledge and take into account such changes to make correct planning, combined with the ability, the expertise and experience of the maxillofacial surgeon for treatment success.

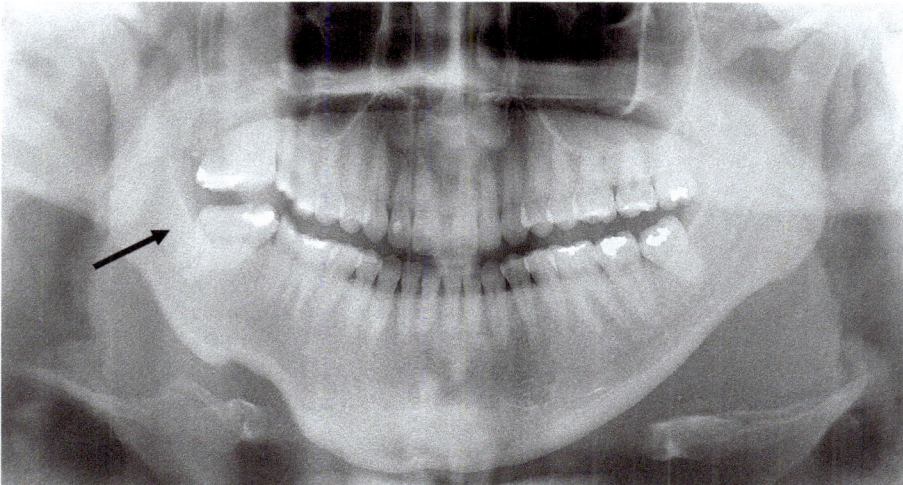

Figure 6: Panoramic Radiograph with patient's movement during the performance of radiography.

Discrepancies in images are recognized by an increasing lack of sharpness and distortion of anatomical structures that appear clearly in other structures. The specific anatomical relationships in radiography allow to distingue positioning errors horizontally, and vertically.

Regarding the location of positioning errors, the discrepancies of the posterior focal point id recognize easily. There is an apparent blurring and widening point behind the stern, while at the front focal point, the structures appear shortened and slightly blurred. Both jaws are also distorted by vertical positioning. Already errors in horizontal placement, they distort more maxilla than the mandible. For example, the positions of lifting and lowering the chin respectively widen and shorten the mandible; however, the maxilla and the upper part of the ascending branch of the mandible are distorted more than the body of the same. The discrepancy between both jaws is higher in the elevated position of the chin than in the dropped position, and reflects the differences in the anatomical arrangement of sectors in the focal plane and the direction of the rays. Thus, the anatomical relationships on radiographs provide a guide to differentiate horizontal from vertical positioning errors (Rushton & Horner, 1996).

According to Gomulka (2000), the most common mistake about position is not positioning the tongue against the palate, which normally produces a radiolucent image, which can occur unilaterally, falsely suggesting a pathological condition. Wrong anterior-posterior positioning is another common error (Figure 7), together with opened lips.

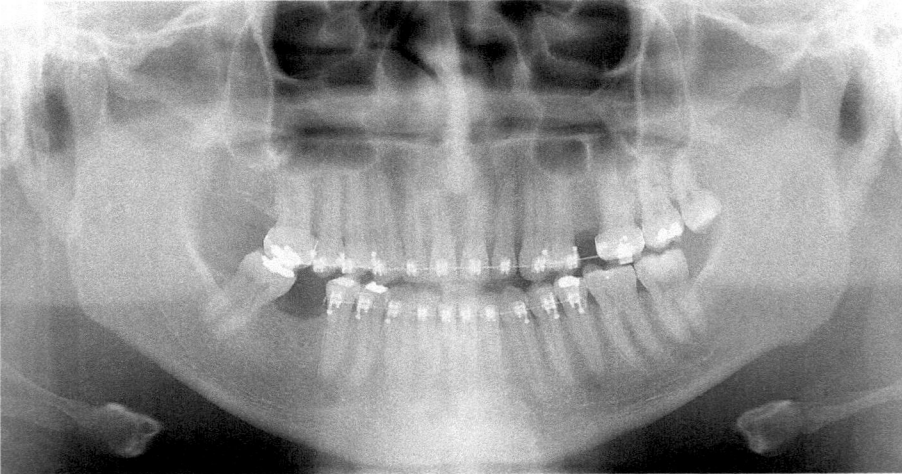

Figure 7: Panoramic Radiographic with wrong anterior-posterior positioning.

Importantly, the severity of the error during radiography can influence more than the amount of these errors. In this context, at the time of an error cripple, in a diagnostic evaluation of radiography, this value shall be an unacceptable diagnosis not contributing to the interpretation of the case. It is possible to say that even if an X-ray contains an error, which may be multiple or not, it can be considered acceptable within the diagnostic value, since this error is small in magnitude; i.e., it is not severe enough to interfere with viewing anatomic structures, allowing us to follow the protocol of interpretation, without having difficulty in reaching the final diagnosis.

In summary, having a correct diagnosis is crucial, and it is associated by clinical, radiographic and laboratory examinations. The panoramic radiograph shows the importance in most diagnosed cases of oral diseases or abnormalities, and even should be an important resource already during childhood, when this radiographic image can detect abnormalities that may influence the development of a correct occlusion of the future adult. Panoramic radiography can be an important tool to aid in the diagnosis and treatment plan; a correct execution of this technique is essential, and, how we saw in this chapter, most errors are under control of the operator and therefore can be completely eliminated by attention to details.

4   Conclusion

In conclusion, patient positioning errors are the type of mistake most frequent in panoramic radiographs, and to decrease them, the professional needs to know them, understand their consequences and then seeking solutions and necessary corrections. Given the importance of this radiograph as a complementary instrument to define an oral diagnosis, it is fundamental to avoid positioning errors of patient during development of radiograph performance. This care can prevent mistakes and the evaluation of possible oral problems, as well, as can avoid an incorrect treatment.

Acknowledgements

The authors would like to thank Radio Center, a dental radiology centerby allowing the performances of the radiographs images presented in this chapter.

References

Akarslan, Z.Z., Erten, H., Güngör, K., Celik, I. (2003). Common errors on panoramic radiographs taken in a dental school. The Journal of Contemporary Dental Practice. 4, 24–34.

Alkurt, M.T., Peker, I., Sanal, O. (2007). Assessment of repeatability and reproducibility of mental and panoramic mandibular indices on digital panoramic images. International Dental Journal, 57(6), 433–438.

Choi, B.R., Choi, D.H., Huh. K.H., Yi, W.J., Heo, M.S., Choi, S.C., et al. (2012). Clinical image quality evaluation for panoramic radiography in Korean dental clinics. Imaging Science Dentistry. 42, 183–190.

Ciftçi, Y., Kocadereli, I., Canay, S., Senyilmaz, P. (2005). Cephalometric evaluation of maxillomandibular relationships in patients wearing complete dentures: a pilot study. Angle Orthodontist. 75(5), 821–825.

Correa, L.R., Spin-Neto, R., Stavropoulos, A., Schropp, L., da Silveira, H.E., Wenzel, A. (2014). Planning of dental implant size with digital panoramic radiographs, CBCT-generated panoramic images, and

CBCT cross-sectional images. Clinical Oral Implants Research. 25(6), 690–695.

Devlin, H., Yuan, J. (2013). Object position and image magnification in dental panoramic radiography: a theoretical analysis. Dentomaxillofacial Radiololy. 42(1), 29951683.

Dhillon, M., Raju, S.M., Verma, S., Tomar, D., Mohan, R.S., Lakhanpal, M., Krishnamoorthy, B. (2012). Positioning errors and quality assessment in panoramic radiography. Imaging Science Dentistry. 42(4), 207–212.

Ezoddini, Ardakani, F., Zangouie Booshehri, M., Behniafar, B. (2011). Evaluation of the distortion rate of panoramic and periapical radiographs in erupted third molar inclination. Iran Journal Radiology. 8(1), 15–21.

Freitas, L., Becker, L. (2000). Natureza e produção dos efeitos biológicos. In: Freitas, A., Rosa, J.E., Souza, I.F. Radiologia odontológica. 5. ed. São Paulo: Artes Médicas. 67–80.

Friedlander, L., Love, R., Chandler, N. A. (2002). Comparison of phosphor-plate digital images with conventional radiographs for the perceived clarity of fine endodontic files and periapical lesions. Oral Surgery Oral Medicine Oral Pathology Oral Radiology Endodontic. 93(3), 321–327.

Gallimidi, J., Brunel, G., Castello, J., Ohnona, M., Tavernier, J.C., Mazza, R. (1989). A practical method for the determination of the available bone height in oral implantology. Revue de Stomatologie et de Chirurgie Maxillo-faciale. 90(5), 357–61.

Gianni, A.B., D'Orto, O., Biglioli, F., Bozzetti, A., Brusati, R. (2002). Neurosensory alterations of the inferior alveolar and mental nerve after genioplasty alone or associated with sagittal osteotomy of the mandibular ramus. Journal of Craniomaxillofacial Surgery. 30(5), 295–303.

Gomolka, K. A. (2000). Identifying and correcting errors for quality panoramic X-rays. CDS Review. Chicago, v.93, n. 4, 50–51.

Kaviani, F.; Johari, M.; Esmaeili, F. (2008). Evaluation of Common Errors of Panoramic Radiographs in Tabriz Faculty of Dentistry. Journal of Dental Research, Dental Clinics, Dental Prospects. 2(3), 99–101.

Langland, O.E., Langlais, R.P. (2002). Principles of Dental Imaging, 2nd Ed., Philadelphia: Lippincott Williams & Wilkins, 311–12.

Larheim, T. A., Westesson, P. L. (2006). Maxillofacial Imaging: Malignant Tumors. 2nd Ed., Springers: Verlag Berlin Heidelberg, 328–33.

Ludlow, J.B., Platin, E. (2000). A comparison of Web page and slide/tape for instruction in periapical and panoramic radiographic anatomy. Journal Dental Education. 64(4), 269–75.

Mahl, C.R., Fontanella, V. (2008). Evaluation by digital subtraction radiography of induced changes in the bone density of the female rat mandible. Dentomaxillofacial Radiology. 37(8), 438–44.

Maloney, P.L., Lincoln, R.E., Coyne, C.P. (2001). A protocol for the management of compound mandibular fractures based on the time from injury to treatment. Journal Oral Maxillofacial Surgery. 59(8), 879–884.

Moreno, M.A. (2011). Advice for patients. Decreasing unnecessary radiation exposure for children. Archives of Pediatric and Adolescent Medicine. 165(5), 480.

Muhammed, A.H., Manson-Hing, L.R., Ala, B. (1982). A comparison of panoramic and intraoral radiographic surveys in evaluating a dental clinic population. Oral Surgery Oral Medicine Oral Pathology. 54(1), 108–17.

Närhi, T.O., Leinonen, K., Wolf, J., Ainamo, A. (2000). Longitudinal radiological study of the oral health parameters in an elderly Finnish population. Acta Odontologica Scandiavica. 58(3), 119–24.

Ohman, A., Kivijärvi, K., Blombäck, U., Flygare, L. (2006). *Pre-operative radiographic evaluation of lower third molars with computed tomography. Dentomaxillofacial Radiology. 35(1), 30–5*

Ono, K., Yoshitake, T., Akahane, K., Yamada, Y., Maeda, T., Kai, M., et al. (2005). *Comparison of a digital flat-panel versus screen-film, photofluorography and storage-phosphor systems by detection of simulated lung adenocarcinoma lesions using hard copy images. The British Journal of Radiology. 78(934), 922–927.*

Passler, F.A., Visser, H. (2006). *Radiologia Odontológica. 1. Ed. Porto Alegre: Artmed.*

Peretz, B., Gotler, M., Kaffe, I. (2012). *Common errors in digital panoramic radiographs of patients with mixed dentition and patients with permanent dentition. International Journal of Dentistry. 2012, 584138.*

Ramesh, A., Tyndall, D.A., Ludlow, J.B. (2001). *Evaluation of a new digital panoramic system: a comparison with film. Dentomaxillcfacial Radiology. 30(2):98–100.*

Royal College of Radiologists, National Radiological Protection Board. (1994). *Guidelines on radiology standards for primary dental care. London: NRPB; 30.*

Rushton, V.E., Horner, K. (1996). *The use of panoramic radiology in dental practice. Journal of Dentistry. 24, 185–201.*

Sewell, J., Drage, N., Brown, J. (2001). *The use of panoramic radiography in a dental accident and emergency department. Dentomaxillofacial Radiology. 30(5), 260–3.*

Sewerin, I. (1990). *Ghost images in rotational panoramic radiography. Tandlaegebladet. 94(8), 314–7.*

Schiff, T., D'Ambrosio, J., Glass, B.J., Langlais, R.P., McDavid, W.D. (1986). *Common positioning and technical errors in panoramic radiography. Journal of American Dental Association. 113(3):422–6.*

Taguchi, A., Ohtsuka. M., Nakamoto. T., Tanimoto. K. (2006). *Screening for osteoporosis by dental panoramic radiographs. Clinical Calcium. 16(2), 291–297.*

Van Ongeval, C. (2007). *Digital mammography for screening and diagnosis of breast cancer: an overview. JBR-BTR. 90(3), 163–166.*

Zubeldia, F.F., Bonomie, J.M., Cloquel, Ale D.A., Padila, A.R., Küstner, E.C., Melcior, B.G. (2003). *La calidad en el servicio de radiologia. Medicine Oral. 8, 311–21.*

White, S.C., Pharaoh, M.J. (2004). *Oral Radiology: principles and interpretation. 5th ed. St. Louis - Missouri: Elsevier Mosby; 200–17.*

White, S.C., Pharaoh, M.J. (2014). *Oral Radiology: principles and interpretation. 7th ed. St. Louis - Missouri: Elsevier Mosby; 63–83.*

212

Chapter 9

The State of HIV Epidemic in Pakistan

Syed H. Abidi[1], Syed S. Ali[2], Muhammad A. Raees[2],
Marcia Kalish[3], Sten Vermund[4], Syed Ali[4]

1 Introduction

With respect to HIV infection, Pakistan is a high-risk, low prevalence country (Figure 1). The prevalence of HIV is low (0.1%) in the country (UNAIDS, 2010), but the infection is concentrated amongst high-risk groups, which mainly include people who inject drugs (PWID), men who have sex with men (MSM), commercial sex workers (CSWs) (Baqi et al., 1999) and Afghan refugees (M. R. Khanani, Ansari et al., 2010; Rajabali et al., 2009). The highest seroprevalence of HIV is seen in PWID (15.4%-18.3%) (M. R. Khanani et al., 2011), followed by MSM (11%) (M. R. Khanani, Somani et al., 2010). The spread of HIV in Pakistan is following the Asian Epidemic Model (Adnan Ahmad Khan, 2010; Brown & Peerapatanapokin, 2004); the epidemic originated among PWID and spread to MSM – the two high risk communities that now form the core of the epidemic (UNAIDS, 2010; Yousaf et al., 2011). Displaced refugees from the neighboring country of Afghanistan have also contributed to the spread of HIV by high risk practices, such as sharing needles, having unsafe sex and selling blood products (Abidi et al., 2012; Rajabali et al., 2009).

The first case of HIV in Pakistan was reported in 1987 in the city of Lahore (R. M. Khanani et al., 1988). The prevalence of the disease has been on the rise since then. During the early and mid-nineties, HIV was initially transmitted in the country by deported

[1] Department of Biological and Biomedical Sciences, Aga Khan University, Karachi, Pakistan
[2] Medical College, Aga Khan University, Karachi, Pakistan.
[3] Vanderbilt Institute of Global Health, Vanderbilt University, Nashville, Tennessee, USA.
[4] Department of Biomedical Sciences, Nazarbayev University School of Medicine, Astana, Kazakhstan.

HIV positive Pakistani workers from the Gulf States (Hub, 2009; Rai et al., 2007; Shah et al., 1999b; USAID, 2010; WHO) (Figure 2). These deportees reportedly seeded the first pockets of the HIV epidemic in Pakistan, initially among the PWID (Rai et al., 2010). One such outbreak occurred in 2004 in a group of PWID in the city of Larkana (Rai et al., 2010; Shah et al., 2004b) where the prevalence reached an alarming 27%, owing to the sharing of contaminated needles amongst the PWID. Following this study, reports of HIV infection were received from major cities of Pakistan (Platt et al., 2009), heralding the emergence of the concentrated epidemics in the years that followed.

Low awareness of sexually-transmitted infections (STI) and poor healthcare standards have contributed to the further proliferation of HIV in Pakistan, now infiltrating the low-risk, general population (UNAIDS, 2010). One such group that has surfaced recently comprises the families, female spouses and children, of PWID and MSM (M. R. Khanani et al., 2011). In a country where the health of pregnant women and newborns is not high priority, vertical transmission of HIV is now likely to expand the epidemic into low-risk groups and general population (Figure 2 and Figure 3).

2 Deported Migrant Workers from the Gulf States

2.1 Deportees from the Gulf – Seeding of the HIV Epidemic in Pakistan

The Gulf States, comprising Qatar, Oman, Saudi Arabia, Bahrain, Kuwait and the United Arab Emirates (Kapiszewski, 2006) have shown one of the highest population growth rates in the last few decades (Kapiszewski, 2006). A large part of this population boom is accounted for by the foreign work force that emigrates to reside in the Gulf States. Since the discovery of oil in this region the respective governments have developed lenient migration policies so as to facilitate foreign nationals to work and reside in these countries, and contribute to the growing economy. According to the latest figures, foreigners account for 37% of the total population of the Gulf States, constituting 70% of the work force in this area. Immigration laws in the Gulf States look favorably on Asian populations (as opposed to foreigners of Arabian descent), since Asians are cheaper to employ, do not pose a threat to the local political setup and are willing to leave their families behind – incurring little liability for their employer (Kapiszewski, 2006). Additionally, many Asians are Muslims and therefore can be easily integrated with the local culture.

In most Gulf States, certain policies are in place to keep the spread of infection and disease amongst foreign nationals in check. One such policy requires foreign workers to volunteer for HIV testing (Kandela, 1994). The process of obtaining or renewing an existing work permit in the Gulf states requires a migrant worker to go through a health screening process (Kandela, 1994). Individuals testing positive for HIV are denied a work permit or the renewal thereof, and are deported to their respective countries immediately (Kandela, 1994; Shah et al., 1999a).

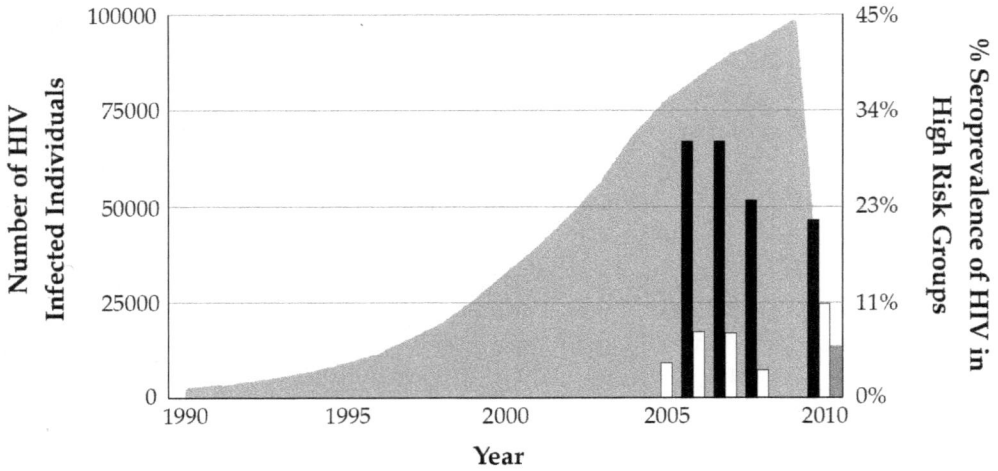

Figure 1: HIV Prevalence in Pakistan: The graph shows rise in the prevalence of HIV in Pakistan from 1990 to 2011 (grey area) (WHO). The bar charts from 2005 to 2008 show percent seroprevalence of HIV in PWID (Red), MSM (Green), and Afghan refugees (Magenta) in Karachi. The data were compiled from the most recent reports published by the NACP (NACP, 2006–2007, 2008), and from the published articles on HIV prevalence (M. R. Khanani, Ansari et al., 2010; M. R. Khanani et al., 2011; Rajabali et al., 2008).

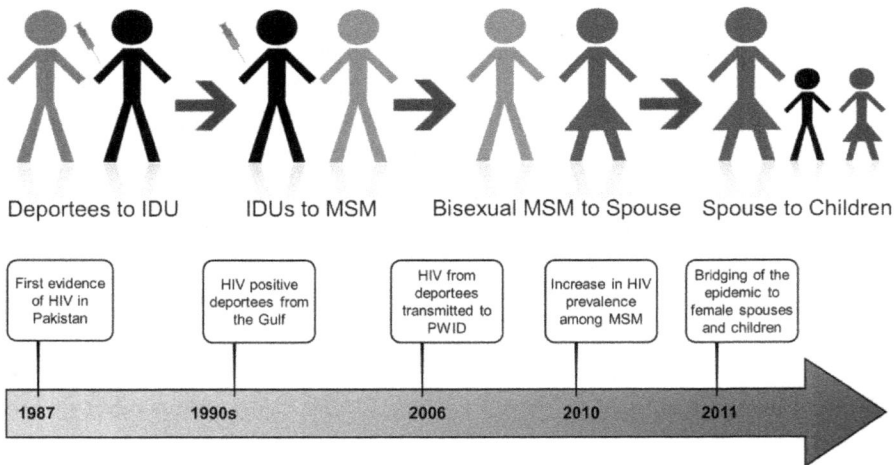

Figure 2: Spread of the HIV Epidemic in Pakistan: A timeline of the reported transmission events that determined the transmission patterns of the HIV epidemic in Pakistan. The virus first infected migrant workers in the Gulf States who on deportation infected PWID via needle sharing (S. Khan et al., 2006). The virus then spread to MSM from PWID via sexual contact between the two groups (M. R. Khanani et al., 2011). Bisexual MSM from the MSM cohort then infected their wives who transmitted the virus vertically to their children.

Figure 3. Evidence of Founder-Effect in the Community of HIV-1 Positive PWID in Pakistan: The Neighbor-Joining (NJ) phylogenetic tree for HIV-1 sequences of the HIV-gag (p24-p7) region (Rai et al., 2010). The tree was constructed by aligning the 26 HIV sequences from PWID (marked grey in the middle) with HIV reference sequences from Los Alamos database. The sequence O.CM.91.MVP5180 was used as out group. Closed squares indicate the nodes representing bootstrap values ≥ 60. The arrow on the right points to the study subject (HIV-GAG35) with a history of contact with commercial sex workers during an extended stay abroad. Reproduced from: Rai et al., 2010.

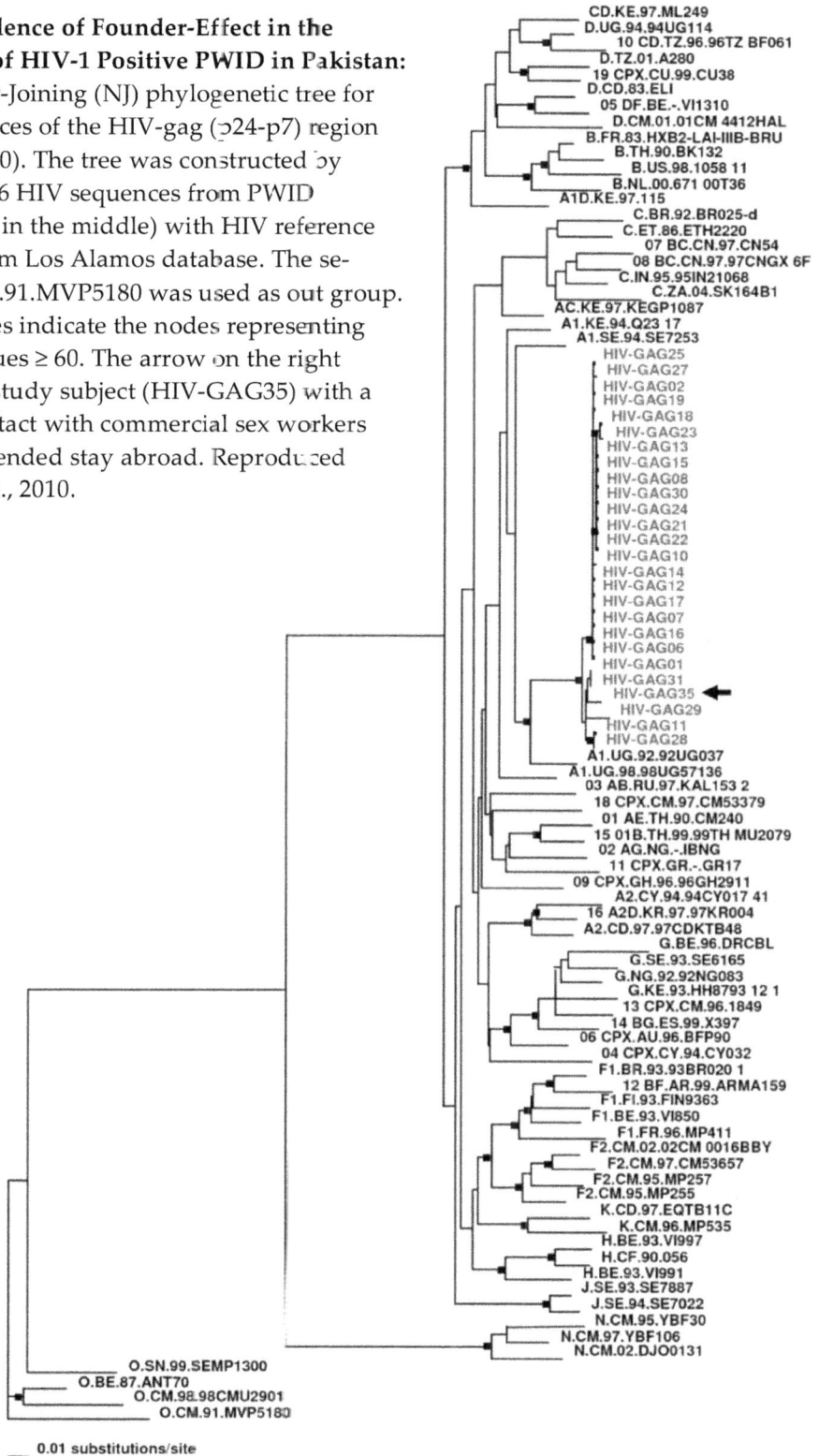

2.2   High Risk Behavior in Migrant Workers

Most Pakistani workers in the Gulf States are young, sexually active men aged between 20 to 40 years, belonging to low socio-economic status. Being isolated from their families predisposes these men to engage in buying and/or selling sex (Hub, 2009; Li et al., 2007; Shah et al., 1999a). Further, due to low level of health awareness, condom use is reported to be low amongst these workers, which puts them at high risk of contracting and transmitting STIs (Shah et al., 1999b). Studies conducted on Asian populations have shown that migrant workers are more likely to have had pre-marital sex and multiple sex partners (Li et al., 2007), and that homelessness drives them to sell sex for food and shelter (M. M. Batool Sharifi-Mood, Masoud Mardani, Bashir Pejman, 2008; M. S. Batool Sharifi-Mood, Esmail Sanei-Moghaddan, Sohila Khosravi, 2006). Homelessness and isolation from their families predispose Pakistani workers in the Gulf States to high-risk sexual behavior. Low literacy and heath awareness level only adds to the risks these workers already face (NACP, 2008). Facing those risk factors, many of the Pakistani migrant workers contracted HIV infection while residing in the Gulf and were deported back to their homeland (Rai et al., 2007; Shah et al., 1999b). While these individuals were allowed to return to and settle in their home-country little attention was paid to the fact that the high-risk behavior that led to their own infection would now facilitate transmission of HIV from these individuals to their immediate contacts. Neither of the governments (Gulf States or Pakistan) anticipated these risks, and therefore no program was put in place to raise awareness among the HIV-positive deportees. They still did not know how HIV transmission occurred, and how the virus could be prevented from further transmission. Consequences were observed in the decade that followed. The HIV positive deportees got involved in the practice of injection drug use and through needle exchange seeded the first HIV epidemics among the PWID in various cities of Pakistan (Rai et al., 2010).

A 2010 study reported a "founder effect" of HIV among a PWID community in Karachi, Pakistan, showing phylogenetic evidence that the epidemic was seeded by a deportee who contracted the virus from a commercial sex worker while employed and residing in the Gulf. Upon his return, the deportee practiced injection drug use and transmitted the infection to fellow PWID through needle-exchange (Rai et al., 2010) (Figures 2 and 3).

2.3   HIV Policy for the Migrant Workers

Government policies in the Gulf States require the employers to make all the necessary arrangements for the deportation of an HIV positive worker. Until such arrangements are made the workers are kept in government controlled medical centers. It is not part of the policy, however, to provide post-test counseling to such individuals (Asia, 2007; Hub, 2009; Kandela, 1993; Shah et al., 1999a; USAID, 2010). Immigration laws in Pakistan, on the other hand, include no special clause for HIV-positive deportees. They are not provided any kind of support upon their return. As the HIV status of these deportees becomes common knowledge, many are shunned by their loved ones and find themselves homeless and unemployed (UNAIDS, 2010). Poverty, social stigma and marginalization then forces them to turn towards selling sex and injecting drugs – turning them into a vector for HIV transmission (Rai et al., 2010).

The immigration laws in Pakistan do take into account certain communicable diseases. Pakistanis traveling to Africa, for instance, are required to get vaccinated for yellow fever. The law, however, still appears to overlook HIV, or STIs in general (Hub, 2009). Given the current status of HIV in the country, it would only be sensible to provide orientation to emigrating Pakistanis about the transmission of STIs but no such practice currently exists (Hub, 2009). It is imperative that the migrant workers be given orientation on safe sex practice. The importance of condom use in all forms of sexual contact should be emphasized. Pakistanis traveling and working abroad should be educated about what to do and whom to contact in case they contract HIV (Rights, 2005). There should also be a mechanism to register HIV-positive deportees with the government so they can receive counseling, care and treatment in a timely fashion. While deported workers are being tested at the port in Pakistan, the country still lacks a strong screening policy at a national level (O. A. Khan & Hyder, 2001).

3   People Who Inject Drugs (PWID)

3.1   Transmission of HIV

The UNAIDS estimates the number of PWID worldwide to be 15.9 million. Nearly 20% (three million) of these PWID are HIV positive (UNAIDS, 2010). The population of PWID has been increasing over the years in Pakistan (WHO). The estimated number of drug users in Pakistan is 650,000 out of which 80,000 to 145,000 are PWID (Adnan Ahmad Khan, 2010). Data from 2008 show that 99.8% of PWID in the country are men and that a majority is illiterate, unmarried and is at a mean age of 33 years (WHO). The average age at which drug users start injecting was reported to be 28 years (WHO). The majority of PWID reside in major cities of Pakistan, such as Karachi, Faisalabad and Lahore (NACP, 2008). PWID form a major high-risk group in Pakistan. This group is considered responsible for the spread of the virus across different high and low risk populations (M. R. Khanani et al., 2011; Niccolai et al., 2009). This group lies at the hubs of the networks that connect the communities at risk of HIV infection (S. Khan et al., 2006). The PWID population shows the highest prevalence of HIV seropositivity in Pakistan. According to the data from the National AIDS Control Program (NACP), 21% of PWID were HIV positive in 2008 (NACP, 2008). In addition, Pakistan is amongst a list of 24 countries where the PWID cohorts make up 20% or more of the total number of people living with HIV/AIDS (UNAIDS, 2010). The rate of spread of the virus within this community is very high because of sharing of needles, a common practice among PWID, and unprotected sex (Adnan Ahmad Khan, 2010; M. R. Khanani et al., 2011; NACP, 2008; Rai et al., 2010; Shah et al., 2004a; UNAIDS, 2010).

Pakistan shares its borders with Afghanistan, the largest producer of poppy (opium) in the region (UNODC, 2011). Afghanistan, Pakistan and Iran are part of the famous "Golden Crescent" area, the hub from where the majority of the world's poppy is produced, exported and trafficked (Taylor, 2006). In 2011, 195, 700 hectare of land was used for opium cultivation in Afghanistan (UNODC, 2011). While a minority of this produce is used locally, the rest is trafficked worldwide through trading routes mainly in the neighboring countries such as Pakistan (Taylor, 2006). Opium is also cultivated in certain areas of Pakistan such as the Federally Administered Areas (FATA) and smaller areas in Baluchistan and Sindh (UNODC, 2011). Areas near the border or trade routes through which the drug is illegally smuggled in the country tend to attract the attention of PWID; this is where a higher percentage of the PWID resides (Bao & Liu, 2009). A majority of drug users use the drug through inhalation (Haque et al., 2004), but as the effects of inhalation diminish over time, a typical drug user looks towards injecting drugs due to the enhanced effect it brings about. In a PWID cohort from Quetta, 58% reported that they preferred to use heroin alone while 42% reported that they preferred a mixture of drugs (Kuo et al., 2006). PWID in Pakistan often use a mixture of different pharmaceutical agents – typically stimulants such as diazepam and amphetamines – to amplify the drug injecting experience (NACP, 2008). A cohort in Lahore also reported use of a mixture of liquid buprenorphine, anti-histamines and tranquilizers. The PWID will normally buy these drugs from the local pharmacies without prescription (Ahmed et al., 2003; Haque et al., 2004).

3.2   High Risk Practices

Most addicts prefer to inject drugs in parks or streets in groups with friends and family (NACP, 2008). Some also ask for help from professional injectors – street doctors, who are PWID themselves and are paid by other PWID to be injected with the drug (NACP, 2008). In the PWID community, a brotherhood-signifying ritual is to load a needle with the drug and pass it on among the fellow PWID sitting in a circle, sharing the same drug-loaded needle (NACP, 2008). "Jerking" is the practice of deliberately drawing blood into the needle while injecting (Figure 4 left). In a PWID cohort in Quetta and Lahore, 92% of the PWID reported to practice jerking (Kuo et al., 2006). As the needle is passed around, jerking will allow it to accumulate, in addition to the drug, a cocktail of contaminating blood from the members of the circle. The practice, evidently, is a sure-fire method to eventually transmit any blood-borne infection from one PWID to the entire injecting group.

It was seen that PWID in 8 major cities around the country used approximately 2 to 3 injections a day (NACP, 2008). With this frequency of injection use, many find it easier to share and re-use needles. A survey conducted by the NACP in 2008 showed that 19.1% of the study participants shared needles (NACP, 2008), while data from 2005 showed that a majority cleaned needles for reuse by a variety of ineffective methods such as boiling or scrubbing with antiseptics (NACP, 2006-2007). As per popular belief, many people still think that such methods of cleaning are sufficient to purge the needles of infective material. Due to unawareness and/or inaccessibility to needle-exchange centers most PWID do not use sterile needles on a regular basis (Bokhari et al., 2007; UN-AIDS, 2010).

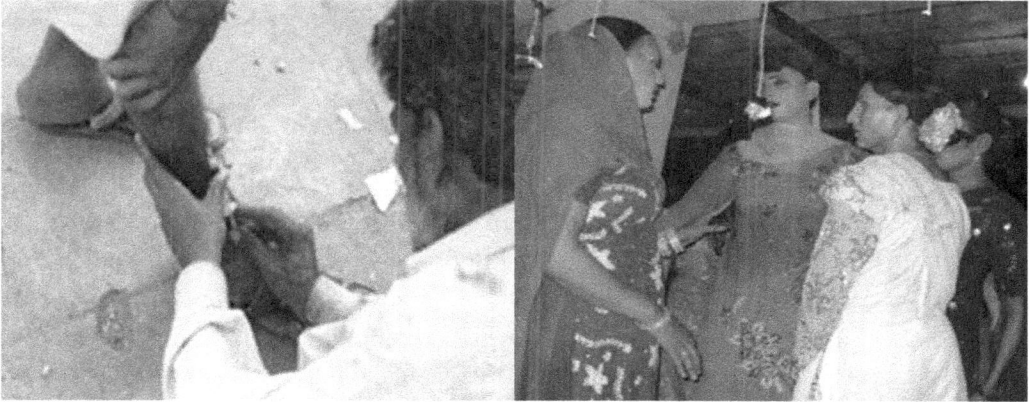

Figure 4. High Risk Groups Where HIV is Most Prevalent in Pakistan: Injection drug users (left) transmit HIV through contaminated needle-exchange within the PWID community and through sexual contact to other high risk groups such as MSM (right).

3.3   Harm Reduction for PWID

The government and the non-governmental organizations have collaborated to establish needle-exchange programs in Pakistan. Some of these needle exchange centers go one step further and provide health care facilities, counseling and even showers to the homeless PWID community. These centers teach the PWID community safe methods of drug injection and raise awareness on HIV prevention (Bokhari et al., 2007). The government's efforts in opening free needle-exchange centers across the country are commendable. Considering, however, that the risk behaviors among the PWID community are multi-layered, the governmental and non-governmental organizations need to collaborate to develop a multi-pronged approach for managing this group. In addition to needle-exchange programs, awareness programs are imperative to educate the PWID regarding safe handling of injectable materials, and the benefits of condom use in protecting against STIs. PWID should be educated about how to recognize signs of blood-borne infections, where to find medical care, and how to protect their sexual partners, spouses and families from getting infected.

Studies from Pakistan have shown transmission of HIV infection, brought into the PWID community by Gulf deportees, and transmitted through the entire PWID group via needle exchange (S. Khan et al., 2006; Rai et al., 2010) (Figure 3). As PWID exhibit multiple high-risk behaviors, they serve as an efficient vector for spreading blood-borne infections within as well as outside the PWID community. In addition to injecting drugs and sharing needles, PWID are also known to practice unsafe sex and have multiple sex partners. PWID also intermingle with other high-risk groups such as CSWs and MSM (Figure 2 and Figure 4). Many have regular sexual contact with sex workers and have multiple sex partners (Adnan Ahmad Khan, 2010; M. R. Khanani et al., 2011; NACP, 2008; Rai et al., 2010; Shah et al., 2004a; UNAIDS, 2010). NACP reports in 2008 showed that only 4.6% PWID had never had sex before (NACP, 2008), while 18% reported that they had sexual contact with female sex workers (FSWs), and 14% said they had sex with men (NACP, 2008). In addition to selling sex, PWID are also known to sell blood in order to support their drug addiction habit. Even though the government of Pakistan has passed legislation at the provincial level to ensure safe blood transfusion practices, the guideline must be effectively enforced in the blood-banks to make sure that all incoming donations are screened thoroughly. The donor population should be monitored as per guidelines to screen out those practicing injection drug use (Kassi et al., 2011).

PWID involve themselves in multiple high risk activities that put them at an increased risk of contracting and spreading HIV. Prime amongst these activities is sharing of needles and unsafe sex with men and women. High frequency of drug injection, lack of awareness about, and of accessibility to, needle exchange centers, and low condom use contribute to the high seroprevalence of HIV in this group, as cited by UNAIDS (UNAIDS, 2010). A recent study showed bridging of HIV infection from PWID to MSM through needle-exchange and sexual contact (Figure 2 and Figure 5). Subsequently, the infection was shown to have further transmitted to female spouses of these PWID and/or MSM through sexual contact (M. R. Khanani et al., 2011) (Figure 5). The PWID group is thus implicated to be the main hub where the HIV epidemics in Pakistan initially expanded and then was bridged into the MSM population through needle exchange and sexual contact (M. R. Khanani et al., 2011).

4   Men Who Have Sex with Men (MSM)

4.1   MSM Demography and Risk Behavior

Men who have sex with men (MSM) include all members of the population who are biologically male but practice sexual relations with other men (Figure 4, right). The term does not describe sexual orientation or preference, since sexual identity and behavior cannot be compiled into clear categories anywhere in the world. While considering risks for STIs, it is important to take into account the gender role adopted by different members of this population. Not all members of this community can be classified as homosexuals or bisexuals, since many men who have sex with men consider themselves heterosexual (UNAIDS, 2006). The individual would therefore categorize his sexual orientation and behavior depending on his own view of his self. The various shades and layers of sexual behavior must be regarded carefully while formulating harm reduction policies for the MSM population. Additionally, social, political and cultural scenario in a country play a role on people's perception and definition of their sexual identity (UNAIDS, 2006). For example, when the AIDS epidemic first started in the 1980s and 1990s in the world it had a definite impact on people's perception and behavior toward homosexuality. These behaviors were remolded as awareness about the virus spread and the availability and efficacy of ART increased (UNAIDS, 2006). The harm reduction policies, therefore, must be reviewed and amended accordingly, in light of the shifting sociopolitical and cultural norms in a given population.

Figure 5. Phylogenetic Analysis of HIV Transmission Between PWID, MSM, and MSM Families: The tree shows a phylogentic relationship between sequences obtained from HIV-1 positive MSM (M. R. Khanani et al., 2011), and IDUs (PWID) sequences, which are bolded in black. The 47 HIV-1 strains from MSM and M-IDU (M-PWID) are shown in highlights, while 15 MSM spouses (MS-) are shown in light grey and 14 MSM children (MC-) are shown in dark grey (M. R. Khanani et al., 2011). Members of each family are assigned identical digit label following the letter prefix. The numbers along the monophyletic branches correspond to bootstrap values. Reproduced from: M. R. Khanani et al., 2011.

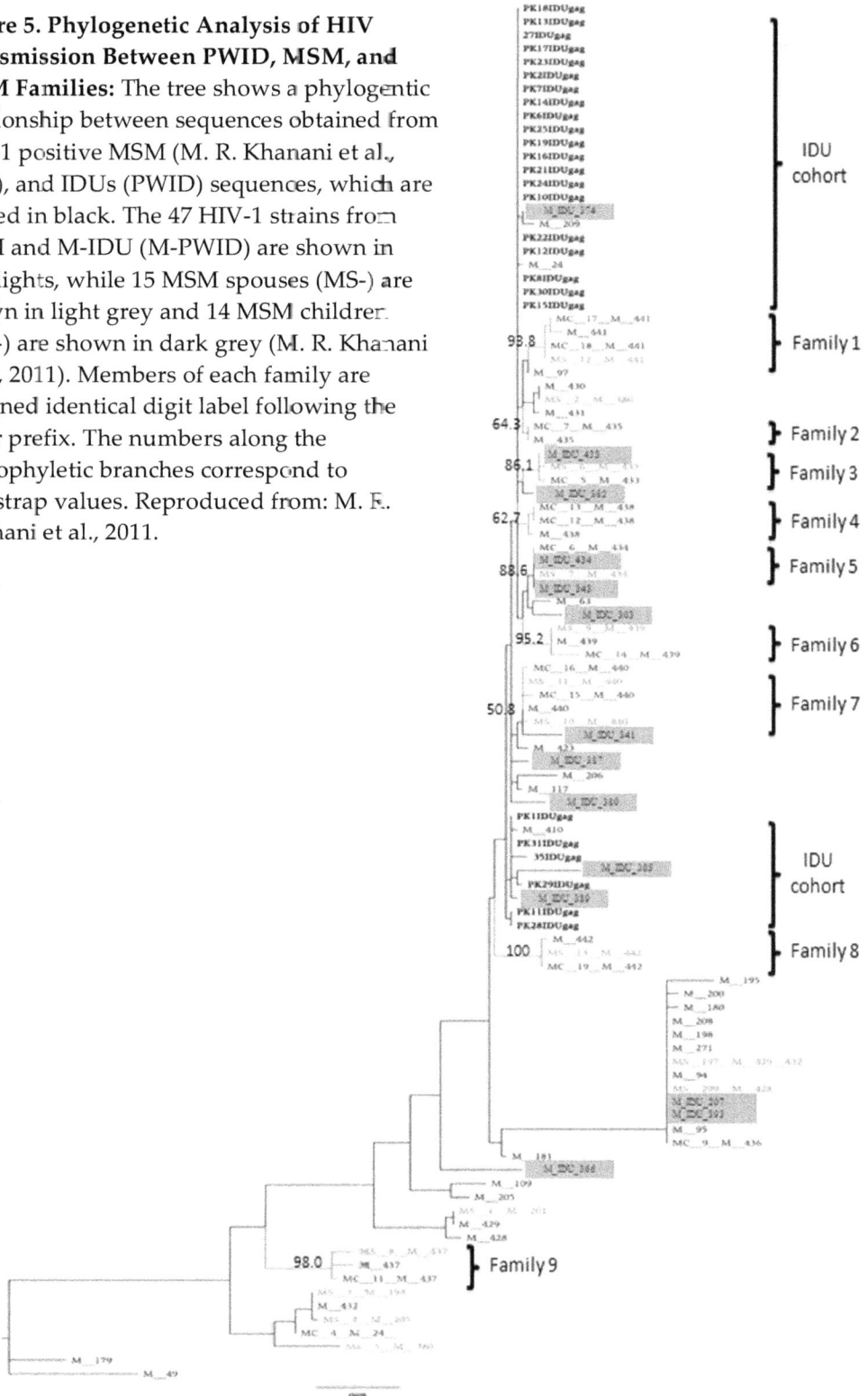

Depending on their behavior, the MSM population may be divided into different sub-groups in Pakistan (Rajabali et al., 2008). This is important because sexual practices and risk behaviors can differ within these subgroups (Rajabali et al., 2008). The risk of transmission for instance depends on whether the individual is a receptive or an insertive partner in anal sex. Compared to vaginal, anal sex is a more efficient mode of transmission of HIV especially for the receptive partner (Rajabali et al., 2008). A survey in Lahore and Karachi showed that 47% of the MSWs in Karachi were insertive partners compared with 2% in Lahore. A majority of the MSWs in Lahore (33%) stated that they were exclusively receptive partners in anal sex (Bokhari et al., 2007)

Hijras, a major subgroup of MSM, are biologically male but identify with the female gender and wear female attire (Figure 4, bottom). Also known as eunuchs, historically they commanded political power because members of this group used to be advisors to the kings. Today, however, Hijras are a marginalized population, driven underground due to social stigma and discrimination. Members of this group associate feminism with spiritual power and hence do not usually marry women, and perform as receptive partners in anal sex. This practice puts them at a higher risk of contracting STIs, especially HIV (Rajabali et al., 2008; UNAIDS, 2006). A majority of Hijras also work as commercial sex workers. A study reported that Hijras had a mean experience of selling sex of 6 years in Lahore and 10 years in Karachi and a majority (96%) reported selling anal sex in the past month (Bokhari et al., 2007). Zenanas and Chavas also identify themselves with the female gender. While the former are receptive partners in anal sex the latter can switch roles. Both groups have families and often marry women. Due to the fear of divorce, marginalization and discrimination Zenanas usually hide their sexual promiscuity from their spouse, which puts their family at a high risk of contracting HIV (Rajabali et al., 2008). Giryas are insertive partners in anal sex and identify with the male gender. They take the role of husbands to Zenanas and Chavas. They may be unaware of their male spouse's promiscuous sex behavior and thus are at an increased risk of being infected (Rajabali et al., 2008; UNAIDS, 2006). Maalishias are masseurs by profession but often sell sex. They can be receptive or insertive partners depending on the situation and the client (Rajabali et al., 2008).

4.2   MSM-PWID

A recently emerged group among the MSM population, this subgroup has a key role in HIV transmission. Members of this group are exposed to two major risk factors for contracting HIV, namely, injection drug use and unsafe sex with other men. Dual risk factors also place this subgroup at a hub that bridges the HIV infection between two subgroups – MSM and PWID (M. R. Khanani et al., 2011; Rajabali et al., 2008; UNAIDS, 2010). PWID are often forced into sex as they need money to buy drugs. They are known to commonly have sex with multiple partners without protection. Unprotected anal sex within PWID was reported by 14% of the study sample in one study (Bokhari et al., 2007). Phylogeny of the HIV virus circulating among the MSM and PWID subgroups living in Karachi has revealed bridging of the virus between the two populations, either via needle-exchange or through sexual contact (Rajabali et al., 2008) (Figure 2 and 5).

4.3   Bisexual MSM

Keeping in mind the fact that the term MSM points to sexual behavior and not sexual preference and that the current social situation in the country forces MSM to marry and hide their homosexuality from the society (M. R. Khanani, Somani et al., 2010; Rajabali et al., 2008) - in fact studies have reported a majority of MSM to be married (M. R. Khanani, Somani et al., 2010; M. R. Khanani et al., 2011). The MSM population in general is at a high risk of transmitting the virus to other groups because many inject drugs and practice unsafe sex accounting for the high seroprevalence of HIV in this group (11%), as reported by studies conducted in 2006 and 2011 (M. R. Khanani, Somani et al., 2010; M. R. Khanani et al., 2011). Multiple risk behaviors of these MSM, coupled with the tendency to hide their promiscuous behavior and HIV status, puts the families of bisexual MSM at a high risk of being infected (Kagimu et al., 1998).

4.4   Male Sex Workers (MSWs)

This subgroup of MSM works in the profession of selling sex. They generally have multiple sex partners and involve in unprotected sex. They may also be married but their promiscuous activity is generally hidden from their families. In addition to promiscuity, MSWs may be exposed to other risk factors as well. In a study, 6.4% of MSWs reported to have had sex with a PWID, while 4.2% reported to be using drugs. Condom use with regular partner (mostly the female spouse) was much higher than that reported for anal sex with a male partner (NACP, 2008). Six-percent of the cohort in a study took part in anal sex, while only 21% of those used a condom. Considering their high risk practices, members of this group can effectively serve as bridging vectors between PWID, MSM, and their own female spouses (Bokhari et al., 2007).

4.5   Truck Drivers

Another minor high risk group is male truck drivers, who are also implicated to have sexual relations with other men. The government estimates the number of truck drivers to be one million in Pakistan (Agha, 2000). Intercity truck drivers remain away from their homes for 2 months at a time and a majority of them is married (Agha, 2000). Truckers usually travels with at least one other person, usually a young helper (Rajabali et al., 2008). A survey on truck drivers from Lahore reports that truck drivers are likely to keep sexual relations with their helper and also buy or sell sex, and inject drugs at truck stops or gathering places (Rajabali et al., 2008). A study from Karachi reports that 22% of the truck drivers admitted to have bought sex from a male or Hijra (Bokhari et al., 2007), while another study reported almost 49% of the truckers to have experienced sex with a man (Agha, 2000).

4.6   High Risk Behavior

High HIV prevalence is reported among the MSM population in Asia: 29% in Myanmar,

5% in Indonesia and 18% in Southern India (UNAIDS, 2010).The MSM population in Pakistan has an HIV seroprevalence of 0.9%, as reported by NACP. Data from Pakistan revealed Karachi to be home to the most MSMs followed closely by Faisalabad (NACP, 2006-2007). A majority of this population was unmarried and aged between 15-19 years (88.9%). As many as 42.4% of the MSM surveyed by NACP were illiterate and a majority (76.9%) lived at home with their families (NACP, 2008). MSMs were found to start sex work at a mean age of 16 years and had been practicing for approximately 5.5 years; individuals from Peshawar tended to start sex work at an earlier age than individuals from Lahore although MSMs in Lahore practiced sex work the longest (NACP, 2008). The survey also found that 15% of the interviewed MSMs were from another city out of which 30% had come to settle permanently while 70% were visiting, whereas 29% of the migrants had moved specifically for sex work. MSM migrants were concentrated the most in Lahore followed by Karachi (NACP, 2008).

Male sex workers entertain on average 2 to 3 clients per night. They get clients either by roaming around in public places, roadsides, parks or bus stops or are referred to by other clients or contacted via cell phones (NACP, 2008). Forty two percent of MSMs in a survey conducted by the NACP, reported to have had a regular non-paying sex partner (male or female) in addition to the clients, while 5% reported paying other members of the same group for anal sex (NACP, 2008), indicating that this subgroup has sex partners spread across both genders and several high risk groups. A non-paying sex partner is likely to be a spouse as well, pointing to the possibility of transmission of infection into the unsuspecting female population. The MSM population is not known to practice exclusivity in their sexual activity; in fact, more often than not, they may also have female sex partners (UNAIDS, 2006). This behavior increases the chance of spreading the virus across genders and into the general low-risk population. Keeping in view the high degree of interactions of this group with female spouses, female sex workers, commercial sex workers, and PWID, this group has a high potential of transmitting the HIV infection across various populations of the country.

4.7   Harm Reduction Policy for MSM

Pakistan is an Islamic republic and according to Islamic law having multiple sex partners, sex outside of marriage, sex with men and any other promiscuous activity is prohibited. Pakistan's penal code states that any form of unnatural or carnal intercourse with man, woman or beast is punishable (Ottosson, 2007; UNAIDS, 2006). These laws impact the social and cultural norms and feed the social stigma against homosexuality. Additionally, these laws are often used as an excuse for the law-enforcing authorities to harass and exploit the MSM population (Rajabali et al., 2008). Furthermore, being ostracized by family members and discrimination by employers alienates these individual, often pushing them into further high risk practices, such as selling sex and injecting drugs. This creates an overall threatening environment for the MSM community, driving them underground and marginalizing them, consequently making them inaccessible to interventions and harm reduction programs.

Low condom use is one of the most important risk factors among Pakistani MSM.

Only 24% of MSMs in a study reported condom use when having sex with other men (NACP, 2008). The most commonly cited reason for low condom use among MSWs is client preference for sex without condom (23%). This is followed by condom unavailability or deeming condom use unnecessary (12%). MSWs are also scared of carrying a condom because they can get arrested and charged for intent of sex if the police found a condom in their possession (Rajabali et al. 2008). Condoms are generally considered a means for preventing conception, their role in providing protection against STIs is largely unappreciated in Pakistan (Haque et al., 2004). The younger members of the MSM population are reported less likely to use condoms (NACP, 2008). Since the majority of the MSM population in Pakistan is young, between the age of 15-19 (NACP, 2008) the risk of acquiring HIV becomes even greater for this group. Low literacy is another factor predisposing these individuals to low condom use. Individuals having had education for at least ten years were found more likely to use condoms than those educated less (NACP, 2008). Since literacy level among the MSM population is reported to be low (NACP, 2008), this further increases their risk of contracting HIV.

Another major factor contributing to low condom use is the lack of effective awareness programs that promote safe sex. Explicit discussion on sexual subjects is taboo is Muslim cultures, including Pakistan (Shafiq & Ali, 2006). Promoting safe sex is especially a sensitive subject in Islamic countries since promotion of safe sex can be viewed as promotion for having sex (Rajabali et al., 2008). It is imperative to address these cultural taboos instead of conceding to this barrier. Appropriate culturally sensitive strategies should be developed for promoting safe sex. There is a scarcity of knowledge on HIV prevention programs and only a few MSM (8.5%) report to visit the centers that have been established to raise awareness (NACP, 2008). The 100% Condom Use Program (CUP) was successful in promoting condom use and reducing STI prevalence in several Asian countries (Zhongdan et al., 2008). A version of condom promotion program, tailored to the cultural and social norms, may be formulated for Pakistan as well. The objectives of this program should be to educate the public about HIV and STD transmission and to promote condom use among the specific high-risk groups. Given the codes of moral standards in Muslim countries, legalization of prostitution or homosexuality will not be accepted here. There are, however, tactfully structured models developed and followed in certain countries that may be applied to Muslim countries. Uganda, for instance, adopted a discreet policy that focused more on destigmatization and open communication (UNAIDS, 2004). Key members of society were encouraged by the program to disclose their HIV status to promote tolerance and acceptance of the diseases by the public. The programs also promoted delaying sexual debut among young members of the population and not having multiple non-regular sex partners (UNAIDS, 2004). The government in Uganda also started another program to educate the Imams, respected religious leaders, on HIV. Imams were recognized as an important resource that could be utilized in relaying information to the general public (Kagimu et al., 1998). In a similar way, the involvement of religious scholars has also proven effective as a harm reduction strategy in Senegal (Diop, 2000). Such socially sensitive programs can be a practical solution in countering the HIV problem in Pakistan as well.

5   Women and Children

5.1   Risk of HIV Infection for Women

Half of the world's HIV-positive population is female, where the infection is growing fastest among the age group of 15-24 years (Gupta, 2004). According to recent estimates, 4.8 million adults are living with HIV in Asia, and 34% of this population comprises women (UNAIDS, 2010). It is generally assumed that women are not at a high risk of HIV, since a majority of them does not practice injecting drugs and does not have multiple sex partners. It is important to appreciate, however, that the male sex partners of these women do in fact involve themselves in high-risk practices which in turn puts the women at risk of acquiring HIV. One study reported that 90% of HIV-positive women in Asia were infected by their husbands or long-term male partners (AVERT). A survey done from Iran reported that 11% of the wives of the men who had worked abroad were HIV positive (M. M. Batool Sharifi-Mood, Masoud Mardani, Bashir Pejman, 2008). In Pakistan, the female population is seriously underrepresented. Women suffer from social marginalization, and in a male-dominated society have little say in life-governing decisions, including those directly concerning themselves.

Studies from Asian societies have revealed serious gender discrimination prevalent in this region. The abortion rate for female babies is much higher than that of male babies (Bunch, 1990), and once born, female babies become victims of neglect. Young girls in these societies may often be less nourished, less educated, and are more likely to be denied proper care when sick compared to young boys (Bunch, 1990). Similarly, young females are often not allowed to make a decision about whom they get married to, or when and if to get pregnant. Compared to their male counterparts, females are more likely to get cheated on and subjected to sexual violence (Bunch, 1990). Indeed, studies from Africa and India show that the risk of HIV transmission to a female may be higher in abusive relationships (Bunch, 1990).

Social taboos in Pakistan make it difficult to discuss STIs or their prevention. Pressures from the society and the male spouse make it impossible for a Pakistani woman to get tested for STIs or openly talk about it (Shafiq & Ali, 2006). A study reports that women who report HIV-related discrimination are more likely to be under high levels of stress, think of suicide as a means of relief from their problems and have a greater number of unprotected sexual episodes (Wingood et al., 2007). Marginalization in this form is likely to drive HIV-positive women to conceal their HIV status and become socially invisible, which creates a barrier for their healthcare. Moreover, if these women become pregnant, they will be inaccessible to proper healthcare that may enable them to prevent HIV transmission to their newborn.

5.2   HIV Transmission to Newborns

Vertical transmission of HIV can happen before, during or after childbirth, depending on viral load, breastfeeding, ART therapy and method of delivery (Newell, 2000) (Figure 2). High Viral Load or low CD4 cell counts are important markers that indicate the probability of transmission of the virus to the fetus. ART therapy is necessary to reduce viral load (Cao et al., 1997; O'Shea et al., 1998; UNAIDS, 2011) and the risk of vertical transmission by 51% in the absence of breastfeeding (Raees et al., 2013). Different methods of delivery affect HIV transmission differently. The risk of transmission is high with vaginal delivery, because during this type of delivery, the baby comes in contact with vaginal secretions and infected blood (Kind et al., 1998). Cesarean sections have been shown to reduce the transmission of HIV to the fetus because they reduce contact with HIV rich reservoirs, and partly because if successful cesarean sections ensure that the delivery occurs before the membranes rupture (McGowan & Shah, 2000).

Breastfeeding has been shown to increase the risk of HIV transmission to newborns (Dunn et al., 1992). The risk of transmission through breastfeeding is shown to be 14% in established maternal infections and 29% in acute maternal infection (Kreiss, 1997). HIV-positive mothers should be counseled to use formulations and not breastfeed infants. Administration of ART has also been shown to reduce the risk HIV transmission through milk (Dabis et al., 1999). This, however, creates a problem for women in developing countries since they cannot afford formulations and have to rely on breast milk to feed their baby (Newell, 2000). Since using formulated milk is highly uncommon in developing countries, HIV-positive mothers are also likely to face social pressure if they try to forgo breastfeeding in order to save their child (de Ruiter & Brocklehurst, 1998). ART, combined with abstinence from breastfeeding and cesarean method of delivery, can be highly effective; reports have shown this combined approach to reduce the risk of delivery to 0% (Kind et al., 1998). Since new standards of therapy started, ART therapy has become affordable and easily available. In fact, the government of Pakistan provides it free of charge for HIV positive individuals, but ART coverage is still very low in the country, owing to poor awareness and limited accessibility of harm reduction programs (UNAIDS, 2010). Since most physicians, health-care providers and HIV-positive mothers are not aware of the benefits of the above-mentioned prevention methods, in most cases, vertical transmission to newborn invariably occurs.

5.3   Prevention and Treatment of HIV in Newborns

UNAIDS reports that 15-20% of women find out their HIV status during neonatal testing (UNAIDS, 2010). There is no proper policy in place in Pakistan that gives guidelines to healthcare practitioners on how to screen or treat HIV positive pregnant women. In the absence of a structured system these mothers are in the dark about their condition and are unaware of the various risk reduction techniques that could save their children from being infected with HIV. Pregnant women need to be given ART therapy for themselves and their fetus (Rights, 2005), and they need to be given this therapy in a timely fashion so that its effect is maximized. ART regimes have been put in place by health ministries in different countries especially after clinical trials in Thailand showed the positive effects of low dose ART therapy for preventing mother to child transmission (Bajunirwe et al., 2004; de Ruiter & Brocklehurst, 1998). If ART therapy for pregnant women is to be successful in Pakistan, proper screening methods need to be in place to diagnose HIV in pregnant women before the baby is born (de Ruiter & Brocklehurst, 1998). Health ministries in Pakistan, however, would have to take the initiative

to educate the obstetricians about these measures. Midwives handle a majority of preg-
nancies and deliveries in Pakistan. The government should focus on educating this
group, as well, about the threats posed by HIV.

Pakistan lacks guidelines for the treatment of not only HIV-positive pregnant
women but also on HIV-positive neonates. While a few pediatricians are trained to
handle HIV-positive children, the majority is not specialized to do so. The immune system is not well-developed in neonates; compared to adults, HIV infection increases susceptibility to other infections in newborns more significantly. Neonates as a result become more vulnerable to opportunistic infections, such as tuberculosis and pneumonia.
The rising cost of medicine in Pakistan has become a significant barrier in ensuring that
neonates with opportunistic infections are provided with antibiotics. In addition to
providing free of cost ART for the HIV patients, the government-run HIV treatment
centers would need to provide medicine and care for opportunistic infections as well.

5.4   HIV Epidemic and the Next Generation

Considering the social structure in Pakistan, the HIV status of children, especially the
male offspring, is kept in secret by the parents. This is an attempt by the parents to protect the children from the prevalent stigma that may hamper their progress later in life.
This well-intentioned mindset, however, also shields the younger HIV positive population from accessibility to intervention and awareness programs. As the ART becomes
more effective, affordable and accessible to this younger HIV-positive generation, the
chances are that they will reach adulthood and live to complete their normal lifespan
(de Martino et al., 2000; Gortmaker et al., 2001). While this may be good news for an
HIV positive patient, considering the current scenario in Pakistan, it can lead to dire
consequences on a larger level: With the ART becoming more effective on one hand,
and the stigma against HIV still robust, the HIV epidemic will have ample chance to
proliferate invisibly into seemingly healthy carriers. Subsequently, the virus may silent-
ly get transmitted horizontally as well as vertically into the next generations. It is necessary to implement measures to eradicate the virus before it turns into a larger insidious
epidemic. This would entail tackling the epidemic in the HIV-positive families. In order
to stop the epidemic from penetrating more deeply into the next generation of individuals, it is imperative for the government to effectively utilize the media and, for the first
time in the country, initiate sex education for young adults. Although cultural and social values will be an obstacle to such efforts, we believe that high-school and college
students can be successfully sensitized about safe sex practices if these recommendations are deployed in culturally sensitive ways.

Before eliminating the virus, however, the stigma against HIV will need to be addressed and eradicated. Only then will it be possible to access the HIV-positive younger
generation and educate them about how to prevent further transmission of the virus.
The government of Pakistan should hold public dialogue about HIV and allow all forms
of media to advertise safe sex and prevention methods. Up till now, the government has
failed to appreciate the potential of electronic and print media in spreading awareness
about HIV (O. A. Khan & Hyder, 2001). As mentioned above, the government could

also educate the Imams, the religious scholars, to spread awareness about HIV. Additionally, empowerment workshops may be organized to motivate the women to come to the forefront and speak for their rights.

6 Conclusion

The HIV epidemic in Pakistan has followed the Asian Epidemic Model: it spread through deportees to PWID and MSM and is now being seen in families and children of infected PWID and bisexual MSMs. The government of Pakistan needs to fine-tune the HIV/AIDS policy, taking into account the new directions the HIV epidemic is taking in the country. Commendable efforts have been made by the National AIDS Control Program, including the establishment of needle-exchange centers, and implementation of awareness programs for high-risk communities. While such programs for the infected PWID and MSM need to be reviewed and improved, new policies should be implemented for empowering the HIV-positive female population (Table 1). Special emphasis must be placed on improving the healthcare and controlling the infection in HIV-positive pregnant women and their offspring.

The provision of free-of-cost ART in Pakistan has also led to improved rates of survival for HIV-infected individuals, so now they can expect to live up to a full lifespan. This, however, comes with added responsibility for the government: HIV infection in Pakistan appears to be entering a new era where the epidemic can expand through generational transmission. The chances are that HIV-positive children of today will, as adults, pass on the legacy of infection to their next generation. In the years to come, the Pakistani government is up for new challenges. The policy makers will have to think of new ways to access and educate the HIV-positive adolescent population of Pakistan. The media needs to be judiciously utilized for this purpose. It is recommended that in a culturally-sensitive manner, high school and college-going youth should be sensitized through sex education about safe sex practice (Table 1).

References

Abidi, S. H., Ali, F., Shah, F., Abbas, F., & Ali. S. (2012). Burden of communicable disease among the native and repatriating Afghans. PLoS Pathog, 8(10), e1002926.

Adnan Ahmad Khan, A. K. (2010). The HIV Epidemic in Pakistan. JPMA.

Agha, S. (2000). Potential for HIV transmission among truck drivers in Pakistan. AIDS, 14(15), 2404–2406.

Ahmed, M. A., Zafar, T., Brahmbhatt, H., Imam, G., Ul Hassan, S., Bareta, J. C., et al. (2003). HIV/AIDS risk behaviors and correlates of injection drug use among drug users in Pakistan. Journal of urban health : bulletin of the New York Academy of Medicine, 80(2), 321–329.

Asia, C. (2007). State of Health of Migrants - Mandatory Testing. Retrieved February 21, 2012, from

High Risk Group	High Risk Behavior and Factors	Initiatives or Recommendations	Harm Reduced
Deportees	Travel and Stay abroad	Migrants should be counseled on STD control and prevention	Transmission of HIV to Pakistani Migrants; Further transmission from HIV-positive deportees to their social contacts and family
	Contact with CSWs while abroad	Condom use should be promoted	
	No screening or post-test counseling	Returning HIV-positive deportees should be enrolled in an awareness, treatment and prevention program	
PWID	Sharing Used Needles	Needle exchange centers have been set up but need to improve coverage	Spread of HIV within the PWID cohort and further transmission to MSM and PWID spouses; Marginalization of PWID community
		PWID should be motivated to visit needle exchange centers	
	Selling Sex to Men		
	Low Condom use	PWID should be educated on the harms of sharing needles and having unprotected sex	
	Lack of Awareness on HIV transmission and Prevention		
	Lack of a proper support system for drug addicts	Rehabilitation and empowerment programs for PWID	

Continued on next page…

…Continued from previous page

High Risk Group	High Risk Behavior and Factors	Initiatives or Recommendations	Harm Reduced
MSM	Inability to bargain for safe sex	The MSM population should be empowered	
	Unprotected anal sex with clients, lack of awareness about safe sex practices	Awareness on the increased risk of HIV transmission during unprotected anal sex	Tendency of the MSM population to hide themselves and their high risk activities; rate of transmission through receptive anal sex; stigmatization of MSM community
	Stigma, marginalization and lack of acceptance of homosexuality by society	Awareness on the increased risk of HIV transmission during unprotected anal sex	
Women	Marginalization and suppression by the male spouse	Promoting women's rights;	
	Having no say in when to get married and get pregnant	Empowerment workshops to motivate women to fight for their rights	Reduced chances of transmission to women and their children; Reduced sexual violence and gender discrimination; ART therapy increased
	Subjected to sexual violence		
	Unawareness about prevention of vertical transmission of HIV	Educating HIV-positive mothers and their healthcare-givers on ART therapy, breastfeeding and cesarean sections.	

Continued on next page…

...Continued from previous page

High Risk Group	High Risk Behavior and Factors	Initiatives or Recommendations	Harm Reduced
	No policy regarding treatment for HIV-positive pregnant women	Maternity clinics and midwives should receive special orientation on managing HIV-positive pregnant women	
Children	Lack of pediatric care for HIV positive children	health policies for HIV positive children should be drafted	
		Awareness and public dialogue	Risk of transmission to children reduced; HIV positive children exposed and intervention made easier; the dangers of the hidden epidemic
	Lack of awareness on child-specific ART therapy	Healthcare professionals should be trained on management of HIV-positive children	
	Stigma and discrimination against HIV-positive children	Awareness and public dialogue should be initiated	
	Lack of awareness about STIs among adolescent youth	Sex education at high school and college level	Risk of further transmission to the next generation

Table 1: HIV in Pakistan: High Risk Groups and Behaviors, And Recommendations for Harm Reduction: The table lists risk behaviors/factors occurring in different high-risk groups and recommendations that may reduce the HIV transmission within and between these groups.

http://www.7sisters.org/pdf/SoH_Report_2007-online_version.pdf

AVERT. Women, HIV and AIDS. Retrieved February 4th 2012, 2012, from http://www.avert.org/women-hiv-aids.htm

Bajunirwe, F., Massaquoi, I., Asiimwe, S., Kamya, M. R., Arts, E. J., & Whalen, C. C. (2004). Effectiveness of nevirapine and zidovudine in a pilot program for the prevention of mother-to-child transmission of HIV-1 in Uganda. Afr Health Sci, 4 (3), 146–154.

Bao, Y. P., & Liu, Z. M. (2009). Systematic review of HIV and HCV infection among drug users in China. International journal of STD & AIDS, 20 (6), 399–405.

Baqi, S., Kayani, N., & Khan, J. A. (1999). Epidemiology and clinical profile of HIV/AIDS in Pakistan. Tropical doctor, 29 (3), 144–148.

Batool Sharifi-Mood, M. M., Masoud Mardani, Bashir Pejman. (2008). Immigration: a potential risk factor for intrafamilial

transmission of HIV infection. Iranian Journal of Clinical Infectious Diseases 3, 3–5.

Batool Sharifi-Mood, M. S., Esmail Sanei-Moghaddan, Sohila Khosravi. (2006). Immigrant Fathers, Mothers and Babies Who are Living with HIV/AIDS. J. Med. Sci, 6 (3), 492–494.

Bokhari, A., Nizamani, N. M., Jackson, D. J., Rehan, N. E., Rahman, M., Muzaffar, R., et al. (2007). HIV risk in Karachi and Lahore, Pakistan: an emerging epidemic in injecting and commercial sex networks. International journal of STD & AIDS, 18 (7), 486–492.

Brown, T., & Peerapatanapokin, W. (2004). The Asian Epidemic Model: a process model for exploring HIV policy and programme alternatives in Asia. Sexually transmitted infections, 80 Suppl 1, i19–24.

Bunch, C. (1990). Women's Rights as Human Rights: Towards a Re-Vision of Human Rights. Human Rights Quarterly, 12 (1990), 486–498.

Cao, Y., Krogstad, P., Korber, B. T., Koup, R. A., Muldoon, M., Macken, C., et al. (1997). Maternal HIV-1 viral load and vertical transmission of infection: the Ariel Project for the prevention of HIV transmission from mother to infant. Nature medicine, 3 (5), 549–552.

Dabis, F., Msellati, P., Meda, N., Welffens-Ekra, C., You, B., Manigart, O., et al. (1999). 6-month efficacy, tolerance, and acceptability of a short regimen of oral zidovudine to reduce vertical transmission of HIV in breastfed children in Cote d'Ivoire and Burkina Faso: a double-blind placebo-controlled multicentre trial. DITRAME Study Group DIminution de la Transmission Mere-Enfant. Lancet, 353 (9155), 786–792.

de Martino, M., Tovo, P. A., Balducci, M., Galli, L., Gabiano, C., Rezza, G., et al. (2000). Reduction in mortality with availability of antiretroviral therapy for children with perinatal HIV-1 infection. Italian Register for HIV Infection in Children and the Italian National AIDS Registry. JAMA : the journal of the American Medical Association, 284 (2), 190–197.

de Ruiter, A., & Brocklehurst, P. (1998). HIV infection and pregnancy. International journal of STD & AIDS, 9 (11), 647–654; quiz 655.

Diop, W. (2000). From government policy to community-based communication strategies in Africa: lessons from Senegal and Uganda. J Health Commun, 5 Suppl, 113–117.

Dunn, D. T., Newell, M. L., Ades, A. E., & Peckham, C. S. (1992). Risk of human immunodeficiency virus type 1 transmission through breastfeeding. Lancet, 340(8819), 585–588.

Gortmaker, S. L., Hughes, M., Cervia, J., Brady, M., Johnson, G. M., Seage, G. R., 3rd, et al. (2001). Effect of combination therapy including protease inhibitors on mortality among children and adolescents *infected with HIV-1. The New England journal of medicine, 345(21), 1522–1528.*

Gupta, G. R. (2004). *Globalization, Women and the HIV/AIDS Epidemic. Peace Review, 16(1), 79–83.*

Haque, N., Zafar, T., Brahmbhatt, H., Imam, G., ul Hassan, S., & Strathdee, S. A. (2004). *High-risk sexual behaviours among drug users in Pakistan: implications for prevention of STDs and HIV/AIDS. International journal of STD & AIDS, 15(9), 601–607.*

Hub, A. D. (2009). *HIV & Migration. Retrieved 17 February, 2012, from http://aidsdatahub.org/dmdocuments/HIV_and_Migration_-_Pakistan.pdf*

Kagimu, M., Marum, E., Wabwire-Mangen, F., Nakyanjo, N., Walakira, Y., & Hogle, J. (1998). *Evaluation of the effectiveness of AIDS health education interventions in the Muslim community in Uganda. AIDS education and prevention : official publication of the International Society for AIDS Education, 10 (3), 215_228.*

Kandela, P. (1993). *Arab nations: attitudes to AIDS. Lancet, 341 (8849), 884_885.*

Kandela, P. (1994). *Gulf states test foreigners for AIDS. BMJ, 308 (6929), 617.*

Kapiszewski, A. (2006, 15-17 May 2006). *Arab versus Asian Migrant Workers in the GCC Countries. United Nations Expert Group meeting on International Migration and Development in the Arab Region, from http://www.un.org/esa/population/meetings/EGM_Ittmig_Arab/P02_Kapiszewski.pdf*

Kassi, M., Afghan, A. K., Khanani, M. R., Khan, I. A., & Ali, S. H. (2011). *Safe blood transfusion practices in blood banks of Karachi, Pakistan. Transfusion medicine, 21 (1), 57–62.*

Khan, O. A., & Hyder, A. A. (2001). *Responses to an emerging threat: HIV/AIDS policy in Pakistan. Health policy and planning, 16 (2), 214–218.*

Khan, S., Rai, M. A., Khanani, M. R., Khan, M. N., & Ali, S. H. (2006). *HIV-1 subtype A infection in a community of intravenous drug users in Pakistan. BMC infectious diseases, 6, 164.*

Khanani, M. R., Ansari, A. S., Khan, S., Somani, M., Kazmi, S. U., & Ali, S. H. (2010). *Concentrated epidemics of HIV, HCV, and HBV among Afghan refugees. J Infect, 61 (5), 434–437.*

Khanani, M. R., Somani, M., Khan, S., Naseeb, S., & Ali, S. H. (2010). *Prevalence of single, double, and triple infections of HIV, HCV and HBV among the MSM community in Pakistan. J Infect, 61 (6), 507–509.*

Khanani, M. R., Somani, M., Rehmani, S. S., Veras, N. M., Salemi, M., & Ali, S. H. (2011). *The spread of HIV in Pakistan: bridging of the epidemic between populations. PloS one, 6 (7), e22449.*

Khanani, M. R., Hafeez, A., Rab, S. M., & Rasheed, S. (1988). *Human immunodeficiency virus-associated disorders in Pakistan. AIDS research and human retroviruses, 4 (2), 149–154.*

Kind, C., Rudin, C., Siegrist, C. A., Wyler, C. A., Biedermann, K., Lauper, U., et al. (1998). *Prevention of vertical HIV transmission: additive protective effect of elective Cesarean section and zidovudine prophylaxis. Swiss Neonatal HIV Study Group. AIDS, 12 (2), 205–210.*

Kreiss, J. (1997). *Breastfeeding and vertical transmission of HIV-1. Acta paediatrica, 421, 113–117.*

Kuo, I., ul-Hasan, S., Galai, N., Thomas, D. L., Zafar, T., Ahmed, M. A., et al. (2006). *High HCV seroprevalence and HIV drug use risk behaviors among injection drug users in Pakistan. Harm reduction journal, 3, 26.*

Li, X., Zhang, L., Stanton, B., Fang, X., Xiong, Q., & Lin, D. (2007). *HIV/AIDS-related sexual risk behaviors among rural residents in China: potential role of rural-to-urban migration. AIDS education and prevention : official publication of the International Society for AIDS Education, 19 (5), 396–407.*

McGowan, J. P., & Shah, S. S. (2000). Prevention of perinatal HIV transmission during pregnancy. J Antimicrob Chemother, 46 (5), 657–668.

NACP. (2006-2007). National Report Round II. from http://www.nacp.gov.pk/library/reports/Surveillance %20&%20Research/HIV-AIDS%20Surveillance%20Project-HASP/HIV%20Second%20Generation %20Surveillance%20in%20Pakistan%20-%20Round%202%20Report%202006-07.pdf

NACP. (2008, 9th October 2008). National Report Round III. from http://www.nacp.gov.pk/library/ reports/Surveillance%20&%20Research/HIV-AIDS%20Surveillance%20Project-HASP/HIV%20 Second%20Generation%20Surveillance%20in%20Pakistan%20-%20National%20report%20Round %20III%202008.pdf

Newell, M. L. (2000). Vertical transmission of HIV-1 infection. Transactions of the Royal Society of Tropical Medicine and Hygiene, 94 (1), 1_2.

Niccolai, L. M., Shcherbakova, I. S., Toussova, O. V., Kozlov, A. P., & Heimer, R. (2009). The potential for bridging of HIV transmission in the Russian Federation: sex risk behaviors and HIV prevalence among drug users (DUs) and their non-DU sex partners. Journal of urban health: bulletin of the New York Academy of Medicine, 86 Suppl 1, 131–143.

O'Shea, S., Newell, M. L., Dunn, D. T., Garcia-Rodriguez, M. C., Bates, I., Mullen, J., et al. (1998). Maternal viral load, CD4 cell count and vertical transmission of HIV-1. Journal of medical virology, 54 (2), 113–117.

Ottosson, D. (2007). State Sposnored Homophobia - A world survey of laws prohibiting same sex activity between consenting adults. from www.ilga.org

Platt, L., Vickerman, P., Collumbien, M., Hasan, S., Lalji, N., Mayhew, S., et al. (2009). Prevalence of HIV, HCV and sexually transmitted infections among injecting drug users in Rawalpindi and Abbottabad, Pakistan: evidence for an emerging injection-related HIV epidemic. Sexually transmitted infections, 85 Suppl 2, ii17–22.

Raees, M. A., Abidi, S. H., Ali, W., Khanani, M. R., & Ali, S. (2013). HIV among women and children in Pakistan. Trends Microbiol, 21 (5,, 213–214

Rai, M. A., Nerurkar, V. R., Khoja, S., Khan, S., Yanagihara, R., Rehman, A., et al. (2010). Evidence for a "Founder Effect" among HIV-infected injection drug users (IDUs) in Pakistan. BMC Infect Dis, 10, 7.

Rai, M. A., Warraich, H. J., Ali, S. H., & Nerurkar, V. R. (2007). HIV/AIDS in Pakistan: the battle begins. Retrovirology, 4, 22.

Rajabali, A., Khan, S., Warraich, H. J., Khanani, M. R., & Ali, S. H. (2008). HIV and homosexuality in Pakistan. The Lancet infectious diseases, 8 (5), 511–515.

Rajabali, A., Moin, O., Ansari, A. S., Khanani, M. R., & Ali, S. H. (2009). Communicable disease among displaced Afghans: refuge without shelter. Nature reviews. Microbiology, 7 (8), 609–614.

Rights, C. f. R. (2005, August). Pregnant Women Living with HIV/AIDS: Protecting Human Rights in Programs to Prevent Mother to Child Transmission of HIV. Center for Reproductive Rights, from http://reproductiverights.org/sites/crr.civicactions.net/files/documents/pub_bp_HIV.pdf

Shafiq, M , & Ali, S. H. (2006). Sexually transmitted infections in Pakistan. The Lancet infectious diseases, 6 (6), 321–322.

Shah, S. A., Altaf, A., Mujeeb, S. A., & Memon, A. (2004a). An outbreak of HIV infection among injection drug users in a small town in Pakistan: potential for national implications. International journal of STD & AIDS, 15 (3), 209.

Shah, S. A., Altaf, A., Mujeeb, S. A., & Memon, A. (2004b). An outbreak of HIV infection among injection drug users in a small town in Pakistan: potential for national implications. Int J STD AIDS, 15 (3), 209.

Shah, S. A., Khan, O. A., Kristensen, S., & Vermund, S. H. (1999a). HIV-infected workers deported from the Gulf States: impact on Southern Pakistan. International journal of STD & AIDS, 10 (12), 812–814.

Taylor, D. L. (2006). The Nexus of Terrorism and Drug Trafficking in the Golden Crescent: Afghanistan. USAWC Strategy Research Project.

UNAIDS. (2004). Making Condoms work for HIV prevention. from http://data.unaids.org/publications/irc-pub06/jc941-cuttingedge_en.pdf

UNAIDS. (2006). HIV and Men who have Sex with Men in Asia and the Pacific. from http://data.unaids.org/publications/irc-pub07/jc901-msm-asiapacific_en.pdf

UNAIDS. (2010). Global Report – UNAIDS Report on the Global AIDS Epidemic. from http://www.unaids.org/globalreport/documents/20101123_GlobalReport_full_en.pdf

UNAIDS. (2011). HIV in Asia and Pacific: Getting to Zero. Retrieved February 8, 2012, from http://www.unaids.org/en/media/unaids/contentassets/documents/unaidspublication/2011/20110826_APGetting ToZero_en.pdf

UNODC. (2011). UNODC World Drug Report 2011. from http://www.unodc.org/documents/data-and-analysis/WDR2011/World_Drug_Report_2011_ebook.pdf

USAID. (2010). Pakistan _ HIV/AIDS Health Profile. Retrieved February 21, 2012, from http://aidsdatahub.org/en/country-profiles/pakistan

WHO. Data Repository. from http://apps.who.int/ghodata/

Wingood, G. M., Diclemente, R. J., Mikhail, I., McCree, D. H., Davies, S. L., Hardin, J. W., et al. (2007). HIV discrimination and the health of women living with HIV. Women & health, 46 (2–3), 99–112.

Yousaf, M. Z., Zia, S., Babar, M. E., & Ashfaq, U. A. (2011). The epidemic of HIV/AIDS in developing countries; the current scenario in Pakistan. Virology journal, 8, 401.

Zhongdan, C., Schilling, R. F., Shanbo, W., Caiyan, C., Wang, Z., & Jianguo, S. (2008). The 100% Condom Use Program: a demonstration in Wuhan, China. Evaluation and program planning, 31 (1), 10–21.

Chapter 10

Population-specific Immuno-evolution of HIV-Subtype A

Syed Hani Abidi[1], Muhammad A. Raees[2], Farhat Abbas[3],
Sarah Rowland-Jones[4], Marcia Kalish[5], Sten H. Vermund[5], Syed Ali[6]

1   Introduction

The Human Immunodeficiency Virus (HIV) has claimed more than 25 million deaths in the past 30 years, and is responsible for over 33 million infections worldwide (Dieffenbach and Fauci 2011). Over time, the virus has diverged into many genetically distinct types and subtypes. HIV-1 subtype A belongs to the group M and has managed to spread globally and establish itself in certain regions of the world including Kenya, Uganda, Japan, Azerbaijan, Belgium, Botswana, Belarus, Congo and recently Afghanistan and Pakistan (Khan, Rai et al. 2006; Ansari, Khanani et al. 2011). Other members of HIV-1 group M, namely, subtypes B, C, D, and circulating recombinant form CRF_AE, together with subtype A are responsible for most of the HIV epidemics worldwide. The first HIV-1 subtype A sequences in the Los Alamos HIV database were deposited in the 1980's and were African in origin. Ever since, the database has amassed subtype A sequences from around the world indicating that this subtype has spread globally and has

[1] Department of Biological and Biomedical Sciences, Aga Khan University, Karachi, Pakistan
[2] Medical College, Aga Khan University, Karachi, Pakistan.
[3] Department of Surgery, Aga Khan University, Karachi, Pakistan.
[4] Nuffield Department of Medicine, University of Oxford, Oxford, UK.
[5] Vanderbilt Institute of Global Health, Vanderbilt University, Nashville, Tennessee, United States of America.
[6] Department of Biomedical Sciences, Nazarbayev University School of Medicine, Astana, Kazakhstan.

now established itself in diverse populations.

HIV evolves rapidly when subjected to host immunological pressures and drug therapy (Moore, John et al. 2002; Hewitt 2003; Brumme and Walker 2009). The virus acquires evolutionary advantage by incorporating escape mutations that prevent detection by human Cytotoxic T cells (CTLs). Each host immune milieu represents unique selection pressures on the virus that drive the mutation of the virus in distinct directions. HIV gag is a highly immunogenic protein that has been studied from different populations to understand selection pressures that are specific to various host immune milieus (Carnero, Li et al. 2009). The gag protein gives rise to distinct epitopes that may be representative of the epitope diversity amongst genetically distinct populations, reflecting evolutionary dynamics of HIV-1 in the backdrop of unique host immune pressures. In this chapter, we will discuss how the changing population immune-genetic pressures might affect HIV-1 subtype A epidemic dynamics, genomic variability and epitope diversity, and steer immuno-evolution of this subtype in new directions.

2   HIV – The Virus and the Disease

2.1   Viral Genome and Morphology

HIV belongs to the lentivirus genus of retroviruses. The viral RNA genome encodes for three structural proteins, two envelope proteins, three enzymes and six accessory proteins (Summers and Karn 2011). As is common with retroviruses, the RNA genome is encoded via a reverse transcriptase to viral DNA that is subsequently integrated into the host cell DNA. The viral genome encodes for several structural proteins, enzymes and surface proteins (Table 1). The gag gene encodes the structural proteins of the virus, namely, the Matrix (MA), Capsid (CA) and Nucleocapsid (NA). The pol gene is responsible for the enzymes: Integrase (IN), Reverse Transcriptase (RT) and Protease (PR). Finally the env gene encodes the envelop proteins, gp120 and gp41 (Summers and Karn 2011).

The virus is enveloped by a lipid bilayer that the virus acquires during replication from the host cell membrane. Inside the envelop is a matrix shell containing 2000 copies of the matrix protein followed by a conical capsid core containing 2000 copies of the capsid protein (Summers and Karn 2011). Embedded in the lipid bilayer are two important proteins that are responsible for the entry of the virus into the cell: gp120 and gp41 (Freed 1998; Summers and Karn 2011). The capsid protein core encloses two copies of the viral RNA attached to 2000 copies of the nucelopcapsid protein, representing a ribonucleoprotein complex. This configuration is said to provide stability to the overall genome structure (Summers and Karn 2011). The core of the virus also contains the three enzymes essential to viral replication and transmission: protease (PR), reverse transcriptase (RT) and integrase (IN). Of the six accessory proteins, nef, Vif and Vpr are packaged in the viral particle while Rev, Tat, and Vpu are translated later in the host cell and are not part of the mature HIV particle.

	Gene	Protein	Function
Structural Proteins	env	SU, TM	gp120 (SU) and gp41 (TM) are envelope proteins responsible for binding to CXCR5 and CCR4 cell surface receptor to initiate viral entry.
	gag	MA	Matrix protein (MA) forms a layer beneath the viral lipid bi-layer and plays a cardinal role in viral budding
		CA	Capsid protein (CA) forms a conical coat around the viral RNA and delivers the viral RNA and accessory proteins to the host cell.
		NC	Nucelocapsid protein (NC) forms a protective complex with the viral RNA that functions to stabilize the structure.
		p6	p6 is involved in the incorporation of viral protein r into new viral particles. The structure of p6 has not been resolved yet.
Enzymes	pol	RT	Reverse transcriptase binds to viral RNA to transcribe viral DNA. The error prone activity of this enzyme leads to mutations.
		IN	Integrase (IN) incorporates viral DNA into the host cell DNA after transporting it to the nucleus.
		PR	Protease (PR) cleaves viral proteins and is essential in viral particle maturation.
Accessory Proteins	vpu	Vpu	Viral protein u (Vpu) aids in viral particle budding from the cell membrane by degrading CD4 proteins thus leading to weakened interaction with env proteins.
	vif	Vif	Viral inhibitory factor (Vif) causes immune evasion of the virus by inhibiting the host cell APOBEC protein.
	vpr	Vpr	Viral protein r (Vpr) is a part of the pre-integration complex and aids in entry of viral DNA, RT and IN into the host cell nucleus.
	nef	nef	Negative regulatory factor (Nef) stops the expression of CD4 thus decreasing T Cell response and quickening disease progression to AIDS.
Regulatory Proteins	rev	rev	Regulator of virion (Rev) is involved in the regulation of splicing and transport of viral RNA.
	tat	tat	Trans-activator of transcription (Tat) functions by binding to viral RNA and increasing viral protein production by elongating the transcription phase

Table 1: HIV Proteins. HIV-encoded proteins and their functions in the viral lifecycle (Bank 2011; Abidi 2013).

2.2   HIV Lifecycle

The lifecycle of HIV can be divided into two distinct phases: the early phase and the late phase. The early phase includes the events of infection and integration of the viral genome into the host DNA, while the late phase includes the replication and budding of the virus to produce mature viral particles.

The early phase starts with the binding of HIV-1 to host cells carrying the CD4 protein on their surface membrane (- 1, step 1). The viral gp120 surface protein interacts with the amino terminal of the CD4 receptor to dock with the host cell. Additional interactions with the CXCR4 and CCR5 receptors are required for membrane fusion and subsequent infection of the host cell (Summers and Karn 2011). Upon successful docking with the CD4 cell, the conical capsid core of the virus enters the cytoplasm of the cell and starts to uncoat. Subsequent to this uncoating, the reverse transcriptase (RT) synthesizes viral DNA strands from viral RNA in the cytoplasm of the host cell (Goff 1990; Freed 1998; Summers and Karn 2011). The next step is the integration of the viral DNA into host chromosomes. For this purpose, a group of proteins escort the viral DNA into the host nucleus in what is referred to as a pre-integration complex. This complex contains Integrase, Matrix protein, Reverse Transcriptase, the accessory protein Vpr as well as the host protein HMG-I(Y) (Miller, Farnet et al. 1997; Summers and Karn 2011). Vpr functions by aiding the entry of the complex through the nuclear membrane and has also been hypothesized to aid in the cell cycle arrest in the G2 phase to aid in integration of the viral and host DNA (Jowett, Planelles et al. 1995). The Integrase finally catalyzes the insertion of viral DNA into the host DNA.

The late phase starts by the transcription (Figure 1, step 2) and translation (Figure 1, step 3) of viral proteins from the viral DNA, taking place in the nucleus of the host cell. The regulatory proteins Tat, Nef and Rev are encoded initially. Tat acts as a regulatory transcription factor that recruits cyclin T and Cyclin dependent protein kinase 9 (Cdk 9) that help in the transcription elongation (Summers and Karn 2011). This is followed by gag and gag-pol synthesis, packaging and export, which is facilitated by the viral protein Rev (Summers and Karn 2011). The env protein is made in the endoplasmic reticulum where it undergoes heavy posttranslational processing before being sent to the cell surface to take part in virus assembly and packaging. The gag-pol Polyprotein and gag protein are synthesized in the cytoplasm on free ribosomes. The gag-pol polyprotein associates with the gag protein. The Matrix domain of this polyprotein interacts directly with the tail of gp41 (from the env group of proteins), and together with two strands of viral mRNA, buds off from the cell. The virus then matures in a multistep process that involves viral protease mediated cleavage of the gag and pol polyproteins into mature MA, CA and NC that rearrange themselves to form an infectious and viable viral particle (Figure 1, step 4) (Summers and Karn 2011).

2.3   HIV Diversity

A high degree of mutational changes in HIV are the result of the error prone viral reverse transcriptase activity. The enzyme has an overall error rate of 1/1700 per detect-

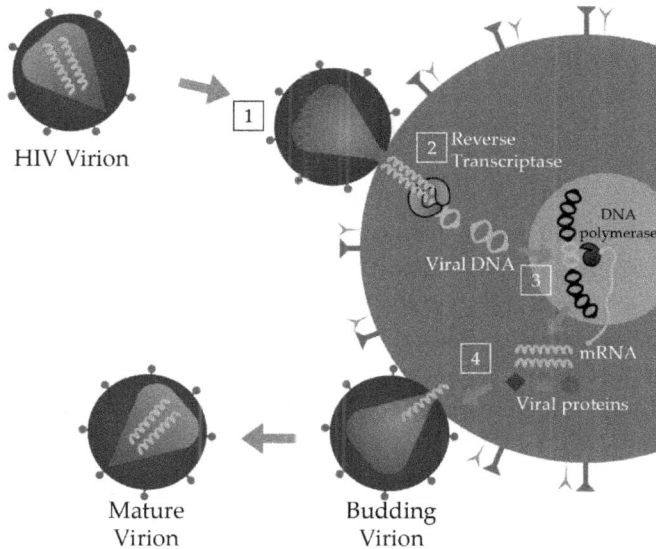

Figure 1: HIV Life Cycle. HIV primarily infects CD4+ T cells by birding to CD4 receptor and co-receptor on the cell surface (1). Following entry into the host cell, the virus reverse transcribes its RNA genome into double-stranded DNA (2), which then gets integrated into host genome (3). The integrated viral DNA encodes for viral proteins and genomic RNA, which assemble into virions, subsequently budding out of the infected cell (4).

able nucleotide incorporation, while in certain regions of the viral genome that are especially susceptible to mutations (mutational hotspots) the error rate can go up to as much as 1 per 70 nucleotides. Genetic analysis of the virus reveals a great deal of heterogeneity, with env diversity amongst different subtypes to be anywhere between 20-50% (Kandathil, Ramalingam et al. 2005). Phylogenetic trees constructed with HIV gene sequences obtained from various sources show these sequences arranged in clusters or clades based on their similarity. Estimation of genetic distances between subtypes within the Group M, using nucleotide or protein sequences, is a good correlate of HIV diversity. Genetic distances measured for different HIV proteins show that the env gene exhibits as much as 25-35% diversity, while the gag gene shows 15% diversity (Kandathil, Ramalingam et al. 2005). This is akin to a tree growing more and more branches with each branch being more different genetically from the parent node it came from. Interestingly, HIV exhibits a great deal of inter- as well as intra-subtype sequence diversity, as reflected, for instance, in the specific sub-clusters observed within subtypes A and F (Takeb, Kusagawa et al. 2004; Kandathil, Ramalingam et al. 2005).

2.4   HIV Epidemiology

The human immune deficiency virus is divided into two types: HIV-1 and HIV-2. HIV-1 is subdivided into Groups M (Main/Major), O (Outlier) and N (New/non M/non O). HIV-1 group M is further divided into subtypes A-H, J and K and is popularly known as the pandemic branch of HIV (Takeb, Kusagawa et al. 2004). HIV-1 is the leading cause of the global HIV epidemic, while HIV-2 is limited to parts of Western Africa with rare cases being reported from Portugal, India, Korea and the Philippines (Kandathil, Ramalingam et al. 2005). The first case of HIV/AIDS was documented in 1981. Following that, the virus has spread across countries and communities and has evolved into the many subtypes mentioned above. The World Health Organization (WHO) estimated a total of 33.4 million people living with AIDS in 2008; with a yearly health burden of 2.7 million new infections and 2 million deaths occurring the same year (Hemelaar, Gouws et al. 2011). The epidemic in 2002 was reported to be growing at an alarming pace with 60 million worldwide infections, a death toll of 25 million and a total of 42 million people living with HIV/AIDS (Takeb, Kusagawa et al. 2004). Age stratified data from the UNAIDS revealed that the epidemic was also strong in the young: a total of 3 million children under the age of 15 were living with HIV/AIDS with 800, 000 new infections and 580, 000 deaths each year (Takeb, Kusagawa et al. 2004).

Phylogenetic analysis has enabled us to better understand the origin of the virus and its evolution into different subtypes. The lineage of HIV has been traced to multiple zoonotic transmissions of simian immunodeficiency virus from non-human primates to humans around the 1900's in west and central Africa. HIV-1 subtype M has been found to originate from SIVcpz, while HIV-2 originated from SIVsm (Takeb, Kusagawa et al. 2004; Hemelaar, Gouws et al. 2011). Molecular clock analyses suggest that HIV group M, while still confined to central and western Africa, diversified into different subtypes in the first half of the 20th century (Worobey, Gemmel et al. 2008; Hemelaar, Gouws et al. 2011). In the second half of the 20th century, the global epidemic of HIV established mainly due to the spread of HIV-1 subtypes (mainly from group M) and recombinant forms to different countries.

HIV-1 Subtype A is the third most common viral subtype and accounts for 7% of the global epidemic. The global proportion of infections caused by subtype A has increased over a period of seven years, from 2000 to 2007. It is interesting to note that the leading subtype of global HIV infections, subtype C, has decreased in prevalence over the same period of time although it still continues to lead the growing epidemic (Hemelaar, Gouws et al. 2011). The global distribution of HIV-1 group M is subtype specific: While Central Africa shows a great diversity of HIV with almost all subtypes found there, the majority of infections in East and West Africa are those of subtypes A and G, respectively. Globally subtype A is found mainly in East Africa, Eastern Europe, Central Asia along with West and Central Africa and South and Southeast Asia (Hemelaar, Gouws et al. 2011).

Certain HIV subtypes are also associated with specific high-risk groups or specific disease scenarios, highlighting the fact that the virus may respond differently to specific immune environments. Subtype B, for example, is associated with male homosexual transmission, while subtype C with heterosexual transmission (Kandathil, Ramalingam et al. 2005); subtypes C, D or G are eightfold more likely to lead to AIDS than subtype A (Takeb, Kusagawa et al. 2004). Interestingly, subtype A is more likely to be transmitted vertically from mother to child. Experiments have shown that subtypes differ in terms of replicative efficiency with subtype A replication being far more efficient than subtype C. This is a surprising finding given that subtype C accounts for the majority of the global epidemic. This reduced efficiency can be accounted for by certain changes in the gp120 protein and the subsequent low affinity for the CD4/CCR5 receptors that are vital for viral infection. The fact that subtype C infections still account for the majority of the HIV epidemic possibly reflects its greater propensity for transmission giving it an overall advantage over other subtypes (Geretti 2006). In summary, subtype-specific data stratified by region is of seminal importance in understanding differences in viral behavior in different host populations (Kandathil, Ramalingam et al. 2005).

3   HIV – The Virus and the Host

3.1   Viral Evolution and Host Immune Response

HIV-1 is a continuously evolving virus. A combination of factors, such as an error-prone reverse transcriptase, viral fitness restriction, and selection pressures from the host immune system drive the virus to acquire mutations in an effort to evade annihilation by the host immune system (Kandathil, Ramalingam et al. 2005; Peters, Mendoza et al. 2008; Cardinaud, Consiglieri et al. 2011). The virus may be perceived as being in a continuous state of change, where the degree and nature of change is dependent on the immune environment of the host. However, not all of the acquired mutations are beneficial for the virus. Escape mutations that compromise the virus' fitness to survive eventually revert to wild type when the particular selection pressure is removed (Peters, Mendoza et al. 2008). Escape mutations give the virus an ability to avoid vital steps of the antigen presentation pathway and eventually escape CTL-mediated extinction (Cardinaud, Consiglieri et al. 2011; Abidi, Shahid et al. 2013).

Mutations can either be intra-epitope or extra-epitope: Intra-epitope mutations have been shown to disable CTL response by disrupting proteasomal processing, HLA binding or altering T-cell receptor interactions (Goulder and Watkins 2004; Cardinaud, Consiglieri et al. 2011). Extra-epitope mutations flank the antigenic regions of the viral protein and can effect processing and generation of viable epitopes by affecting trimming of viral proteins by proteasomes and/or aminopeptidases (Milicic, Price et al. 2005; Tenzer, Wee et al. 2009; Cardinaud, Consiglieri et al. 2011).

The magnitude of the immune response is highly dependent on the viral protein from which the epitope is derived. CTLs are responsible for controlling the infection in the initial stages, and it is a known fact that certain viral peptides mount a stronger immune response than others (Betts, Ambrozak et al. 2001; McMichael and Rowland-Jones 2001; Addo, Yu et al. 2003; Carnero, Li et al. 2009). Gag, pol and nef are highly immunogenic proteins of HIV, while Vpu is the least immunogenic. In chronically untreated HIV infections the main protein targeted by the immune system is p17 gag, while Vpr is most targeted in untreated acute infections (Addo, Yu et al. 2003). Gag is a highly conserved protein that plays an integral role in viral transmission and replication. It has been seen that viral escape mutations that lead to a decrease in viral fitness most commonly arise in p24 gag (Goulder and Watkins 2008). Analysis of mutations in the gag gene is therefore important for studying immune evasion as well as the development of viable vaccine options (Carnero, Li et al. 2009).

3.2   Host Immune Machinery

The host cell immune response to HIV infection is mediated by antigen presenting cells (APCs) and Cytotoxic T Cells (CTLs); CD 8+ T cell in particular. The human body handles pathogens (bacteria and viruses) using the innate and the adaptive arm of the immune system (Cooper, Fehniger et al. 2004). While the innate arm has limited specificity, and is the first line of defense against attack on the body, the adaptive arm is evolutionarily newer and more apt at recognizing specific pathogens and mounting an attack against them. The adaptive arm is further divided into Humoral and Cell-Mediated immunity. The former includes B Cells and involves the production of antibodies while the latter includes CTLs (CD 8+) and helper T Cells (CD 4+), which work via recognition of antigens on APCs. Antigens are presented in association with the Major Histocompatibility protein (MHC) which in humans is known as Human Leukocyte Antigen (HLA) (Medzhitov and Janeway 1998; Gromme and Neefjes 2002; Peters, Mendoza et al. 2008).

CTLs, in order to mount an immune response against the virus, require the antigen to be presented (by the MHC proteins) on the surface of the antigen presenting cells (APCs). The MHC-antigen complex formation is essential to the recognition of antigen by CTLs, since studies have shown that free antigens or MHC molecules cannot stimulate a T cell response. Antigens may be presented by either of the two types of MHC proteins, class I and II; these antigen-MHC complexes are recognized by, respectively, CD8+ CTLs and CD4+ CTLs. It is important to note that class I presentation is reserved for proteins that undergo intracellular (cytoplasmic or nucleic) synthesis and processing, while proteins that are ingested by the cell from the extracellular matrix and then process by APCs internally are presented by class II MHC proteins (Monaco 1995).

3.3   Antigen Processing and Presentation

3.3.1   Proteasomal Degradation

The first step in the processing of antigen is the proteasomal degradation of proteins (Figure 2, step 1). These proteins can be either pathogen or self-based (Rock, York et al. 2004). Majority of the viral epitopes presented to the T cells are generated by C terminal cleavage of viral antigenic proteins. Although, N terminal cleavage can also lead to epitope production, majority of the epitopes generated in this fashion are N terminally extended. These N terminally extended epitopes are further processed or trimmed by the aminopeptidases in the endoplasmic reticulum, producing epitopes of appropriate length (Abidi, Shahid et al. 2013). The protein to be degraded is marked by ubiquitin and is broken down to peptides of varying lengths (Rock, York et al. 2004). Under the influence of interferon gamma, the proteasome starts cleaving peptides into 8-10 amino acid long fragments – length that is efficiently recognized by the MHC class I molecules (Yewdell, Reits et al. 2003). This particular manner of proteasomal cleavage produces peptide fragments with length that is favored for binding by the transporter associated with antigen processing (TAP) protein, and eventually by the MHC molecule (Monaco 1995).

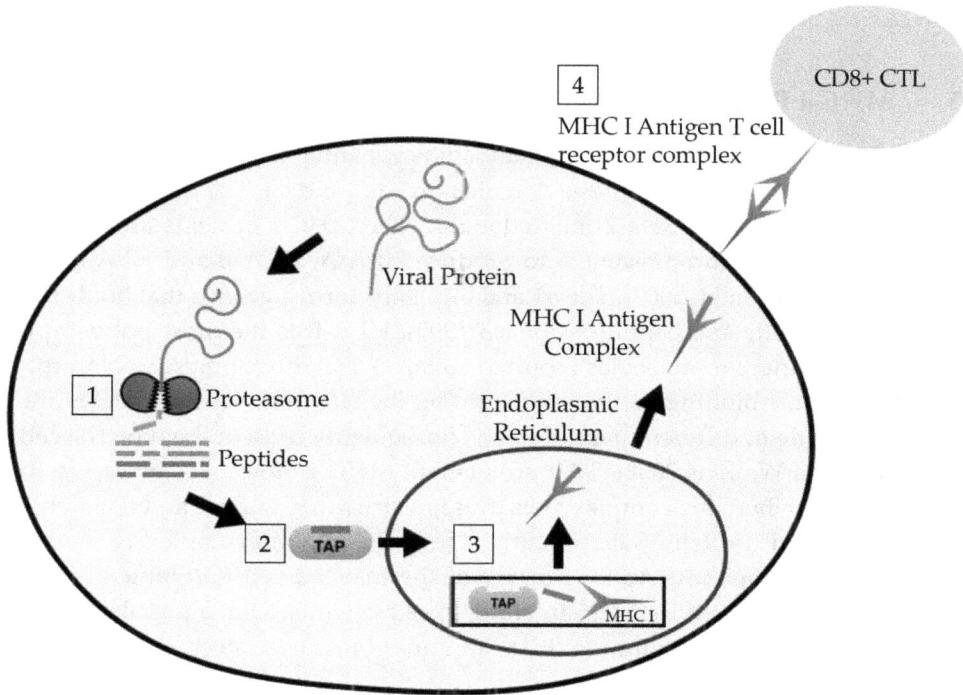

Figure 2: The MHC Class I Antigen Presentation Pathway. Major steps involved in antigen presentation are proteasomal degradation of viral proteins (1), TAP binding (2), peptide binding to MHC-I (3), and peptide display and binding to CD8+ T cells (4).

3.3.2   Transporter Associated with Antigen Processing (TAP)

The TAP transport protein is found on the membrane of the endoplasmic reticulum (ER) and aids in the transport of MHC compatible peptides into the ER (Figure 2, step 2) (Monaco 1995; Rock, York et al. 2004). It is a part of the ATP binding cassette (ABC) family of proteins and works in an energy dependent manner. This protein not only forms the transportation framework but is also a part of a peptide-loading complex that loads the antigen onto the MHC protein (Yewdell, Reits et al. 2003). Without functional TAP proteins, MHC class I molecules are inappropriately folded and are physiologically unstable on the cell membrane (Monaco 1995). TAP protein is selective in its choice of peptides to transport. While it can transport peptides 7-20 amino acids in length, in reality a majority of peptides are either smaller or larger than this and are further processed by proteasomes in the cytoplasm before being transported by the TAP protein (Momburg, Roelse et al. 1994). It has also been shown that peptides that end in hydrophobic and basic residues are preferentially transported by the TAP proteins (Monaco 1995). HIV uses this to its advantage by selectively accumulating escape mutations that lower peptide affinity for TAP binding that eventually leads to errors in epitope production (Abidi, Shahid et al. 2013).

3.3.3   MHC-I Presentation

The MHC-I proteins, also called the human leukocyte antigen (HLA) class I in humans, occur as an α chain composed of three domains—α1, α2, and α3. The α1 rests upon a unit of the non-MHC molecule Beta 2 microglobulin. The MHC-I proteins are encoded by the A, B and C loci of chromosome 6 to produce HLA-A, HLA-B and HLA-C, respectively (Yewdell, Reits et al. 2003). The α1 and α2 chains form a groove that holds the 8-10 amino acid long antigenic peptide (Monaco 1995). HLA-B is the most polymorphic of the lot with 817 different molecules reported so far. A majority of these polymorphisms occur in the peptide binding groove, highlighting the fact that these molecules are able to bind a multitude of different peptides and subsequently present them on the cell surface (Goulder and Watkins 2008). TAP protein and MHC 1 molecules interact in the ER (Figure 2, step 3), where the complex goes through structural folding and is finally separated from the TAP protein. Subsequently, the MHC-peptide complex is transported through the Golgi apparatus to the surface of the infected cell (Gromme and Neefjes 2002). It has been observed that certain HLA types are enriched in a population specific manner; supporting the argument that immune pressures steer the evolution of epitopes in a population-specific manner.

3.3.4   T Cell Immune Response

T cell receptors engage with the MHC class I molecules on the APCs (Figure 2, step 4), activating a myriad of pathways that ultimate destroy the infected cell along with the virus. T cell-mediated death of APC is facilitated by the T-cell initiated production of cytokines and chemokines (McMichael and Rowland-Jones 2001). Cytokines such as Interferon gamma have been known to work by inhibiting viral replication, while chemokines competitively bind to the CCR5 receptor thus inhibiting viral entry into cells (McMichael and Rowland-Jones 2001). During an acute infection the viral load of HIV goes up before decreasing again. The initial increase in viral load can be accounted for by the fact that CTLs take a while to be selected and differentiated. As the population of HIV specific CTLs increases the viral load goes down. It is hypothesized that the viral load is inversely proportional to CTL population, although different authorities offer differing opinions on this subject (Betts, Ambrozak et al. 2001; McMichael and Rowland-Jones 2001; Carnero, Li et al. 2009). Nevertheless, it is important to note that there is an active interaction between the virus and CTLs at the cellular level.

3.4   Host Innate factors

In addition to the cellular immunity, host innate factors also play a crucial role in controlling HIV infection. One such factor, Apolipoprotein B mRNA editing enzyme catalytic polypeptide (APOBEC) is a family of cytidine deaminases. It is composed of 3 proteins, namely APOBEC1, APOBEC2 and APOBEC3 encoded from chromosomes 6, 12 and 22, respectively. APOBEC3 is composed of a series of 7 sub members, labelled A through G (Goila-Gaur and Strebel 2008). The APOBEC family of proteins is responsible for providing immunity against retroviruses (Cullen 2006; Goila-Gaur and Strebel 2008). APOBEC3G, the most widely studied member of APOBEC family, for example, functions as an activation-induced deaminase. It provides antiretroviral immunity by interfering with the reverse transcription process by mutating deoxycytidine to deoxyuridibe residue in the negative strand of primary HIV DNA (Cullen 2006; Donahue, Vetter et al. 2008).This activity results in G to A hypermutations in the proviral DNA, which disrupts the coding and replicative capacity of HIV, resulting in the generation of nonviable virions (Donahue, Vetter et al. 2008; Sadler, Stenglein et al. 2010). APOBEC3G gets packaged into new virion particles and inhibits viral transmission after the virus enters a new host cell (Stopak, de Noronha et al. 2003). G to A substitutions can thus be used to measure the degree of APOBEC-mediated mutations within the viral genome.

The fact that HIV-1, despite the obstacle presented by APOBEC, can still cause an active infection in the host cell is due to the protection provided by the viral infectivity factor (Vif). Encoded by HIV, Vif is a 27 KD protein that is essential to viral replication and infectivity. Virions that lack the Vif protein cannot survive in cells containing the APOBEC3G system (Goila-Gaur and Strebel 2008). Although the exact method of immune evasion by Vif is not clear, studies have postulated that it uses a multipronged approach to ensure viral escape from the APOBEC system. Vif prevents incorporation of APOBEC3G into the budding virion and increases post translational degradation of APOBEC by 26s proteasome. This leads to low levels of APOBEC in the cytoplasm and in the nucleus of the host cell (Stopak, de Noronha et al. 2003).

4   Population-Dependent Viral Dynamics

4.1   Population-Dependent Diversity of HIV Subtype A

Phylogenetic analyses have elucidated not only the relationships between HIV sequences but have also provided an understanding about the degree of diversity brought about by mutations in the viral genome. These phenomena are illustrated by phylogenetic trees that are composed of clusters of closely linked genes sequences, while the unrelated sequences are observed to be dispersed throughout the tree. The trees can be rooted using a sequence less closely related to the sequences of interest. This sequence serves as a reference and forms the base to which all other sequences are compared. More a sequence has diversified, the further will it branch out from the root sequence.

Phylogenetic analysis conducted using gag sequences from the HIV Los Alamos

Database revealed that majority of subtype A sequences were diverse and appeared scattered throughout the phylogenetic tree, without any apparent relationship between the branching topology and the time of sampling (Figure 3) (Abidi, Kalish et al. 2014).

Figure 3: Maximum Likelihood Phylogenetic Tree of HIV-1 Subtype A Gag Sequences. The tree was constructed using 1893 sequences submitted to the Los Alamos HIV database from 1985 to 2005. Gag sequence from SIVcpz was used to root the tree and compare the genetic diversity of and the relationships between sequences. Sequences from year-groups, 1985–1990, 1990–1995, 1995–2000, 2000–2005, and 2005–2010 are shown in red, blue, orange, pink and green color, respectively.[1] The green shaded area highlights Pakistani and Afghani sequences clustered together. The green boxes with arrows point to samples from Afghanistan (AFG) and Pakistan (PK). Red, green and orange circles indicate nodes with bootstrap values of >90, >80 and >70, respectively. The tree was reproduced from Abidi, Kalish et al. 2014. The colored figure can be found in: https://iconceptpress.com

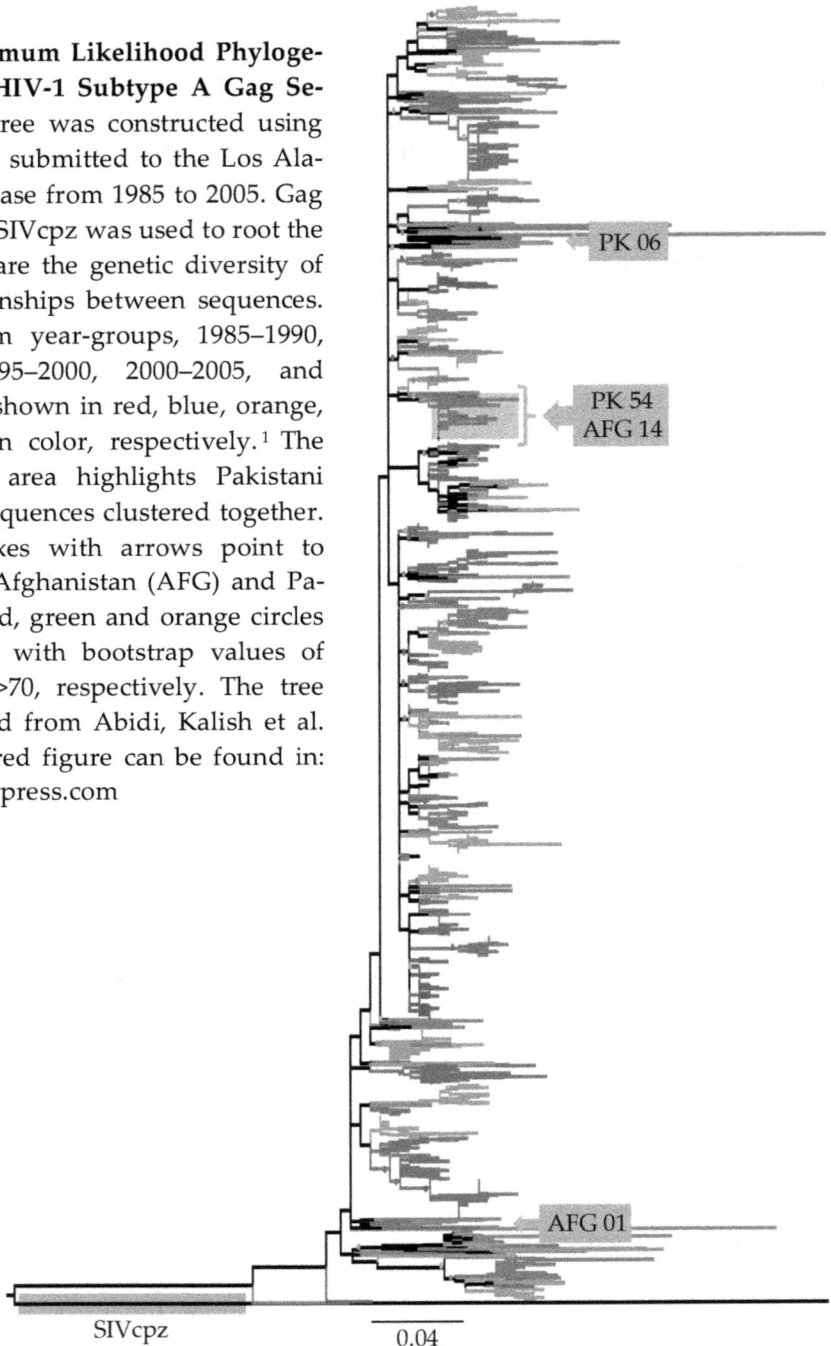

Since most of these sequences were Kenyan in origin, majority of the clusters observed in the tree represented Kenya transmission networks (Figure 3). The tree revealed one significant cluster that comprised sequences from only Pakistan and Afghanistan (Figure 3, green shaded square), indicating that the HIV epidemic in the two countries is phylogenetically related (Abidi, Kalish et al. 2014). The political turmoil in Afghanistan has been ongoing since the past 30 years and has displaced a large number of Afghans into the neighboring countries of Pakistan and Iran. The lack of proper health care and weak government policies have led to the propagation of infectious diseases, including HIV and other sexually transmitted infections, in the refugee population. Afghan refugees have been reported to partake in high risk behaviors that are similar to those exhibited by Pakistani high risk communities. The high risk groups in the Pakistan and Afghan populations include People who inject drugs (PWID), Men who have sex with men (MSM), and individuals with multiple sex partners that may include commercial sex workers. As corroborated by the phylogenetic analyses, the HIV epidemic in this region is thought to have spread from PWID to MSM and then to Afghan Refugees (Ansari, Khanani et al. 2011). Currently, it has been reported that the HIV epidemic in Pakistan has bridged into the female spouses and children of MSM and PWID (Raees, Abidi et al. 2013) (Khanani, Somani et al. 2011). These examples of phylogenetic analyses illustrate that transmission networks may also play a significant role in determining the spread and prevalence of particular viral subtypes and mutational variants in a region. For instance, frequent travel among the Afghan refugees is thought to be one of the reasons for the transmission of HIV in Afghanistan, Pakistan, and Iran. It is possible that the introduction of diverse HIV subtypes to and from new geographical locations has contributed to the increase in the genetic diversity of HIV under selection from the ever-changing host immune pressures.

4.2   Temporal Dynamics of HIV-1 Subtype A Divergence and Spread

Bayesian analysis can help us form associations between viral divergence and epidemic dynamics (Abidi, Kalish et al. 2014). This provides us with insight into the effect of selection pressures on the virus over time, and allows us to make inferences regarding the trend of active infections based on viral fitness and replicative ability. It has been shown that HIV subtype A epidemic may have originated in 1956 (±1 year), dating back to the most recent common ancestor of subtype A (Figure 4, black dotted line) (Abidi, Kalish et al. 2014). The HIV subtype A epidemic remained stable till the mid 1980's, which was followed by an increase in transmissibility as shown by the 10-fold growth in effective population size (Figure 4, Area A). The growth of the epidemic continued to occur after that reaching a plateau phase during the late 80's to the early 2000 (Figure 4, Area B). This plateau phase was characterized by a high but stable number of HIV transmissions worldwide. The effective population size then decreased from early 2000 to 2004 leading to another plateau in the epidemic's growth (Figure 4, Area C) (Abidi, Kalish et al., 2014). The sharp rise in the mid 1980's to early 2000 was preceded by a stable phase during which the virus might have been accumulating different mutations under the influence of new selection pressures. The subsequent decline in the viral transmission ability

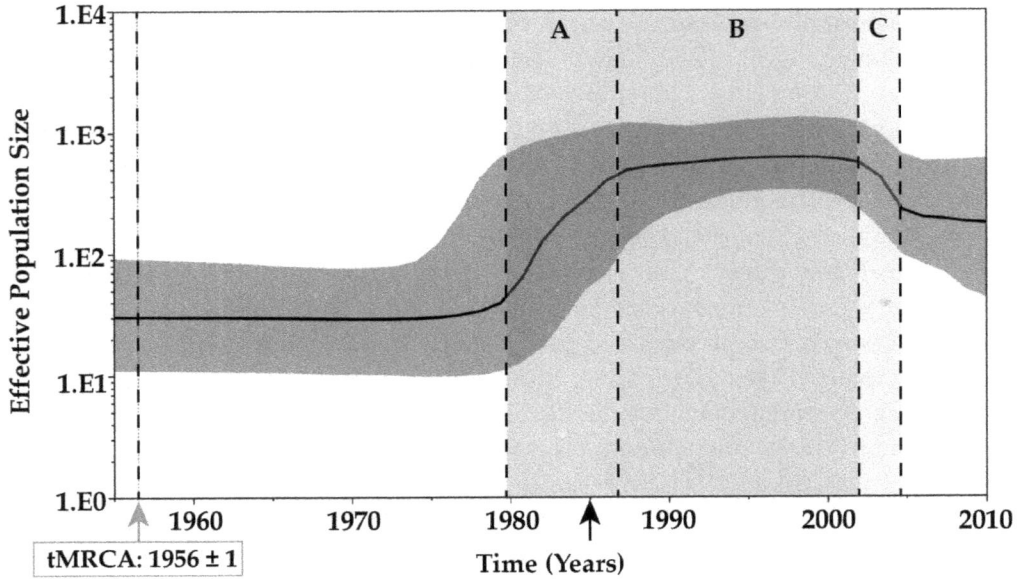

Figure 4: Temporal Dynamics of Subtype-A Divergence and Spread. This Bayesian Skyline plot was constructed using 113 sequences that best represented the years and countries studied. X-axis represents time in years while the Y-axis represents the effective population size. The thick black line describes the median, and the gray bands represent the 95% highest posterior density intervals. The dotted black line represents tMRCA in 1956±1 year. The black arrow represents the oldest reported sequence in the Los Alamos HIV database (1985). Area A, B and C represent periods of increase in viral population size, a plateau phase and decline in the population size, respectively. The figure was reproduced from Abidi, Kalish et al. 2014.

might be a reflection of decreased viral fitness as the virus struggled to adjust to the newly encountered host immune pressures (Abidi, Kalish et al. 2014). This decline in effective transmission might also be attributable to other factors in the patient population, such as successful prevention programs, and/or effective antiviral therapy.

4.3   Time-Dependent Evolution of HIV-1 Subtype A

Shannon entropy and G to A substitution analyses provide us with a method to analyze the time dependent evolution of HIV. Shannon entropy is a measure of the probability of acquisition of mutations in a given set of viral genomic sequences (Abidi, Shahid et al. 2014). High Shannon entropy values for a given position in a gene sequence indicate higher probability of mutation at that point. G to A substitutions in the viral genome is a measure of mutations under host APOBEC mediated immune pressures. These data, when analyzed together with the Bayesian analysis (discussed above), gives insight into the relationship between escape mutations and viral infectivity on a temporal scale. The Shannon entropy values of HIV gag sequences taken from 1985 to 2010 have shown a consistent rise in entropy and G to A substitutions every five years with the rise during 2005 to 2010 being markedly high (Figures 5a and 5b) (Abidi, Kalish et al. 2014). Superimposing Bayesian analysis findings on these data reveals that the period of high degree of Shannon entropy and G to A substitutions corresponds to a decreasing trend in the effective population size or effective transmission of the virus (Figure 4, Area C). This might indicate that under strong immune pressures the virus rapidly accumulates escape mutations, which likely occurs at the cost of viral fitness. It is possible that these mutations are transitory, and with the passage of time the virus might undergo refinement, selecting escape mutations more favorable to viral transmission and survival.

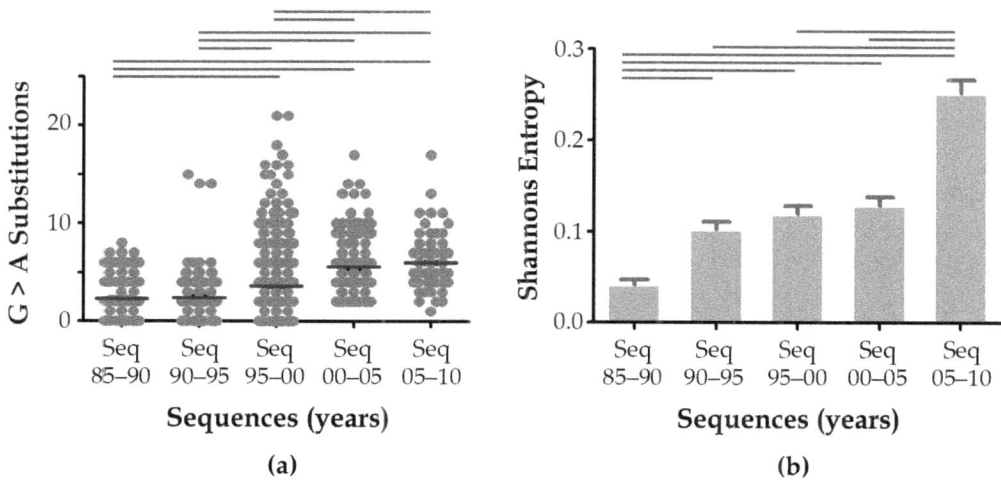

(a)   (b)

Figure 5: Time-Bound Changes in HIV-1 Subtype A Genomic Variability. HIV-1 subtype A gag variability was measured for sequences from 1985-2010, divided in five year-groups: 1985–1990, 1990–1995, 1995–2000, 2000–2005, and 2005–2010. The sequence variability was measured in terms of a) G→A substitutions and b) Shannon entropy. a) G→A substitutions: Small circles represent number of substitutions for each sequence; grey lines show the mean for a particular year-group. The line over the scatter plot represents statistically significant ($p<0.001$) differences between groups. b) Shannon entropy analysis: The vertical axis represents mean entropy scores, while the horizontal axis shows sequences from 1985-2010, divided in five year-groups. The lines over bars represent a statistically significant difference between the groups ($p<0.001$). Error bars represent the standard error of the mean. The figure was reproduced from Abidi, Kalish et al. 2014.

4.4   Population-Specific Immune Evolution

Viral response to host immune pressures can be specific to a given population (Abidi,

Shahid et al. 2013). Predominantly occurring HLA alleles represent one of the population-specific selection pressures that may determine the evolution of HIV within a population. Small differences in HLA makeup of host populations can reflect in significant impacts on viral evolution as well as on the overall host immune response to the virus. An example of this is seen between HLA- B*3502/B*3503 versus HLA-B*3501, all restricting HIV gag epitopes. While HLA-B*3502 and B*3503 only differ from HLA-B*3501 in three and one amino acid, respectively, the former two are associated with rapid disease progression, while the latter is not (Goulder and Watkins 2008). The existence of a variable response to polymorphic HLA molecules highlights the complex immune dynamics between the host and HIV. HLA-B*27 mediated immune response, for instance, has a clear association with slow disease progression to AIDS. Patients with HLA-B*27 mount a stronger CTL response against the vi rus and are thus able to better control the viral load and disease progression (Goulder and Watkins 2008). Similarly, patients with HLA-B*57 have been reported to maintain lower viral load and exhibit delayed progression to AIDS. When HIV is transmitted to HLA-B*57 negative subjects, for example, it has been observed that the virus reverts to the wild type, exhibiting improved replicative fitness, and survival capability (Goulder and Watkins 2008). This results in rapid disease progression to AIDS.

Recent studies on comparative analysis of population-specific immunogenetic (HLA) pressures on HIV subtype A epitope processing and presentation, showed that highly similar HIV subtype A strains accumulate gag epitope mutations in a population-specific manner (Abidi, Shahid et al. 2013; Abidi, Kalish et al. 2014). The study, conducted on HIV subtype A-infected Pakistani, Afghan and Kenyan cohorts, showed that among these populations the differences in HIV gag are specifically observed at the amino acids 303, 332, 339, 362, 370, 376 and 388. At these positions, the Pakistani version of HIV gag exhibited amino acids Threonine, Threonine, Valine, Alanine, Methionine and Arginine, respectively, whereas at the same positions, the Kenyan version showed the amino acids Threonine, Serine, Alanine, Isoleucine, Valine, Isoleucine and Lysine (Figure 6). The Afghan sequences exhibited mutation patterns identical to Pakistani sequences. The Pakistani version of HIV gag also showed insertion of an extra Glutamine at position 372, which was absent in the Kenyan sequences (Abidi, Shahid et al. 2013; Abidi, Kalish et al. 2014). These differences show intra-subtype genomic diversity in HIV gag most likely reflecting population-based unique selection pressures.

In silico analyses have shown that the mutations in the gag gene affect its proteasomal degradation into antigenic peptides, TAP binding of the resulting peptides, and eventually epitope presentation. Pakistani HIV gag shown to carry unique proteasomal degradation sites at positions: 362, 367, 392 and 396, while the Kenyan gag are sequences showed a unique site at position 370. TAP protein binding sites also differed between the two groups; Pakistani gag version showed TAP binding sites at positions: 295, 296, 298, 325, 368, 388, 392 and 394 whereas Kenyan version at: 295, 296, 298, 326, 329, 335 and 376 (Figure 7). It is interesting to note that the gag epitope profile of HIV subtype A strain infecting Afghan cohort was exactly similar to that of Pakistan subtype A strains, probably because of the close geographical association of these two populations, overlapping transmission networks, and the fact that the HIV epidemic in these

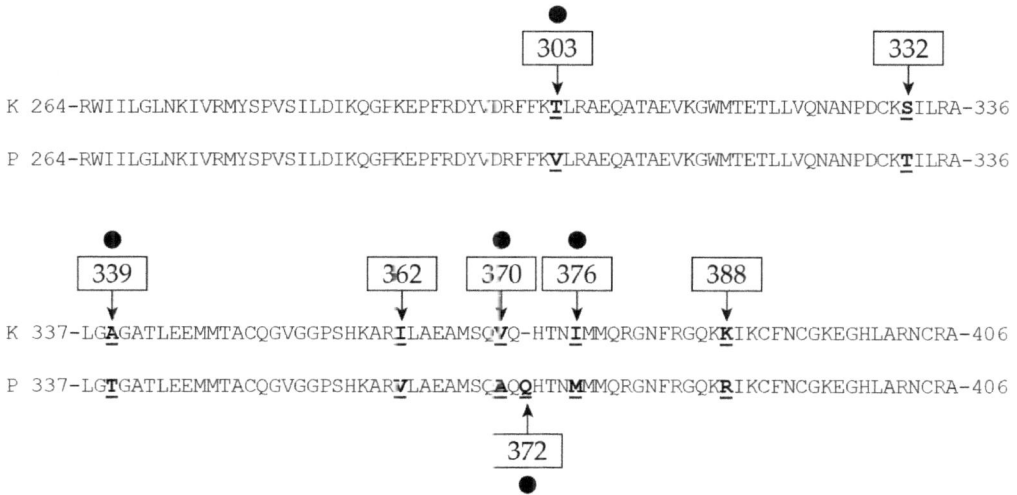

Figure 6: **Alignments of Pakistani and Kenyan Gag Sequences.** Alignment of HIV-1 consensus gag sequences from Pakistani (P) and Kenyan (K) samples. Mutations uniquely observed in each study population are shown as bold and underline characters. Above each unique amino acid, its position is marked, while asterisk on the mutation represents a significant difference (p<0.05) between the two study populations with the respect to that mutation. Positions of the first and last amino acids in each row are also marked. The figure was reproduced from Abidi, Shahid et al. 2013.

populations is not old enough for the viral genes to exhibit mutations evolved under population-specific selection pressures (Abidi, Kalish et al. 2014). HIV subtype A epitope variability has been shown to have increased in the Afghan, Pakistani and Kenyan populations since 2005. This, together with high Shannon entropies and a declining trend in effective viral population size shows that the virus is accumulating mutations at a fast pace, and that these mutations may be detrimental to viral fitness. As more subtype A sequences become available, similar analyses will give a better understanding of how the genetic and immunological pressures will shape the HIV epidemic in these populations in the upcoming years. A year-wise analysis of epitope sequences from the same populations will help in deciphering the true nature of this phenomenon. Further analyses will also provide a better understanding of the directions in which the HIV-1 epidemics may evolve in the future. This information will be crucial in anticipating prevention and control strategies for sub type A-infected patients, especially in populations where the epidemic is newly emerging.

6   Conclusion

HIV/AIDS is a growing epidemic that represents a significant health burden on the

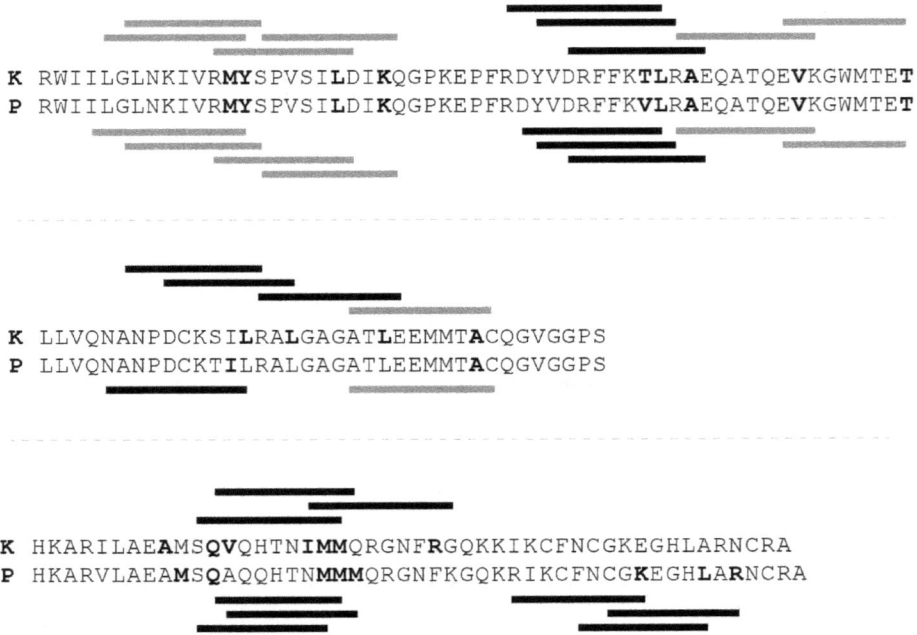

K RWIILGLNKIVR**MY**SPVSI**L**DI**K**QGPKEPFRDYVDRFFK**TLRA**EQATQEVKGWMTE**T**
P RWIILGLNKIVR**MY**SPVSI**L**DI**K**QGPKEPFRDYVDRFFK**VLRA**EQATQEVKGWMTE**T**

K LLVQNANPDCKS**I**LRALGAGAT**L**EEMMT**A**CQGVGGPS
P LLVQNANPDCKT**I**LRALGAGATLEEMMT**A**CQGVGGPS

K HKARILAE**A**MS**QV**QHTN**IMM**QRGNF**R**GQKKIKCFNCGKEGHLARNCRA
P HKAR**V**LAE**A**MS**Q**A**Q**QHTN**MMM**QRGNF**K**GQKR**I**KCFNCGK**E**GHLARNCRA

Figure 7: Map of Sites of Proteasomal Degradation, TAP Binding, HLA-Binding, And CTL Epitopes in HIV-1 Gag from Pakistan and Kenya. The figure shows a map of proteasomal degradation sites, TAP and HLA binding sites as well as CTL epitopes form Kenya (K) and Pakistan (P). Bold letters represent proteasomal degradation sites, while grey and black lines represent common and unique TAP and HLA binding sites and CTL epitopes, respectively. The figure was reproduced from Abidi, Shahid et al. 2013.

world population. The virus has disseminated on a global level with different subtypes dominating the HIV epidemics in specific geographical locations. With each host population providing a unique set of immune selection pressures, the virus is incorporating genetic mutation patterns in a population- specific manner. Phylogenetic analysis of HIV subtype A sequences from Kenya, Pakistan and Afghanistan show how population-specific pressures may lead to diversity within the same subtype. This mutational diversity can be traced over the course of history and related to the intracellular pathways involved in epitope production, HLA selection and disease progression. A deeper understanding of these mechanisms helps in subtype-specific drug and vaccine design.

References

Abidi, S. H., M. L. Kalish, et al. (2014). HIV-1 subtype A Gag variability and epitope evolution. PLoS One 9(6): e93415.

Abidi, S. H., A. Shahid, et al. (2013). Population-specific evolution of HIV Gag epitopes in genetically *diverged patients. Infect Genet Evol 16: 78-86.*

Abidi, S. H., A. Shahid, et al. (2014). *HIV-1 progression links with viral genetic variability and subtype, and patient's HLA type: analysis of a Nairobi-Kenyan cohort. Med Microbiol Immunol 203(1): 57-63.*

Abidi, S. H. H. (2013). *Immunodynamics of HIV-1 in genetically diverse cohorts Ph.D., The Aga Khan University.*

Addo, M. M., X. G. Yu, et al. (2003). *Comprehensive epitope analysis of human immunodeficiency virus type 1 (HIV-1)-specific T-cell responses directed against the entire expressed HIV-1 genome demonstrate broadly directed responses, but no correlation to viral load. J Virol 77(3): 2081-2092.*

Ansari, A. S., M. R. Khanani, et al. (2011). *Patterns of HIV infection among native and refugee Afghans. AIDS 25(11): 1427-1430.*

Bank, T. R. P. D. (2011). *The structural Biology of HIV. 2014, from http://www.pdb.org/pdb/education_discussion/educational_resources/struct_bio_hiv_hires.pdf.*

Betts, M. R., D. R. Ambrozak, et al. (2001). *Analysis of total human immunodeficiency virus (HIV)-specific CD4(+) and CD8(+) T-cell responses: relationship to viral load in untreated HIV infection. J Virol 75(24): 11983-11991.*

Brumme, Z. L. and B. D. Walker (2009). *Tracking the culprit: HIV-1 evolution and immune selection revealed by single-genome amplification. J Exp Med 206(6): 1215-1218.*

Cardinaud, S., G. Consiglieri, et al. (2011). *CTL escape mediated by proteasomal destruction of an HIV-1 cryptic epitope. PLoS Pathog 7(5): e1002049.*

Carnero, E., W. Li, et al. (2009). *Optimization of human immunodeficiency virus gag expression by newcastle disease virus vectors for the induction of potent immune responses. J Virol 83(2): 584-597.*

Cooper, M. A., T. A. Fehniger, et al. (2004). *NK cell and DC interactions. Trends Immunol 25(1): 47-52.*

Cullen, B. R. (2006). *Role and mechanism of action of the APOBEC3 family of antiretroviral resistance factors. J Virol 80(3): 1067-1076.*

Dieffenbach, C. W. and A. S. Fauci (2011). *Thirty years of HIV and AIDS: future challenges and opportunities. Ann Intern Med 154(11): 766-771.*

Donahue, J. P., M. L. Vetter, et al. (2008). *The HIV-1 Vif PPLP motif is necessary for human APOBEC3G binding and degradation. Virology 377(1): 49-53.*

Freed, E. C. (1998). *HIV-1 gag proteins: diverse functions in the virus life cycle. Virology 251(1): 1-15.*

Geretti, A. M. (2006). *HIV-1 subtypes: epidemiology and significance for HIV management. Curr Opin Infect Dis 19(1): 1-7.*

Goff, S. P. (1990). *Retroviral reverse transcriptase: synthesis, structure, and function. J Acquir Immune Defic Syndr 3(8): 817-831.*

Goila-Gaur, R. and K. Strebel (2008). *HIV-1 Vif, APOBEC, and intrinsic immunity. Retrovirology 5: 51.*

Goulder, P. J. and D. I. Watkins (2004). *HIV and SIV CTL escape: implications for vaccine design. Nat Rev Immunol 4(8): 630-640.*

Goulder, P. J. and D. I. Watkins (2008). *Impact of MHC class I diversity on immune control of immunodeficiency virus replication. Nat Rev Immunol 8(8): 619-630.*

Gromme, M. and J. Neefjes (2002). *Antigen degradation or presentation by MHC class I molecules via classical and non-classical pathways. Mol Immunol 39(3-4): 181-202.*

Hemelaar, J., E. Gouws, et al. (2011). Global trends in molecular epidemiology of HIV-1 during 2000-2007. AIDS 25(5): 679-689.

Hewitt, E. W. (2003). The MHC class I antigen presentation pathway: strategies for viral immune evasion. Immunology 110(2): 163-169.

Jowett, J. B., V. Planelles, et al. (1995). The human immunodeficiency virus type 1 vpr gene arrests infected T cells in the G2 + M phase of the cell cycle. J Virol 69(10): 6304-6313.

Kandathil, A. J., S. Ramalingam, et al. (2005). Molecular epidemiology of HIV. Indian J Med Res 121(4): 333-344.

Khan, S., M. A. Rai, et al. (2006). HIV-1 subtype A infection in a community of intravenous drug users in Pakistan. BMC Infect Dis 6: 164.

Khanani, M. R., M. Somani, et al. (2011). The spread of HIV in Pakistan: bridging of the epidemic between populations. PLoS One 6(7): e22449.

McMichael, A. J. and S. L. Rowland-Jones (2001). Cellular immune responses to HIV. Nature 410(6831): 980-987.

Medzhitov, R. and C. A. Janeway, Jr. (1998). Innate immune recognition and control of adaptive immune responses. Semin Immunol 10(5): 351-353.

Milicic, A., D. A. Price, et al. (2005). CD8+ T cell epitope-flanking mutations disrupt proteasomal processing of HIV-1 Nef. J Immunol 175(7): 4618-4626.

Miller, M. D., C. M. Farnet, et al. (1997). Human immunodeficiency virus type 1 preintegration complexes: studies of organization and composition. J Virol 71(7): 5382-5390.

Momburg, F., J. Roelse, et al. (1994). Peptide size selection by the major histocompatibility complex-encoded peptide transporter. J Exp Med 179(5): 1613-1623.

Monaco, J. J. (1995). Pathways for the processing and presentation of antigens to T cells. J Leukoc Biol 57(4): 543-547.

Moore, C. B., M. John, et al. (2002). Evidence of HIV-1 adaptation to HLA-restricted immune responses at a population level. Science 296(5572): 1439-1443.

Peters, H. O., M. G. Mendoza, et al. (2008). An integrative bioinformatic approach for studying escape mutations in human immunodeficiency virus type 1 gag in the Pumwani Sex Worker Cohort. J Virol 82(4): 1980-1992.

Raees, M. A., S. H. Abidi, et al. (2013). HIV among women and children in Pakistan. Trends Microbiol 21(5): 213-214.

Rock, K. L., I. A. York, et al. (2004). Post-proteasomal antigen processing for major histocompatibility complex class I presentation. Nat Immunol 5(7): 670-677.

Sadler, H. A., M. D. Stenglein, et al. (2010). APOBEC3G contributes to HIV-1 variation through sublethal mutagenesis. J Virol 84(14): 7396-7404.

Stopak, K., C. de Noronha, et al. (2003). HIV-1 Vif blocks the antiviral activity of APOBEC3G by impairing both its translation and intracellular stability. Mol Cell 12(3): 591-601.

Summers, M. F. and J. Karn (2011). Special issue: Structural and molecular biology of HIV. J Mol Biol 410(4): 489-490.

Takeb, E. Y., S. Kusagawa, et al. (2004). Molecular epidemiology of HIV: tracking AIDS pandemic. Pediatr Int 46(2): 236-244.

Tenzer, S., E. Wee, et al. (2009). Antigen processing influences HIV-specific cytotoxic T lymphocyte immunodominance. Nat Immunol 10(6): 636-646.

Worobey, M., M. Gemmel, et al. (2008). Direct evidence of extensive diversity of HIV-1 in Kinshasa by 1960. Nature 455(7213): 661-664.

Yewdell, J. W., E. Reits, et al. (2003). Making sense of mass destruction: quantitating MHC class I antigen presentation. Nat Rev Immunol 3(12): 952-961.

www.ingramcontent.com/pod-product-compliance
Lightning Source LLC
Chambersburg PA
CBHW061808210326
41599CB00034B/6926